For Further Review Visit:

www.SurgicalTechReview.com

Individual Code for 50% off site on page 250

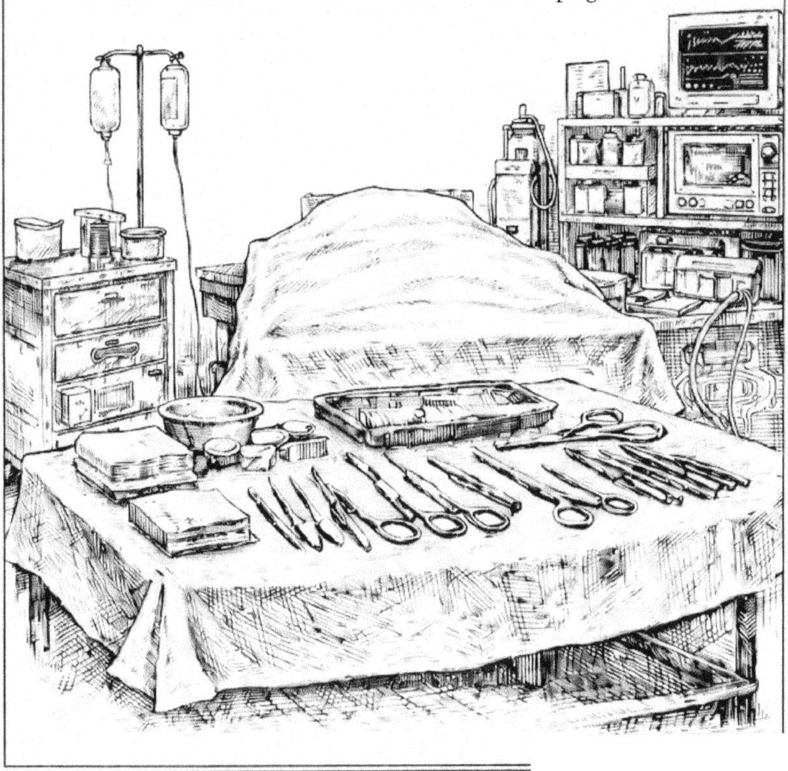

AF719549

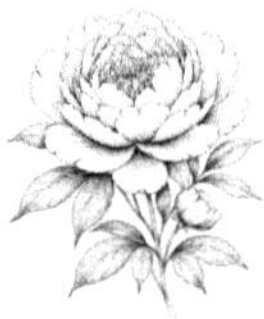

Dedicated to my Inna,
who has supported & encouraged me
through all of my ideas and adventures

The Surgical Technologist's Guide: Procedure Steps & Anticipation Tips
ISBN: 979-8-90271-654-9

Author:
Nikki Davidson, CST

Published by:
Surgical Tech Review, LLC
Vero Beach, Florida
2026

Disclaimer

The information contained in this book is intended for educational purposes only. Surgical procedures, procedural steps, and instrumentation may vary based on the surgeon's preference, the patient's condition, institutional protocols, and available equipment.
This guide is not intended to replace formal education, institutional training, or clinical judgment. The steps and instruments described represent general practices commonly used in surgical procedures and are provided as a reference to support learning and anticipation in the operating room. Readers are responsible for adhering to their facility's policies and the direction of the operating surgeon at all times.

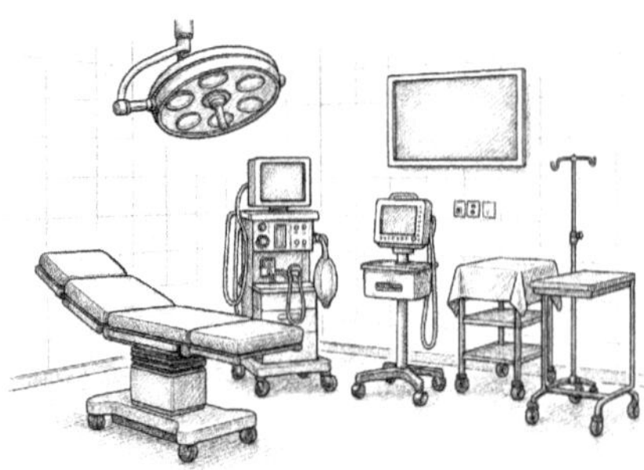

Section III: Ophthalmic Procedures

Section IV: Otorhinolaryngologic Procedures

Section V: Oral and Maxillofacial Procedures

Section VI: Plastic and Reconstructive Procedures

Section VII: Genitourinary Procedures

Section VIII: Orthopedic Procedures

Section IX: Cardiothoracic Procedures

Section IX: Cardiothoracic Procedures

Section X: Peripheral Vascular Procedures

Section XI: Neurosurgery Procedures

Section I: General Procedures

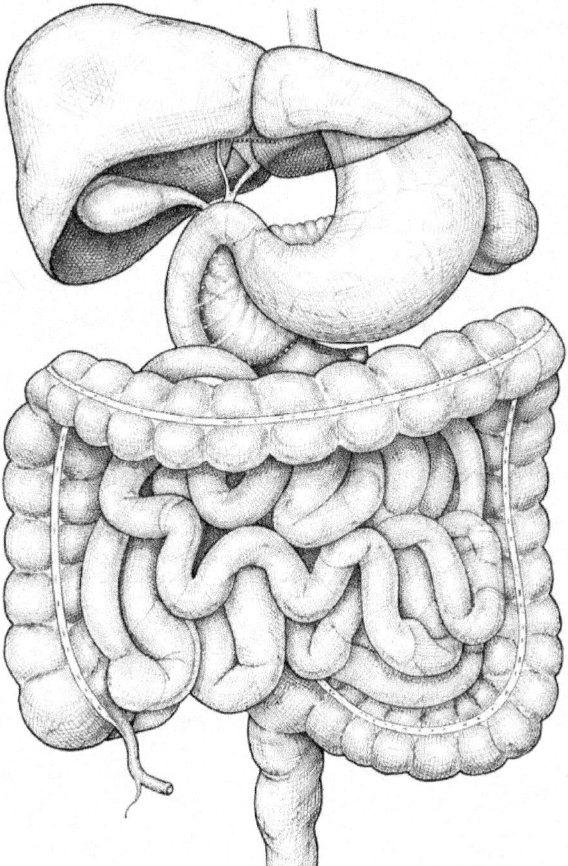

Appendectomy (Open)

Step 1 – Incision & initial exposure
Instruments: #10 blade on 3 handle, Adsons w/ teeth, Metzenbaum scissors, Bovie, Army Navy retractor, Yankauer suction. RLQ McBurney Incision
Anticipation: Have Bovie tested and suction on before incision. Hand small retractors as soon as skin is opened. Be ready to switch to deeper retraction (Richardson) when fascia is reached.

Step 2 – Enter peritoneum & locate cecum/appendix
Instruments: Debakey forceps, Richardson retractors, Metzenbaum, moist laps.
Anticipation: As the peritoneum is tented using Adsons with teeth, have Metzenbaum scissors ready, then immediately pass Yankauer suction, and moist laps; there may be fluid/pus.Assist with exposure and retraction to allow the surgeon to orient toward the cecum in the RLQ.

Step 3 – Deliver appendix & protect bowel
Instruments: Babcock(s) for appendix, Debakeys, small Malleable, moist laps.
Anticipation: Be ready to pass Babcock, not toothed clamps, for the appendix/cecum. Keep field dry and bowel wrapped in moist laps to prevent desiccation.

Step 4 – Divide mesoappendix
Instruments: Kelly clamps, Metzenbaum scissors, 2-0 Vicryl or 2-0 Silk sutures.
Anticipation: Pre-load ties on Curved Criles/Kellys and have several ready. Expect a clamp–cut–tie rhythm; follow it with your pass pattern and keep suction near the mesoappendix.

Step 5 – Ligate & divide appendix at base
Instruments: Crile or right-angle clamp, absorbable ligature, Mayo scissors; possible purse-string suture 2-0 absorbable & atraumatic forceps if inversion used.
Anticipation: Have base ligature, 3-0 synthetic absorbable suture, and any purse-string sutures cut to length and loaded. Anticipate the specimen coming off, open the specimen cup before division.

Step 6 – Irrigation & hemostasis
Instruments: Irrigation set, Suction, laps, hemostatic agents.
Anticipation: Offer warm irrigation proactively after stump secured. Start closing count with circulator while surgeon irrigates.

Step 7 – Layered closure
Instruments: Needle driver, Mayo scissors, fascial suture, 3-0/4-0 skin suture or stapler, Adsonss.
Anticipation: Know surgeon's usual fascial and skin sutures. Pre-load fascial stitch before they ask; have dressing and skin adhesive or staples on the field when skin closure starts.

Mayo Stand Suggestion:

- Scalpel handle #3 with #10 blade
- Metzenbaum scissors
- Mayo scissors (curved or straight)
- Debakey forceps
- Adsons forceps with teeth
- Babcock forceps (1–2)
- Kelly or Crile clamps (2–4)
- Right Angle Clamp (1-2)
- Small Malleable retractors
- Army Navy retractors
- Richardson retractor

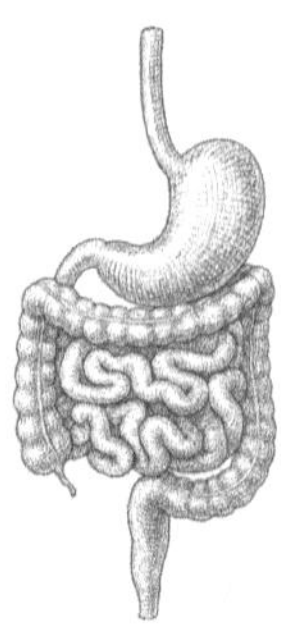

Breast Biopsy

Step 1 – Confirm site, position, prep, and mark incision
Instruments: Skin marker, ruler, marking pen, #15 blade, Adsons w/ teeth.
Anticipation: Verify correct side and lesion with surgeon and team. If a localization wire is present, ensure it is secured, not kinked, and always visible during draping.

Step 2 – Incise skin and access subcutaneous tissue
Instruments: #15 blade, Bovie, Adsonss, Debakeys, Metzenbaum scissors.
Anticipation: Anticipate frequent cautery use due to fatty breast tissue, keep Bovie clean and suction available. Hand small retractor such as skin hooks or Senns early to maintain exposure.

Step 3 – Deepen dissection toward palpable or imaged lesion
Instruments: Metzenbaum, Debakey, small Weitlaner, Ray-Tecs.
Anticipation: Maintain gentle retraction to avoid skin-edge ischemia. Be ready to blot frequently as bleeding can obscure the dissection plane.

Step 4 – Circumferential dissection and mobilization of mass
Instruments: Metzenbaum scissors, #15 blade, Allis or Babcock for traction, Debakeys.
Anticipation: Understand surgeon's margin technique, some want wide circumferential margins. Have orientation sutures or colored clips ready before the mass is freed.

Step 5 – Excise specimen and orient margins as required
Instruments: Allis/Babcock, marking sutures or clips, specimen cup, Ray-Tecs.
Anticipation: Confirm margin labeling sequence (e.g., long = lateral, short = superior). Speak each labeled margin clearly for circulator documentation. Avoid crushing tissue with forceful instruments. Have Ink, colored clips or suture for specimen marking

Step 6 – Inspect cavity, achieve hemostasis
Instruments: Bovie, suction, irrigation, hemostatic agents (Surgicel, Floseal).
Anticipation: Expect oozing from adipose tissue; keep suction quiet and ready. Anticipate surgeon needing to cauterize multiple small bleeders stay ahead with Bovie and Debakeys.

Step 7 – Evaluate cosmetic contour and approximate tissue planes
Instruments: Metzenbaum, needle driver, 3-0 absorbable sutures.
Anticipation: Many surgeons reshape cavity to prevent postoperative deformity, anticipate request for interrupted absorbable sutures to reapproximate deep tissue.

Step 8 – Consider drain placement (surgeon preference)
Instruments: JP or Blake drain, scissors, 3-0 nylon or silk for securing drain.
Anticipation: If surgeon routinely uses drains, have it primed early. Keep the trocar tip safe when handing. Prepare a drain exit site before closure begins.

Step 9 – Skin closure
Instruments: Needle driver, 4-0 Monocryl or Vicryl, Adsonss, skin adhesive or steri-strips.
Anticipation: Be prepared for subcuticular closure for cosmetic result. Have steri-strips and a nonadherent breast dressing ready.

Mayo Stand Suggestion:

- #15 blade on scalpel handle
- Adsons forceps with teeth
- Debakey forceps
- Metzenbaum scissors
- Mayo scissors (straight)
- 4 Curved hemostat
- Senn retractor
- Army Navy retractor (pair)
- Skin Hooks
- Allis clamps
- Babcock forceps
- Needle driver

Colon Resection (Open)

Step 1 – Midline laparotomy & initial exploration
Instruments: #10 blade, Bovie, Debakeys, Metzenbaum scissors, Army Navy retractor, Richardson retractor, Moist laps.
Anticipation: As soon as the peritoneum is opened, prepare suction; fluid often escapes. Hand moist laps quickly for quadrant packing. Anticipate a switch to deep retraction (Richardson) as exposure develops. Keep Optional Lap Sponge Stick prepared.

Step 2 – Identify target colon segment
Instruments: Debakeys, Metzenbaums, Deavers or Malleable retractor, laparotomy sponges.
Anticipation: Help the surgeon locate the diseased segment by retracting small bowel out of the operative quadrant. Use moist laps to maintain bowel hydration and prevent injury.

Step 3 – Mobilize colon by incising lateral peritoneal attachments
Instruments: Bovie, long Metzenbaums, Debakeys, Malleable retractor
Anticipation: Anticipate the white line of Toldt dissection; prepare long cautery tips for deep fields. Maintain steady, gentle retraction so the surgeon can follow the avascular plane safely.

Step 4 – Mobilize mesentery & identify vascular pedicle
Instruments: Debakeys, right-angle clamp, Metzenbaums, long retractor, vascular clips or ligature ties.
Anticipation: Know whether the surgeon plans high ligation (e.g., IMA, middle colic). Pre-load several 2-0/3-0 silk ties on right-angle clamps. Expect suction need when dissecting near major vessels.

Step 5 – Control and ligate vascular pedicle
Instruments: Right-angle clamps, Kellys, silk ties, clip applier, vascular stapler (if used), Metzenbaums.
Anticipation: Have ties on sticks ready in sequence, this part of surgery follows a clamp–tie–cut rhythm. Confirm vascular stapler type and reload color before passing it.

Step 6 – Transect bowel proximally and distally
Instruments: Doyen (atraumatic bowel) clamps, GIA or TA stapler with cartridges, Mayo scissors.
Anticipation: Moisture to protect bowel before clamping; anticipate surgeon's preference: stapled vs hand division. Open and test staplers ahead of time; confirm correct reload sizes, have available.

Step 7 – Remove specimen & confirm orientation
Instruments: Specimen basin, marking sutures/clips, long Deavers, Debakeys.
Anticipation: Mark orientation if requested. Confirm with circulator for pathology labeling. Prepare a basin and towel before specimen leaves the field.

Step 8 – Prepare for anastomosis (stapled or hand-sewn)
Instruments: Bowel clamps (Doyen), GIA/EEA stapler sets, anvil, lubricating jelly, sizers (for EEA).
Anticipation: If using EEA stapler, open full system early, verify that anvil, shaft, and staple height match. Assist with passing anvil into bowel and protect tissue edges during coupling.

Step 9 – Construct anastomosis
Instruments: EEA stapler (GIA/TA), needle drivers, 3-0/4-0 absorbable sutures for reinforcement.
Anticipation: For stapled anastomosis, anticipate alignment of tissue ends and assist with exposure. Expect leak test, prepare saline-filled syringe and clamps to occlude bowel segments when requested.

Colon Resection (Open)

Step 10 – Inspect anastomosis for hemostasis and integrity
Instruments: Bovie, bipolar, suction, irrigation.
Anticipation: Keep suction quiet and open; surgeons frequently blot and irrigate during this phase. Maintain exposure and suction so the surgeon can identify small staple-line bleeders. and anticipate hemostatic agents.

Step 11 – Irrigate abdomen and place drains if needed
Instruments: Irrigation setup, Poole suction, JP or Blake drain(s), 3-0 nylon/silk for drain stitch.
Anticipation: Confirm whether surgeon wants pelvic drain or no drain. Prime drain before placement; provide appropriate suture for securing drain to skin.

Step 12 – Close fascia and skin
Instruments: Needle driver, Mayo scissors, #1 or #0 fascial suture, 3-0/4-0 skin sutures or staples, Adsonss.
Anticipation: Pre-load fascial stitch before surgeon finishes irrigation. Start closing counts early. Prepare the correct skin closure tools—many surgeons switch between staples and subcuticular sutures.

Mayo Stand Suggestion:

- #10 blade on scalpel handle
- Metzenbaum scissors (standard length)
- Long Metzenbaum scissors (if deep abdomen)
- Mayo scissors (straight or curved)
- Debakey forceps (standard)
- Debakey forceps (long)
- Adsons with teeth (for skin/fascia)
- Kelly or Crile clamps (4–6)
- Right-angle clamps (2–3)
- Babcock forceps (2)
- Doyen bowel clamps (2)
- Army Navy retractor (pair)
- Malleable retractors (small or medium)
- Needle driver (Mayo-Hegar)
- Ties on sticks (silk preloaded on Kellys)

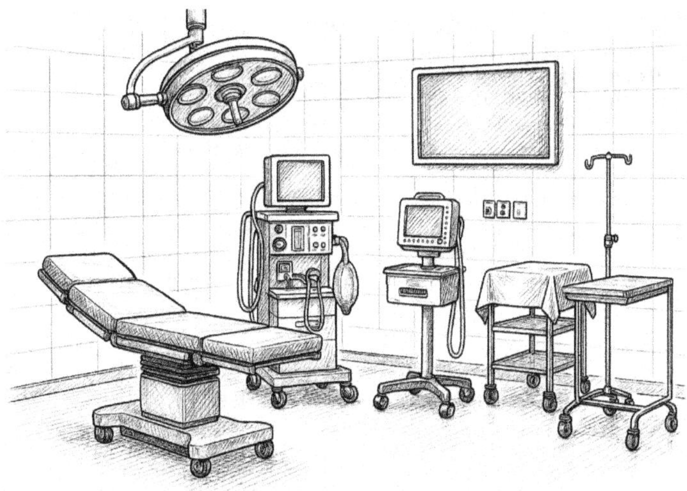

Gastrostomy (Open)

Step 1 – Upper midline or left subcostal incision
Instruments: #10 blade, Adsons w/ teeth, Bovie, Metzenbaum and Mayo scissors, Army Navy retractor, suction.
Anticipation: Expect quick transition from superficial to deep retraction: prepare Richardson retractors. Ensure suction is ready before peritoneum is entered; upper abdomen often releases fluid on entry.

Step 2 – Enter peritoneum & expose stomach
Instruments: Debakey forceps, Metzenbaum scissors, Poole suction, moist laps.
Anticipation: When the peritoneum is tented, have Metzenbaums ready for safe entry. Immediately pass moist laps to protect bowel and improve visualization. Assist with gentle retraction of left lobe of liver possibly with Deaver retractor, if needed.

Step 3 – Identify and mobilize anterior gastric wall
Instruments: Debakeys, Babcocks, Malleable retractors, moist laps.
Anticipation: Use Babcocks only (no toothed clamps) on stomach. Keep stomach moist to prevent serosal injury. Anticipate surgeon needing traction on the greater omentum to gain access.

Step 4 – Place stay sutures on stomach
Instruments: Needle driver, 2-0 absorbable or silk sutures, Mayo scissors.
Anticipation: Pre-cut 3–4 stay sutures before surgeon requests them. Load the first suture early and keep tails organized; these sutures will later secure the stomach to the abdominal wall.

Step 5 – Create gastrotomy
Instruments: #11 blade or cautery, Metzenbaum scissors, suction, Ray-Tecs.
Anticipation: Small gastric vessels may bleed, have suction ready and anticipate frequent Bovie use along with Debakeys. Prepare to stabilize stomach with stay sutures while surgeon makes opening.

Step 6 – Insert G-tube and verify position
Instruments: Selected G-tube (Malecot, Foley, or balloon-type), syringe for balloon inflation, lubricant, clamps.
Anticipation: Test balloon or patency before giving the tube to the surgeon. Lubricate tip and have the syringe prefilled. Confirm the surgeon's preferred tube type before opening packaging.

Step 7 – Secure tube to gastric wall (Stamm technique)
Instruments: Needle driver, 2-0 absorbable sutures for purse-string or fixation sutures.
Anticipation: Pre-load sutures and anticipate sequence: purse-string tightening → reinforcing sutures → test pull on tube. Keep traction on stay sutures steady to keep stomach in position.

Step 8 – Anchor stomach to peritoneum/abdominal wall
Instruments: Needle driver, absorbable sutures, Metzenbaums.
Anticipation: This step prevents leakage, expect surgeon to request multiple interrupted sutures. Pass sutures with consistent pattern; ensure tube isn't twisted or kinked while stomach is secured.

Step 9 – Irrigate, check hemostasis, and trim tube
Instruments: Irrigation set, Poole suction, scissors, hemostatic agents.
Anticipation: Offer warm irrigation to check for leaks. Have hemostatic agents available, minor gastric oozing is common. Prepare to trim tubing to surgeon's preferred external length.

Step 10 – Close incision & dress tube site
Instruments: Needle driver, Mayo scissors, fascial suture, 3-0/4-0 skin sutures or stapler, dressing supplies (split gauze for tube).

Gastrostomy (Open)

Anticipation: Pre-load fascial suture. Have split gauze and tube stabilization device ready. Assist with careful dressing placement to avoid traction on the fresh stoma.

Mayo Stand Suggestion:

- #10 blade on handle
- Metzenbaum scissors
- Mayo scissors
- Debakey forceps
- Adsons with teeth
- Babcock forceps (2)
- Hemostats
- Malleable retractors
- Army Navy retractor
- Richardson retractor
- Stay sutures (2-0) pre-loaded
- G-tube (Malecot/Foley) + prefilled syringe

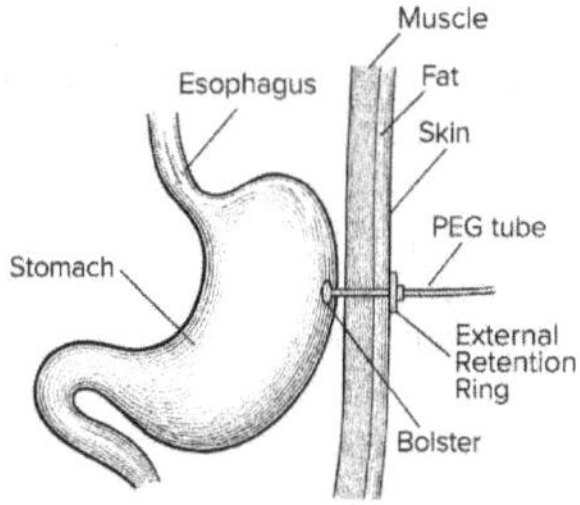

Hemorrhoidectomy

Step 1 – Position patient and expose anal canal
Instruments: Anal retractor (Hill-Ferguson, Pratt, or Fansler), lubricating jelly, light source.
Anticipation: Confirm lithotomy or jackknife position and protect all pressure points. Apply lubricant to retractor before passing. Prepare cottonoids and small sponges early for meticulous hemostasis.

Step 2 – Identify hemorrhoidal columns and plan excision
Instruments: Debakey or Adsons forceps, marking pen, suction.
Anticipation: Know typical hemorrhoid positions (3, 7, 11 o'clock). Provide gentle suction to clear small amounts of blood. Avoid excessive manipulation which can cause mucosal tears.

Step 3 – Grasp hemorrhoid and elevate tissue
Instruments: Allis clamps (1–2), Debakey forceps.
Anticipation: Hand Allis first to control the hemorrhoidal complex. Ensure traction is steady but not crushing. Prepare the Bovie for immediate use once mass is elevated.

Step 4 – Dissect hemorrhoid from underlying sphincter
Instruments: Bovie, Metzenbaum scissors, fine hemostats.
Anticipation: Maintain perfect visualization: adjust retractors angle frequently without being asked. Anticipate surgeon wanting precise cautery, provide smoke evacuation and keep Bovie tip clean.

Step 5 – Skeletonize and ligate vascular pedicle
Instruments: Needle driver, 2-0 or 3-0 absorbable suture, fine forceps.
Anticipation: Pre-load multiple sutures on the needle driver; this step can be repeated for each column. Keep the anal mucosa and internal sphincter protected to avoid postoperative complications.

Step 6 – Excise hemorrhoid
Instruments: Bovie or Metzenbaum scissors, Ray-Tecs, suction.
Anticipation: Expect oozing once excision occurs, anticipate suction and hemostatic agents. Keep track of Allis clamps so they don't over-rotate or drag tissue unintentionally.

Hemorrhoidectomy

Step 7 – Close mucosal defect (Ferguson) or leave open (Milligan-Morgan)
Instruments: Needle driver, fine absorbable sutures (3-0/4-0), small scissors.
Anticipation: Confirm closure style with surgeon before opening sutures. Offer fine, well-cut lengths. Keep tissue under minimal tension to avoid mucosal tearing.

Step 8 – Repeat for remaining hemorrhoidal columns
Instruments: Allis clamps, Bovie, Metzenbaums, suture material.
Anticipation: Anticipate surgeon's sequence: typically largest hemorrhoid first. Ensure good visualization by adjusting retractor between columns to prevent sphincter stretch.

Step 9 – Achieve final hemostasis
Instruments: Bovie, bipolar, hemostatic agents (Gelfoam, Surgicel), suction.
Anticipation: Maintain suction and retraction to assist the surgeon, as the anal canal bleeds easily. Offer bipolar for pinpoint bleeding. Have small hemostatic agents cut to size for quick placement.

Step 10 – Apply dressing and packing (if used)
Instruments: Ointment, lubricated gauze or commercial anal packing, abdominal pad.
Anticipation: Confirm surgeon preference, many avoid heavy packing. Apply ointment to the anal area gently. Prepare external gauze that will not adhere to perianal skin.

Mayo Stand Suggestion:

- Scalpel #15 Blade
- 2 curved Hemostats
- 2 Allis
- 2 Pennington
- Metzenbaum scissors
- Debakey forceps
- Adsons with teeth
- Self-retaining retractors
- handheld retractors

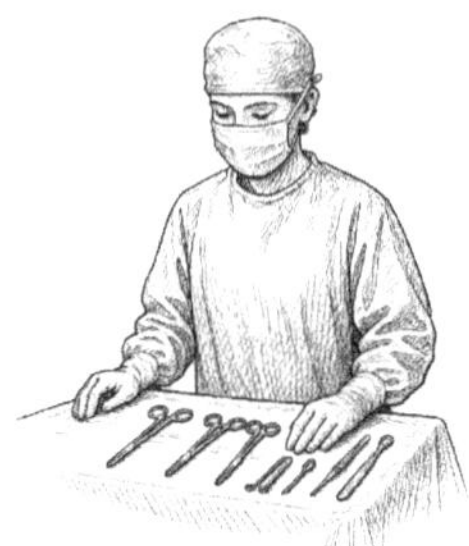

Laparoscopic Appendectomy

Step 1 – Establish pneumoperitoneum and place trocars
Instruments: Veress needle or Hasson trocar, 10–12 mm trocar (umbilical), two 5 mm trocars, insufflation tubing, camera.
Anticipation: Confirm insufflator settings and CO_2 flow before insertion. Ensure camera is white-balanced and focused. Hand trocars in correct order and orient angles for the surgeon's preferred port placement. 5mm in RUQ, 5mm midline Suprapubic

Step 2 – Diagnostic laparoscopy and identification of appendix
Instruments: 30° laparoscope, atraumatic bowel grasper, suction-irrigator.
Anticipation: Assist with camera movements: anticipate needs by keeping the appendix centered and horizon stable. Have suction ready for obscuring fluid or debris.

Step 3 – Expose appendix using atraumatic graspers
Instruments: Atraumatic graspers (Maryland or Babcock), laparoscopic suction-irrigation, laparoscopic dissector.
Anticipation: Appendix is grasped at the tip, never at the inflamed base. Anticipate surgeon needing tension/counter-tension, be proactive with retraction angles and instrument swapping.

Step 4 – Create window in mesoappendix
Instruments: Maryland dissector, hook cautery or Maryland cautery, suction-irrigator.
Anticipation: Prepare to control small bleeders with cautery quickly. Keep suction near but not obstructing the field. If appendix is retrocecal, expect difficult exposure—prepare an additional retractors or switch grasper positions.

Step 5 – Divide mesoappendix
Instruments: Laparoscopic bipolar, harmonic scalpel, or vascular stapler depending on surgeon preference.
Anticipation: If stapler is used, open and assemble with correct reload BEFORE the surgeon asks. Ensure harmonic tips stay clean. Monitor smoke accumulation and anticipate activation pauses for camera clarity.

Step 6 – Secure and divide the appendiceal base
Instruments: Endoloop (2–3 total), or linear stapler with appropriate load, laparoscopic scissors.
Anticipation: If using endoloops, load the loop guider correctly and have 2 loops ready (one for base, one for backup). If stapler is used, ensure CO_2 pressure remains stable before firing. Open specimen bag early if surgeon uses stapler for base.

Step 7 – Transect appendix and retrieve specimen
Instruments: Laparoscopic scissors or stapler, endoscopic specimen retrieval bag, suction-irrigator.
Anticipation: Open specimen bag before the surgeon requests it; keep the mouth open and accessible. Assist with angling the camera as the appendix is placed in the bag. Keep suction ready, abscess cases often release pus at removal.

Step 8 – Irrigate and inspect right lower quadrant
Instruments: Suction-irrigator, laparoscopic grasper, hemostatic agents.
Anticipation: Anticipate surgeon wanting irrigation under the cecum and around the pelvis. Keep camera steady to identify small bleeding points. Prepare hemostatic agents in anticipation of surgeon request during inspection.

Step 9 – Remove trocars and close port sites
Instruments: Needle driver, 0 or 2-0 absorbable sutures for fascia (if >10–12 mm port), skin sutures or Dermabond.
Anticipation: Prepare fascial closure suture before the last trocar is removed. Pass skin closure materials immediately. Confirm final instrument count matches post-specimen removal count.

Mayo Stand Suggestion:

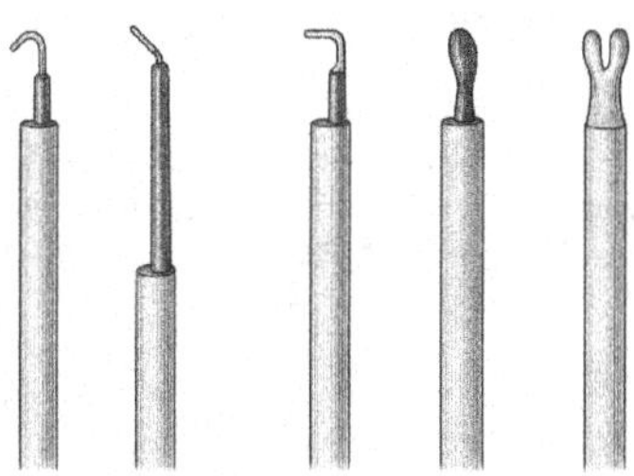

- 30° laparoscope
- Maryland dissector
- Atraumatic fenestrated grasper
- Laparoscopic scissors
- Suction-irrigation handpiece
- Hook cautery or Maryland cautery
- Endoloops (2–3) OR stapler with reloads
- Specimen retrieval bag
- Needle driver (laparoscopic)
- Port closure device (if used by surgeon)
- Laparoscopic suction tubing & irrigation extension
- Extra graspers for retraction

Laparoscopic Cholecystectomy

Step 1 – Establish pneumoperitoneum and place trocars
Instruments: Veress/Hasson, 10–12 mm trocar, 5 mm trocars, insufflation tubing, 30° scope.
Anticipation: Confirm insufflation setup and camera readiness; hand trocars in correct sequence for surgeon's preferred layout.

Step 2 – Explore abdomen and expose gallbladder
Instruments: 30° scope, atraumatic grasper, suction-irrigator.
Anticipation: Keep horizon level and anticipate traction needs; use suction early if fluid obscures RUQ.

Step 3 – Retract gallbladder for exposure
Instruments: Atraumatic graspers (2).
Anticipation: Maintain steady cephalad traction at fundus; anticipate adjustments to expose Calot's triangle.

Step 4 – Dissect peritoneum over Calot's triangle
Instruments: Maryland dissector, hook cautery, suction-irrigator.
Anticipation: Clear smoke promptly and maintain exposure so the surgeon can safely identify cystic duct and artery.

Step 5 – Achieve the Critical View of Safety
Instruments: Maryland dissector, atraumatic grasper.
Anticipation: Provide traction and counter-traction to fully expose hepatocystic triangle. Provide steady traction and exposure to allow the surgeon to confirm that only two structures enter the gallbladder.

Step 6 – Clip and divide the cystic duct
Instruments: Clip applier with clips, laparoscopic scissors.
Anticipation: Open correct clip size and have reloads ready; stabilize view and be prepared for suction if bile leaks.

Step 7 – Clip and divide the cystic artery
Instruments: Clip applier, scissors.
Anticipation: Pass clips cleanly and quickly; anticipate minor bleeding along artery and have suction positioned near—but not in—the field.

Step 8 – Dissect gallbladder off liver bed
Instruments: Hook cautery, suction-irrigator, atraumatic grasper.
Anticipation: Expect oozing from liver bed; be proactive with suction and keep camera steady to avoid losing depth perception.

Step 9 – Remove gallbladder through port
Instruments: Specimen bag, grasper, suction.
Anticipation: Open bag before requested; help orient camera for bag insertion. Prepare for suction if gallbladder is perforated.

Step 10 – Irrigate and inspect RUQ and liver bed
Instruments: Suction-irrigator, hemostatic agents.
Anticipation: Irrigate under liver edge and along cystic duct stump; assist in identifying small bleeders.

Laparoscopic Cholecystectomy

Step 11 – Remove trocars and close port sites
Instruments: Needle driver, absorbable sutures, skin closure materials.
Anticipation: Prepare fascial closure for ≥10–12 mm ports; have skin closure supplies ready and complete counts before final closure.

Mayo Stand Suggestion:

- 30° laparoscope
- Maryland dissector
- Hook cautery
- Atraumatic graspers (2)
- Laparoscopic scissors
- Suction-irrigator handpiece
- Clip applier + extra clips
- Specimen retrieval bag
- Laparoscopic needle driver
- Port closure device (if used)
- Extra atraumatic grasper
- Defogger for Scope

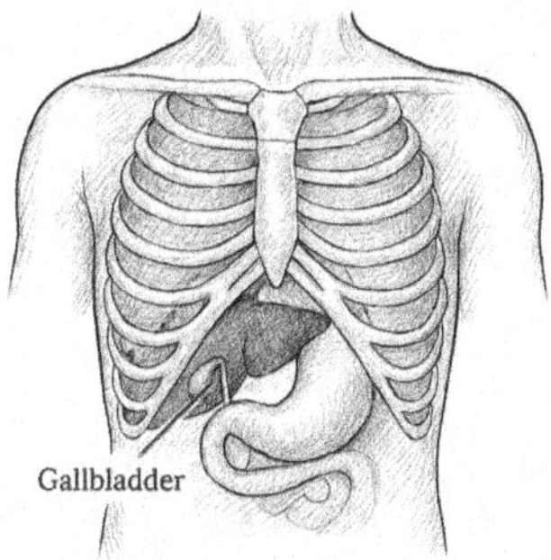

Laparoscopic Nissen Fundoplication

Step 1 – Establish pneumoperitoneum and place trocars
Instruments: Veress/Hasson setup, 30° scope, 10–12 mm and 5 mm trocars.
Anticipation: Ensure insufflation and camera are fully ready before trocar placement. Hand trocars in the correct sequence for the surgeon's preferred foregut layout.

Step 2 – Retract liver and expose the esophageal hiatus
Instruments: Nathanson liver retractors (or fan-type), atraumatic grasper.
Anticipation: Secure and adjust liver retractors for stable exposure of the hiatus. Expect the surgeon to reposition it frequently to improve visualization.

Step 3 – Divide gastrohepatic ligament
Instruments: Maryland dissector, hook cautery or harmonic scalpel, suction-irrigator.
Anticipation: Keep suction ready for small venous bleeders. Assist with counter-traction to avoid injuring the caudate lobe or aberrant left hepatic artery if present.

Step 4 – Dissect and mobilize the esophagus
Instruments: Maryland dissector, atraumatic graspers, blunt dissector.
Anticipation: Maintain gentle, steady traction on the esophagus. Anticipate surgeon wanting increased mediastinal exposure, adjust scope angle and graspers as requested.

Step 5 – Divide the short gastric vessels
Instruments: Harmonic scalpel or bipolar energy device, atraumatic grasper, suction-irrigator.
Anticipation: These vessels bleed easily, have suction close and keep the camera steady. Anticipate multiple energy activations and be proactive about smoke clearance.

Step 6 – Create posterior window behind esophagus
Instruments: Maryland dissector, blunt dissector, atraumatic graspers.
Anticipation: Assist with careful traction to avoid tearing the esophageal wall. When surgeon reaches posterior plane, be ready to pass graspers through the window to help pull the stomach behind the esophagus.

Laparoscopic Nissen Fundoplication

Step 7 – Bring fundus posteriorly and wrap around esophagus
Instruments: Atraumatic graspers (2), Maryland dissector.
Anticipation: Anticipate need for precise alignment, keep fundus tension balanced. Watch orientation to ensure the wrap is smooth and not twisted.

Step 8 – Construct the 360° fundoplication (Nissen wrap)
Instruments: Needle driver, 2-0 nonabsorbable sutures, atraumatic forceps.
Anticipation: Pre-load sutures and have 3–4 ready. Assist with holding fundus steady as sutures approximate left and right sides of the wrap. Keep tension gentle to avoid tearing gastric tissue.

Step 9 – Secure wrap to esophagus and crura (if surgeon prefers)
Instruments: Needle driver, sutures, atraumatic graspers.
Anticipation: Be prepared to pass interrupted sutures quickly; soft tissue bites require careful handling. Anticipate request to place a stitch anchoring wrap to esophagus or hiatus to prevent migration.

Step 10 – Final inspection, irrigation, and removal of trocars
Instruments: Suction-irrigator, hemostatic agents, needle driver for port closure.
Anticipation: Irrigate and suction near spleen, liver bed, and wrap. Prepare fascial closure for ≥10–12 mm port. Confirm counts before skin closure.

Mayo Stand Suggestion:

- Maryland dissector
- Atraumatic graspers (2–3)
- Hook cautery
- Harmonic scalpel (or bipolar device)
- Suction-irrigation handpiece
- Needle driver
- Right-angle or curved-tip dissector
- 5 Trocars (4x5mm, 1x10-12mm)
- Endoscopic scissors
- Liver retractors (Nathanson)
- Scope defog/anti-fog system
- Extra graspers for retraction
- Long atraumatic forceps for wrap manipulation

Laparoscopic Splenectomy

Step 1 – Establish pneumoperitoneum and place trocars
Instruments: Veress/Hasson setup, 30° scope, 10–12 mm trocar, three or four 5 mm trocars.
Anticipation: Confirm insufflator and camera readiness. Hand trocars in correct sequence: left upper quadrant ports must allow safe approach to hilum and splenic attachments.

Step 2 – Retract stomach and mobilize splenic flexure
Instruments: Atraumatic graspers, suction-irrigator, harmonic scalpel or bipolar device.
Anticipation: Retract stomach medially to expose spleen. Anticipate tension adjustments as surgeon frees splenic flexure; suction helps maintain a clear field when colonic attachments bleed.

Step 3 – Divide splenocolic ligament
Instruments: Harmonic scalpel or bipolar sealing device, atraumatic grasper.
Anticipation: The splenocolic ligament often has small vessels, keep suction close and the camera steady. Provide counter-traction to prevent tearing colon or capsule.

Step 4 – Mobilize spleen by dividing splenorenal and splenophrenic ligaments
Instruments: Energy device (harmonic, bipolar), atraumatic graspers.
Anticipation: Maintain gentle retraction as these ligaments can be thick. Watch for the tail of pancreas near the hilum; avoid traction that obscures it.

Laparoscopic Splenectomy

Step 5 – Identify and expose splenic hilum
Instruments: Maryland dissector, atraumatic graspers, suction-irrigator.
Anticipation: Keep field dry, visibility here is crucial. Anticipate need for precise camera movements and controlled retraction as surgeon isolates artery and vein.

Step 6 – Control splenic artery and vein
Instruments: Laparoscopic clip applier, vascular stapler (Endo GIA), laparoscopic scissors.
Anticipation: Prepare appropriate clip sizes and verify stapler reload compatibility. Be ready to clear smoke or fluid quickly, hilum bleeding becomes serious fast.

Step 7 – Complete mobilization of superior spleen and release remaining attachments
Instruments: Energy device, atraumatic graspers.
Anticipation: Spleen is fragile, anticipate extremely gentle handling. The short gastric vessels can bleed briskly; keep suction near and irrigate to maintain visibility.

Step 8 – Place spleen into retrieval bag
Instruments: Endoscopic retrieval bag, atraumatic graspers.
Anticipation: Open bag early and hold wide for insertion. Once spleen is inside, expect need for morcellation, ensure bag integrity and camera positioning allow safe fragmentation.

Step 9 – Remove spleen via enlarged port site
Instruments: Retrieval bag (loaded), Kelly or ring forceps, suction.
Anticipation: Monitor the extraction port, protect fascia from tearing. Anticipate surgeon needing suction for small blood collections forming during splenic removal.

Step 10 – Irrigate and inspect left upper quadrant
Instruments: Suction-irrigator, hemostatic agents.
Anticipation: Assist with irrigation and suction so the surgeon can inspect the diaphragm, pancreatic tail, and hilum for bleeding. Keep hemostatic agents ready slight oozing is common after splenic bed mobilization.

Step 11 – Remove trocars and close port sites
Instruments: Needle driver, 0 or 2-0 absorbable suture for fascia, skin closure supplies.
Anticipation: Prepare fascial closure for ≥10–12 mm ports, especially extraction site. Complete counts before final closure.

Mayo Stand Suggestion:

- #11 blade on scalpel handle
- Veress needle
- Trocars: 10–12 mm trocar and 5 mm trocars (2–3)
- Maryland dissector
- Atraumatic graspers (2–3)
- Harmonic scalpel or bipolar sealing device
- Laparoscopic scissors
- Suction–irrigation handpiece
- Clip applier with medium-large clips
- Specimen retrieval bag (large

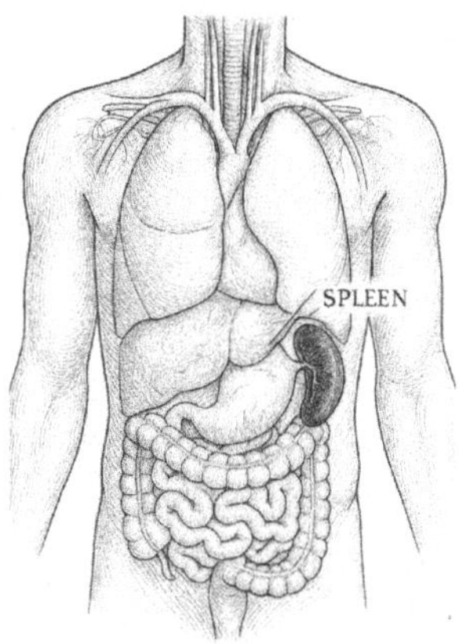

Exploratory Laparotomy

Step 1 – Midline incision
Instruments: #10 blade, Adsons with teeth, Bovie, Army Navy retractor.
Anticipation: Have Bovie tested and ready; hand retractor early for initial exposure. Expect deepening of incision quickly—prepare Richardson retractor.

Step 2 – Enter peritoneum safely
Instruments: Metzenbaum scissors, Debakey forceps, suction.
Anticipation: As peritoneum is tented, be ready with Metzenbaums. Anticipate sudden fluid escape —have suction positioned before entry.

Step 3 – Pack quadrants and expose pathology
Instruments: Moist laps, long Deaver or Malleable retractor, Poole suction.
Anticipation: Pass moist laps quickly for four-quadrant packing. Assist with systematic visualization —upper abdomen, pelvis, paracolic gutters.

Step 4 – Conduct systematic abdominal exploration
Instruments: Debakeys, long instruments, suction-irrigator.
Anticipation: Follow surgeon's order of exploration (stomach → liver → spleen → bowel → pelvis). Be ready to reposition retractors frequently to expose each region.

Step 5 – Identify and assess pathology
Instruments: Debakeys, Bovie, Metzenbaums.
Anticipation: Stabilize camera-like visualization with consistent retraction. Be ready to suction small bleeding points that obscure evaluation.

Step 6 – Perform indicated procedure (biopsy, repair, resection, control bleeding)
Instruments: Vary—fine needle driver, Metzenbaums, Kellys, clips, staplers, specimen cup.
Anticipation: Anticipate what the surgeon will likely need based on finding:
- mass → biopsy supplies
- bleeding → hemostats, clips
- perforation → suture, irrigate

Stay proactive and adapt quickly.

Step 7 – Irrigate operative field
Instruments: Irrigation system, Poole suction.
Anticipation: Prepare warm irrigation; anticipate surgeon needing repetitive irrigate–suction cycles for contamination or bleeding control.

Step 8 – Remove packs and re-inspect all quadrants
Instruments: Debakeys, suction, moist laps.
Anticipation: Count laps carefully as they leave the cavity. Maintain visualization as surgeon inspects bowel, liver, and pelvis for missed pathology.

Step 9 – Close fascia
Instruments: Needle driver, #1 or #0 sutures, Mayo scissors.
Anticipation: Pre-load the fascial suture and anticipate prolonged continuous suture—manage tension and suture tails carefully.

Step 10 – Close skin and apply dressing
Instruments: Skin stapler or suture, Adsons, dressing supplies.
Anticipation: Provide closure materials; prepare sterile dressing before skin closure is complete.

Exploratory Laparotomy

Mayo Stand Suggestion:

- #10 blade on scalpel handle
- Metzenbaum scissors
- Mayo scissors (curved or straight)
- Debakey forceps
- Adsons with teeth
- Army Navy retractor
- Richardson retractor
- Kelly/Crile clamps (4–6)
- Poole suction handpiece
- Needle driver (Mayo-Hegar)

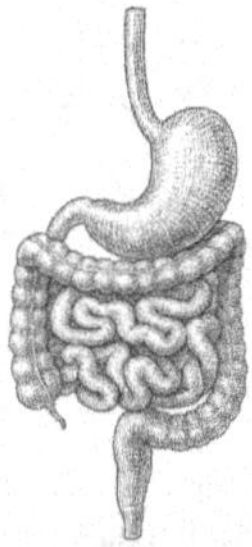

Liver Resection

Step 1 – Upper abdominal incision and exposure
Instruments: #10 blade, Adsons w/ teeth, Bovie, Army Navy retractor, Richardson/Deaver retractor.
Anticipation: Prepare deep retractor early; exposure escalates quickly. Ensure suction is ready—liver is highly vascular.

Step 2 – Enter peritoneum and pack abdomen
Instruments: Metzenbaum scissors, Debakeys, moist laps, Poole suction.
Anticipation: As peritoneum is tented, be ready for fluid release. Pack quadrants to isolate liver and protect bowel.

Step 3 – Mobilize liver by dividing ligamentous attachments
Instruments: Bovie, Metzenbaums, long Deavers, Malleable retractor.
Anticipation: Expect division of falciform, coronary, and triangular ligaments. Maintain steady retraction; avoid capsular tears.

Step 4 – Identify resection margins and target anatomy
Instruments: Debakeys, marking pen, intraoperative ultrasound probe (if used).
Anticipation: Be ready to adjust retractor repeatedly for visualization. If ultrasound is used, ensure probe cover and gel are prepared.

Step 5 – Control inflow (Pringle maneuver if used)
Instruments: Vascular tape/umbilical tape, right-angle clamp, Rumel tourniquet.
Anticipation: Have tape and tourniquet assembled before request. Be aware of clamp placement and be prepared to respond if the surgeon or anesthesia requests time confirmation.

Step 6 – Transect liver parenchyma
Instruments: CUSA, harmonic scalpel, bipolar device, suction-irrigator.
Anticipation: This is a bleeding-prone phase—keep suction active and camera-like visualization steady. Anticipate frequent instrument exchanges.

Step 7 – Identify and ligate intrahepatic vessels and ducts
Instruments: Right-angle clamps, clips, silk ties, laparoscopic or open vascular stapler (if used).
Anticipation: Pre-load ties and have clip reloads open. Maintain clear field—small ducts and veins are easily obscured.

Liver Resection

Step 8 – Complete specimen division and remove specimen
Instruments: Scalpel or scissors, specimen basin, marking sutures/clips.
Anticipation: Prepare specimen container early and confirm orientation requirements for pathology.

Step 9 – Achieve hemostasis of liver bed
Instruments: Argon beam coagulator, bipolar cautery, hemostatic agents (Surgicel, Floseal).
Anticipation: Expect prolonged hemostasis. Offer topical agents proactively and keep suction gentle to avoid disrupting clots.

Step 10 – Irrigate and inspect operative field
Instruments: Irrigation system, Poole suction.
Anticipation: Irrigate along cut surface and subphrenic space. Be alert for bile leakage—surgeon may request additional clips or sutures.

Step 11 – Place drains if indicated
Instruments: JP/Blake drain, scissors, 3-0 nylon or silk.
Anticipation: Prime drains early and prepare exit site. Ensure drain does not rest directly on raw liver surface unless surgeon prefers.

Step 12 – Close abdominal wall and skin
Instruments: Needle driver, #1 or #0 fascial sutures, Mayo scissors, skin stapler or sutures.
Anticipation: Pre-load fascial sutures. Start closing counts early; liver cases often have numerous sponges.

Mayo Stand Suggestion:

- #10 blade on scalpel handle
- Metzenbaum scissors
- Mayo scissors (curved)
- Debakey forceps
- Adsons with teeth
- Right-angle clamps (2–3)
- Kelly/Crile clamps (4–6)
- Long Deaver or Malleable retractors
- Needle driver (Mayo-Hegar)
- Umbilical/vascular tape with Rumel tourniquet

McVay Inguinal Herniorrhaphy (Cooper's Ligament)

Step 1 – Inguinal incision and superficial dissection
Instruments: #10 blade, Adsons w/ teeth, Bovie, Metzenbaum scissors, Army Navy retractor.
Anticipation: Prepare for quick transition to deeper exposure. Control superficial bleeders early to maintain a clean field.

Step 2 – Expose external oblique aponeurosis
Instruments: Metzenbaums, Debakeys, Army Navy retractor.
Anticipation: Identify and protect ilioinguinal and iliohypogastric nerves. Anticipate careful retraction to avoid nerve injury.

Step 3 – Incise external oblique and open inguinal canal
Instruments: Metzenbaums, Bovie, Debakeys, self-retaining retractors (Weitlaner).
Anticipation: As the canal opens, anticipate need for a self-retainer. Maintain orientation of cord structures throughout.

Step 4 – Isolate and protect spermatic cord
Instruments: Penrose drain or vessel loop, Debakeys, Babcock.
Anticipation: Pass Penrose early to gently retract the cord. Avoid excessive traction that could compromise cord contents.

McVay Inguinal Herniorrhaphy (Cooper's Ligament)

Step 5 – Identify hernia type and reduce hernia sac
Instruments: Metzenbaums, Debakeys, Babcock, suction.
Anticipation: Femoral hernias may be subtle—maintain exposure of the femoral canal. Anticipate opening sac carefully to avoid bowel injury.

Step 6 – Excise or ligate hernia sac
Instruments: Metzenbaums, Kelly clamps, absorbable ties.
Anticipation: Have ties pre-cut and ready. Expect clamp-tie-cut sequence; keep suction nearby for small bleeders.

Step 7 – Identify Cooper's (pectineal) ligament
Instruments: Debakeys, right-angle clamp, Malleable retractors.
Anticipation: Cooper's ligament lies deep and medial—anticipate need for strong lighting and retraction. Avoid femoral vein injury.

Step 8 – Approximate transversus abdominis/conjoint tendon to Cooper's ligament
Instruments: Needle driver, nonabsorbable sutures (e.g., 0 or 1), Mayo scissors.
Anticipation: Sutures are placed under tension—assist by maintaining exposure and controlling suture tails. Watch closely for femoral vessel proximity.

Step 9 – Continue repair laterally to inguinal ligament
Instruments: Needle driver, sutures, Debakeys.
Anticipation: Expect multiple interrupted sutures. Anticipate surgeon checking tension to avoid postoperative pain or recurrence.

Step 10 – Reposition spermatic cord and close inguinal canal
Instruments: Metzenbaums, Debakeys, absorbable sutures.
Anticipation: Ensure cord lies without twisting or compression. Maintain clear visualization during layered closure.

Step 11 – Close external oblique and superficial layers
Instruments: Needle driver, absorbable sutures, Mayo scissors.
Anticipation: Prepare sutures early; layered closure proceeds quickly once repair is complete.

Step 12 – Skin closure and dressing
Instruments: Skin stapler or sutures, Adsonss, dressing supplies.
Anticipation: Provide closure materials promptly. Prepare pressure dressing if surgeon prefers to reduce seroma formation.

Mayo Stand Suggestion:

- #10 blade on scalpel handle
- Metzenbaum scissors
- Mayo scissors (curved)
- Debakey forceps
- Adsons with teeth
- Kelly clamps (4)
- Right-angle clamp
- Babcock forceps
- Needle driver (Mayo-Hegar)
- Penrose drain or vessel loop

Modified Radical Mastectomy

Step 1 – Skin marking and incision
Instruments: Skin marker, #10 blade, Adsons w/ teeth, Bovie, Army Navy retractor.
Anticipation: Confirm side and incision pattern (elliptical). Hand retractor early and keep Bovie ready skin flaps require meticulous hemostasis.

Step 2 – Elevate superior and inferior skin flaps
Instruments: Bovie, Metzenbaum scissors, Debakey forceps, Army Navy or Richardson retractor.
Anticipation: Maintain even flap thickness to preserve vascularity. Anticipate frequent cautery for diffuse bleeding in subcutaneous tissue.

Step 3 – Dissect breast tissue off pectoralis major
Instruments: Bovie, Metzenbaums, Debakeys, moist laps.
Anticipation: Protect pectoralis fascia if surgeon preserves it. Keep laps moist to protect muscle and reduce tissue trauma.

Step 4 – Identify and preserve pectoralis major; expose axilla
Instruments: Debakeys, long Metzenbaums, Malleable or Deaver retractor.
Anticipation: Exposure shifts toward axilla, anticipate deeper retraction. Maintain clear visualization as anatomy becomes more complex.

Step 5 – Identify axillary vein and landmarks
Instruments: Debakeys, right-angle clamp, suction.
Anticipation: The axillary vein is fragile, keep suction quiet and field dry. Be ready to adjust retractor frequently to avoid vessel injury.

Step 6 – Perform axillary lymph node dissection (Levels I–II)
Instruments: Metzenbaums, right-angle clamps, clips or ties, suction.
Anticipation: Watch for thoracodorsal nerve, long thoracic nerve, and vessels. Anticipate repeated clamp–tie–cut sequence; have ties and clips ready.

Step 7 – Control bleeding and complete breast removal
Instruments: Bovie, bipolar, hemostatic agents, suction.
Anticipation: Axillary dissection often oozes, offer hemostatic agents proactively. Maintain gentle suction to avoid disrupting clots.

Step 8 – Orient and remove specimen
Instruments: Specimen basin, marking sutures/clips.
Anticipation: Confirm orientation requirements for pathology. Prepare basin before specimen leaves field to avoid delays.

Step 9 – Irrigate operative field and reassess hemostasis
Instruments: Irrigation system, suction.
Anticipation: Expect surgeon to inspect axilla closely. Be ready to suction pooled fluid and identify small bleeders.

Step 10 – Place drains (usually two)
Instruments: JP or Blake drains, scissors, 3-0 nylon or silk.
Anticipation: Prime drains early and prepare exit sites. Ensure drains are positioned to cover both breast bed and axilla.

Modified Radical Mastectomy

Step 11 – Close deep tissue and skin
Instruments: Needle driver, absorbable sutures, Mayo scissors, skin stapler or sutures.
Anticipation: Anticipate layered closure; have sutures pre-loaded. Coordinate with circulator for drain count and final counts.

Step 12 – Apply dressing and secure drains
Instruments: Nonadherent dressing, gauze, tape, drain bulbs.
Anticipation: Secure drains without tension. Prepare bulky dressing or breast binder if surgeon prefers.

Mayo Stand Suggestion:

- #10 blade on scalpel handle
- Metzenbaum scissors
- Mayo scissors (curved)
- Debakey forceps
- Adsons with teeth
- Army Navy retractor
- Right-angle clamps (2)
- Kelly clamps (4)
- Needle driver (Mayo-Hegar)
- JP or Blake drains

Open Chole with Cholangiogram

Step 1 – Right subcostal incision and exposure
Instruments: #10 blade, Adsons with teeth, Bovie, Army Navy retractor, Richardson retractor, suction.
Anticipation: Anticipate rapid need for deep retraction. Have suction ready before entering the peritoneum as bile stained fluid may be present.

Step 2 – Enter peritoneum and expose gallbladder
Instruments: Metzenbaum scissors, Debakey forceps, moist laps, Poole suction.
Anticipation: As the peritoneum is tented, be ready with Metzenbaums. Pack bowel away from the right upper quadrant promptly with moist laps.

Step 3 – Retract gallbladder and expose Calots triangle
Instruments: Babcock forceps, Debakeys, Malleable or Deaver retractor.
Anticipation: Use atraumatic traction on the gallbladder fundus. Maintain steady exposure to clearly visualize cystic duct and artery.

Step 4 – Dissect tissue in Calots triangle
Instruments: Metzenbaum scissors, Bovie, right angle clamp, suction.
Anticipation: Maintain a clean field to prevent misidentification of structures. Anticipate frequent suction and careful blunt dissection.

Step 5 – Isolate cystic duct for cholangiogram
Instruments: Right angle clamp, vessel loop or silk tie.
Anticipation: Pass ties early and be prepared to partially occlude the cystic duct without transecting it. Confirm cholangiogram equipment readiness.

Step 6 – Perform intraoperative cholangiogram
Instruments: Cholangiogram catheter, syringe with contrast, C arm drape, clamps.
Anticipation: Coordinate with anesthesia and radiology for imaging. Flush catheter to remove air before insertion to avoid false filling defects.

Step 7 – Clip or ligate and divide cystic duct
Instruments: Clips or silk ties, Metzenbaum or Mayo scissors.
Anticipation: Confirm cholangiogram completion before division. Anticipate bile leakage and have suction positioned.

Open Chole with Cholangiogram

Step 8 – Clip or ligate and divide cystic artery
Instruments: Right angle clamp, clips or ties, scissors.
Anticipation: Cystic artery may retract after division. Maintain exposure and be ready to control bleeding immediately.

Step 9 – Dissect gallbladder from liver bed
Instruments: Bovie, Metzenbaum scissors, suction irrigation.
Anticipation: Expect oozing from the liver bed. Offer gentle suction and hemostatic agents as needed.

Step 10 – Remove gallbladder and inspect field
Instruments: Specimen basin, Debakeys, suction.
Anticipation: Prepare specimen container early. Inspect liver bed and ductal stumps for bleeding or bile leakage.

Step 11 – Irrigate and place drain if indicated
Instruments: Irrigation system, Poole suction, JP or Blake drain, scissors, suture.
Anticipation: Prime drain early and prepare exit site. Confirm surgeon preference regarding drain placement.

Step 12 – Close incision and apply dressing
Instruments: Needle driver, #1 or #0 fascial suture, Mayo scissors, skin staples or sutures.
Anticipation: Preload fascial sutures. Coordinate counts and prepare dressing before skin closure begins.

Mayo Stand Suggestion:

- #10 blade on scalpel handle
- Metzenbaum scissors
- Mayo scissors curved
- Debakey forceps
- Adsons with teeth
- Babcock forceps
- Right angle clamp
- Kelly clamps
- Needle driver
- Cholangiogram catheter and syringe

Pancreatectomy

Step 1 – Upper abdominal incision and exposure
Instruments: #10 blade, Adsons with teeth, Bovie, Army Navy retractor, Richardson or Deaver retractor, suction.
Anticipation: Exposure escalates quickly. Prepare deep retractor early and keep suction ready due to vascular tissue.

Step 2 – Enter peritoneum and pack abdomen
Instruments: Metzenbaum scissors, Debakey forceps, moist laps, Poole suction.
Anticipation: As peritoneum is tented, anticipate fluid release. Pack bowel away from upper abdomen to isolate the pancreas.

Step 3 – Expose pancreas and identify anatomy
Instruments: Debakeys, long Metzenbaums, Malleable retractor.
Anticipation: Identify stomach, transverse colon, and pancreas orientation. Expect frequent retractors adjustments for visualization.

Step 4 – Open lesser sac
Instruments: Bovie, Metzenbaums, Debakeys, suction.
Anticipation: Dissection near gastrocolic ligament may bleed. Maintain gentle traction to avoid gastric injury.

Step 5 – Mobilize pancreas from surrounding structures
Instruments: Metzenbaums, Debakeys, right angle clamp, suction.
Anticipation: Be alert for splenic vessels in distal resections. Maintain a clear field and anticipate careful blunt dissection.

Step 6 – Identify and control splenic artery and vein if applicable
Instruments: Right angle clamps, clips or silk ties, vascular stapler if used.
Anticipation: Have multiple ties and clip reloads ready. Vascular control is critical before pancreatic division.

Step 7 – Transect pancreas
Instruments: Scalpel or stapler, Mayo scissors, suction.
Anticipation: Anticipate pancreatic fluid leakage. Suction and hemostatic agents should be immediately available.

Step 8 – Secure pancreatic remnant
Instruments: Needle driver, nonabsorbable or absorbable sutures, hemostatic agents.
Anticipation: Surgeons may oversew or staple the stump. Prepare sutures early and manage suture tails carefully.

Step 9 – Remove specimen and orient for pathology
Instruments: Specimen basin, marking sutures or clips.
Anticipation: Confirm specimen orientation requirements before removal to avoid delays.

Step 10 – Irrigate operative field and inspect for leaks
Instruments: Irrigation system, Poole suction.
Anticipation: Maintain exposure and suction so the surgeon can inspect for pancreatic duct leakage and bleeding. Be ready to assist with additional sutures or sealants.

Step 11 – Place drains near pancreatic stump
Instruments: JP or Blake drain, scissors, silk or nylon sutures.
Anticipation: Prime drains early and ensure correct positioning to monitor pancreatic output.

Step 12 – Close abdominal wall and skin
Instruments: Needle driver, #1 or #0 fascial sutures, Mayo scissors, skin closure supplies.
Anticipation: Start closing counts early. Ensure drains are secured and functioning before final closure.

Mayo Stand Suggestion:

- #10 blade on scalpel handle
- Metzenbaum scissors
- Mayo scissors curved
- Debakey forceps
- Right angle clamps
- Kelly clamps
- Needle driver
- Vascular clips or ties
- Malleable retractors

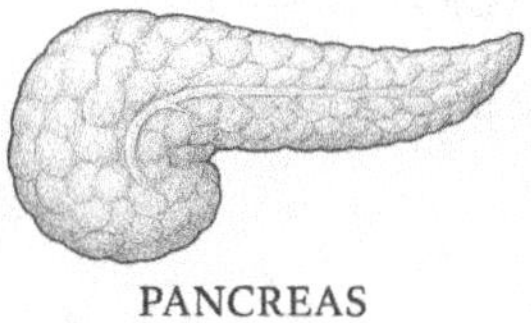

PANCREAS

Pancreaticduodenectomy (Whipple)

Step 1 – Upper abdominal incision and exposure
Instruments: #10 blade, Adsons with teeth, Bovie, Army Navy retractor, Richardson or Deaver retractor, suction.
Anticipation: This is a long case with escalating exposure needs. Prepare deep retractor early and confirm suction and cautery function before proceeding.

Step 2 – Enter peritoneum and perform initial exploration
Instruments: Metzenbaum scissors, Debakey forceps, moist laps, Poole suction.
Anticipation: As peritoneum is tented, be ready for fluid release. Assist with systematic exploration to rule out metastatic disease before proceeding.

Step 3 – Mobilize duodenum Kocher maneuver
Instruments: Metzenbaums, Debakeys, long Malleable or Deaver retractor.
Anticipation: Maintain steady medial retraction of the duodenum. Be alert for inferior vena cava and portal structures during deep dissection.

Step 4 – Expose pancreas and identify major vascular structures
Instruments: Debakeys, right angle clamps, suction.
Anticipation: Maintain a dry field to visualize portal vein superior mesenteric vein and artery. Expect frequent suction use and careful retraction.

Step 5 – Divide stomach or duodenum depending on technique
Instruments: GIA or TA stapler with appropriate reloads, bowel clamps, Mayo scissors.
Anticipation: Confirm whether a pylorus preserving approach is planned. Have correct stapler loads opened and tested before division.

Step 6 – Transect common bile duct
Instruments: Right angle clamp, Metzenbaum scissors, silk ties or clips.
Anticipation: Anticipate bile spillage. Keep suction ready and maintain clear visualization of ductal anatomy.

Step 7 – Transect pancreas at neck
Instruments: Scalpel or stapler, suction, hemostatic agents.
Anticipation: Expect pancreatic juice leakage. Keep suction close and be ready to assist with suture control of the pancreatic stump.

Step 8 – Control and divide pancreaticoduodenal vessels
Instruments: Right angle clamps, clips or silk ties, vascular stapler if used.
Anticipation: This is a critical bleeding risk phase. Pre load ties and have clip reloads immediately available.

Step 9 – Remove specimen and orient for pathology
Instruments: Specimen basin, marking sutures or clips.
Anticipation: Confirm orientation before specimen leaves field. Communicate clearly with circulator for pathology documentation.

Step 10 – Reconstruct pancreaticojejunostomy
Instruments: Needle driver, fine absorbable sutures, atraumatic forceps.
Anticipation: This anastomosis is delicate. Prepare multiple fine sutures early and manage suture tails carefully to prevent tangling.

Pancreaticduodenectomy (Whipple)

Step 11 – Reconstruct hepaticojejunostomy
Instruments: Needle driver, fine absorbable sutures, Debakey forceps.
Anticipation: Keep bile duct edges moist and visible. Anticipate slow deliberate suturing and maintain optimal exposure.

Step 12 – Reconstruct gastrojejunostomy or duodenojejunostomy
Instruments: Stapler or needle driver and sutures, bowel clamps.
Anticipation: Confirm reconstruction sequence with surgeon. Prepare staplers or sutures well in advance.

Step 13 – Irrigate and inspect all anastomoses
Instruments: Irrigation system, Poole suction.
Anticipation: Carefully inspect for bleeding or leaks. Be ready to assist with reinforcement sutures or sealants.

Step 14 – Place drains near anastomoses
Instruments: JP or Blake drains, scissors, silk or nylon sutures.
Anticipation: Prime drains early and confirm placement near pancreatic and biliary anastomoses.

Step 15 – Close abdominal wall and skin
Instruments: Needle driver, #1 or #0 fascial sutures, Mayo scissors, skin closure supplies.
Anticipation: Begin closing counts early. Ensure drains are secured and functioning before final closure.

Mayo Stand Suggestion:

- #10 blade on scalpel handle
- Metzenbaum scissors
- Mayo scissors curved
- Debakey forceps
- Adsons with teeth
- Right angle clamps
- Kelly clamps
- Needle driver
- Vascular clips or ties
- Malleable retractors

Sentinel Node Biopsy

Step 1 – Confirm injection site and patient positioning
Instruments: Skin marker, towels, sterile gauze.
Anticipation: Verify laterality and injection site before prep. Confirm time of dye injection since lymphatic uptake timing affects node visualization.

Step 2 – Inject Isosulfan blue dye
Instruments: Syringe with Isosulfan blue dye, fine needle, gauze.
Anticipation: Inject slowly to avoid tissue necrosis. Be aware of possible allergic reaction including hypotension or rash and communicate any changes immediately.

Step 3 – Massage injection site to promote lymphatic flow
Instruments: Sterile gauze or gloved hands.
Anticipation: Gentle massage improves dye migration. Time management matters here since sentinel node staining is time dependent.

Step 4 – Make incision over nodal basin
Instruments: #15 blade, Adsons with teeth, Bovie, Army Navy retractor.
Anticipation: Incision is often small and precise. Hand retractor early and maintain meticulous hemostasis for visibility.

Sentinel Node Biopsy

Step 5 – Dissect through subcutaneous tissue
Instruments: Metzenbaum scissors, Debakey forceps, Bovie, suction.
Anticipation: Blue stained lymphatic channels may be delicate. Avoid aggressive traction that could tear vessels and obscure the sentinel node.

Step 6 – Identify blue stained lymphatic channels
Instruments: Debakey forceps, Metzenbaums, suction.
Anticipation: Maintain a dry field. Use gentle blunt dissection to follow dye to the sentinel node.

Step 7 – Identify sentinel lymph node
Instruments: Debakeys, Metzenbaums, small retractor.
Anticipation: The node may be partially blue or only lightly stained. Anticipate surgeon palpating for firmness while visually confirming dye uptake.

Step 8 – Excise sentinel lymph node
Instruments: Metzenbaums, small hemostats, specimen cup.
Anticipation: Avoid crushing the node. Open specimen container before excision and confirm correct labeling immediately.

Step 9 – Inspect wound for additional blue nodes
Instruments: Debakeys, suction, Bovie.
Anticipation: More than one sentinel node may be present. Maintain exposure while surgeon reassesses the field.

Step 10 – Achieve hemostasis
Instruments: Bovie, bipolar, suction.
Anticipation: Bleeding can obscure small lymphatics. Keep suction gentle to avoid disrupting fragile tissue.

Step 11 – Close incision
Instruments: Needle driver, absorbable sutures, Mayo scissors, skin closure supplies.
Anticipation: Closure is typically cosmetic. Have fine sutures ready and assist with layered approximation.

Step 12 – Apply dressing and monitor patient
Instruments: Nonadherent dressing, gauze, tape.
Anticipation: Blue dye may discolor urine and skin temporarily. Ensure anesthesia and recovery staff are aware of dye administration.

Mayo Stand Suggestion:

- #15 blade on scalpel handle
- Metzenbaum scissors
- Mayo scissors curved
- Debakey forceps
- Adsons with teeth
- Small hemostats
- Army Navy retractor
- Needle driver
- Syringe with Isosulfan blue dye
- Specimen cup

SENTINEL NODE BIOPSY

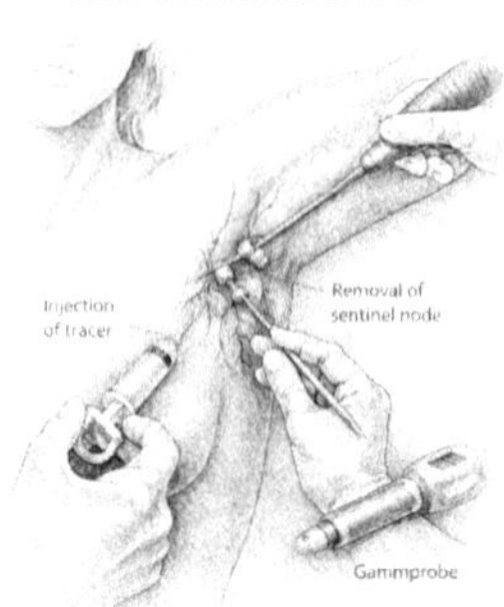

Splenectomy Open

Step 1 – Upper abdominal incision and exposure
Instruments: #10 blade, Adsons with teeth, Bovie, Army Navy retractor, Richardson or Deaver retractor, suction.
Anticipation: Exposure deepens quickly in the left upper quadrant. Prepare long retractor early and keep suction ready due to vascular tissue.

Step 2 – Enter peritoneum and pack abdomen
Instruments: Metzenbaum scissors, Debakey forceps, moist laps, Poole suction.
Anticipation: As the peritoneum is tented, anticipate fluid release. Pack abdomen with moist laparotomy sponges to protect it and isolate the spleen.

Step 3 –The costal margin is retracted upward
Instruments: Bovie, Metzenbaums, Debakeys, Malleable retractors.
Anticipation: Gentle traction prevents injury.

Step 4 – Divide splenocolic ligament
Instruments: Bovie or energy device, Debakeys, suction.
Anticipation: This ligament may contain small vessels. Keep suction close and the field dry.

Step 5 – Divide splenorenal and splenophrenic ligaments
Instruments: Metzenbaums, Bovie or harmonic device, long retractor.
Anticipation: Maintain steady retraction. Be mindful of the diaphragm and tail of the pancreas during dissection.

Step 6 – Identify and control short gastric vessels
Instruments: Right angle clamps, clips or silk ties, Metzenbaums.
Anticipation: Short gastrics bleed easily. Preload ties and anticipate clamp tie cut rhythm.

Step 7 – Identify splenic artery and vein
Instruments: Debakey forceps, right angle clamp, suction.
Anticipation: Clear visualization is critical. Maintain gentle handling to avoid avulsion of vessels.

Step 8 – Ligate and divide splenic vessels
Instruments: Right angle clamps, vascular clips or ties, scissors or vascular stapler if used.
Anticipation: Confirm complete control before division. Be ready to manage brisk bleeding if vessel retracts.

Step 9 – Remove spleen from operative field
Instruments: Specimen basin, moist laps.
Anticipation: Handle spleen gently to avoid capsular rupture. Prepare specimen basin early.

Step 10 – Inspect splenic bed and tail of pancreas
Instruments: Suction irrigation, Debakeys, hemostatic agents.
Anticipation: Look specifically for bleeding and pancreatic injury. Anticipate additional clips or sutures if oozing persists.

Step 11 – Irrigate and place drain if indicated
Instruments: Irrigation system, Poole suction, JP or Blake drain, scissors, sutures.
Anticipation: Prime drain early and position near splenic bed if used. Confirm surgeon preference.

Splenectomy Open

Step 12 – Close abdominal wall and skin
Instruments: Needle driver, #1 or #0 fascial sutures, Mayo scissors, skin closure supplies.
Anticipation: Begin closing counts early. Ensure drains are secured before final skin closure.

Mayo Stand Suggestion:

- #10 blade on scalpel handle
- Metzenbaum scissors
- Mayo scissors curved
- Debakey forceps
- Adsons with teeth
- Right angle clamps
- Kelly clamps
- Long Deaver or Malleable retractors
- Needle driver
- Vascular clips or silk ties

TEP Laparoscopic Inguinal Hernia Repair

Step 1 – Infraumbilical incision and access to preperitoneal space
Instruments: #11 blade, Veress needle or balloon dissector, 10 mm trocar, camera.
Anticipation: Confirm correct plane before balloon inflation. Maintain midline orientation to avoid peritoneal violation.

Step 2 – Create preperitoneal working space
Instruments: Balloon dissector, insufflation tubing, 30 degree laparoscope.
Anticipation: Watch for loss of space from peritoneal tears. Keep insufflation pressure controlled to maintain workspace.

Step 3 – Place additional trocars under direct vision
Instruments: Two 5 mm trocars, trocar obturators.
Anticipation: Trocar placement must stay within preperitoneal space. Anticipate need to reposition if peritoneum balloons inward.

Step 4 – Identify key anatomical landmarks
Instruments: Maryland dissector, atraumatic graspers.
Anticipation: Clearly identify pubic tubercle, Cooper ligament, inferior epigastric vessels, and spermatic cord structures before dissection.

Step 5 – Reduce hernia sac
Instruments: Maryland dissector, atraumatic grasper, suction if needed.
Anticipation: Indirect sacs may be long and adherent. Apply gentle traction to avoid tearing peritoneum or cord structures.

Step 6 – Dissect cord structures free of hernia sac
Instruments: Maryland dissector, blunt dissector.
Anticipation: Protect vas deferens and testicular vessels. Maintain clear separation between sac and cord.

Step 7 – Identify and reduce direct hernia defect if present
Instruments: Atraumatic grasper, Maryland dissector.
Anticipation: Direct defects appear as bulges in Hesselbach triangle. Maintain gentle pressure to fully reduce sac contents.

Step 8 – Prepare space for mesh placement
Instruments: Maryland dissector, suction irrigation if needed.
Anticipation: Ensure wide dissection extends beyond myopectineal orifice. Poor space preparation leads to mesh folding.

TEP Laparoscopic Inguinal Hernia Repair

Step 9 – Insert and position mesh
Instruments: Pre shaped mesh, graspers.
Anticipation: Orient mesh correctly to cover indirect direct and femoral spaces. Keep mesh flat and untwisted.

Step 10 – Fix mesh if surgeon prefers
Instruments: Tack device or sutures.
Anticipation: Avoid tacking near nerves or vessels. Confirm surgeon preference since many TEP repairs are non fixation.

Step 11 – Desufflate preperitoneal space and inspect mesh position
Instruments: Camera, suction.
Anticipation: Watch mesh remain flat during desufflation. Adjust if migration occurs.

Step 12 – Remove trocars and close port sites
Instruments: Needle driver, absorbable sutures, skin closure supplies.
Anticipation: Close fascia at larger ports. Complete counts before skin closure.

Mayo Stand Suggestion:

- #11 blade on scalpel handle
- Veress needle or balloon dissector
- 10 mm trocar
- Two 5 mm trocars
- Maryland dissector
- Atraumatic graspers
- Laparoscopic scissors
- Pre shaped mesh
- Tack device if used
- Needle driver

Thyroidectomy

Step 1 – Transverse cervical incision and exposure
Instruments: #15 blade, Adsons with teeth, Bovie, Army Navy retractor, suction.
Anticipation: Incision is cosmetic and precise. Maintain meticulous hemostasis early to keep the field clear and avoid obscuring small vessels.

Step 2 – Elevate subplatysmal flaps
Instruments: Bovie, Metzenbaum scissors, Debakey forceps, Army Navy retractor.
Anticipation: Preserve flap thickness to protect blood supply. Anticipate frequent cautery for small bleeding vessels.

Step 3 – Separate strap muscles
Instruments: Metzenbaums, Debakeys, self retaining retractors if used.
Anticipation: Gentle midline separation avoids muscle damage. Maintain exposure without excessive lateral traction.

Step 4 – Expose thyroid gland
Instruments: Debakeys, Babcock forceps, Malleable retractors.
Anticipation: Use atraumatic graspers on thyroid tissue. Anticipate need for steady medial and inferior traction.

Step 5 – Control superior pole vessels
Instruments: Right angle clamp, silk ties or clips, Metzenbaums.
Anticipation: Stay close to the gland to protect the external branch of the superior laryngeal nerve. Preload ties and control vessels sequentially.

Step 6 – Identify and preserve recurrent laryngeal nerve
Instruments: Debakeys, suction, nerve monitor probe if used.
Anticipation: Maintain a dry field and minimal traction. Alert surgeon immediately if nerve monitor signals change.

Step 7 – Identify and preserve parathyroid glands
Instruments: Debakeys, Metzenbaums, moist laps.
Anticipation: Keep glands moist and intact. Be prepared for autotransplant if gland viability is compromised.

Step 8 – Control inferior thyroid vessels
Instruments: Right angle clamps, clips or ties, Metzenbaums.
Anticipation: These vessels are close to the recurrent laryngeal nerve. Maintain clear visualization and controlled dissection.

Step 9 – Remove thyroid lobe or entire gland
Instruments: Babcock forceps, Metzenbaums, specimen basin.
Anticipation: Handle specimen gently. Prepare basin early and confirm orientation requirements if malignancy is suspected.

Step 10 – Inspect field and achieve hemostasis
Instruments: Bovie, bipolar cautery, suction, hemostatic agents.
Anticipation: Even small bleeders can cause postoperative airway compromise. Inspect thoroughly before closure.

Step 11 – Place drain if indicated
Instruments: JP drain, scissors, silk or nylon suture.
Anticipation: Prime drain early. Confirm placement does not compress airway structures.

Step 12 – Close strap muscles skin and apply dressing
Instruments: Needle driver, absorbable sutures, Mayo scissors, skin closure supplies.
Anticipation: Ensure no bleeding before closure. Prepare pressure dressing if surgeon prefers.

Mayo Stand Suggestion:

- #15 blade on scalpel handle
- Metzenbaum scissors
- Mayo scissors curved
- Debakey forceps
- Adsons with teeth
- Babcock forceps
- Needle driver
- Suction tip
- Hemostatic agents
- Right Angle Clamps

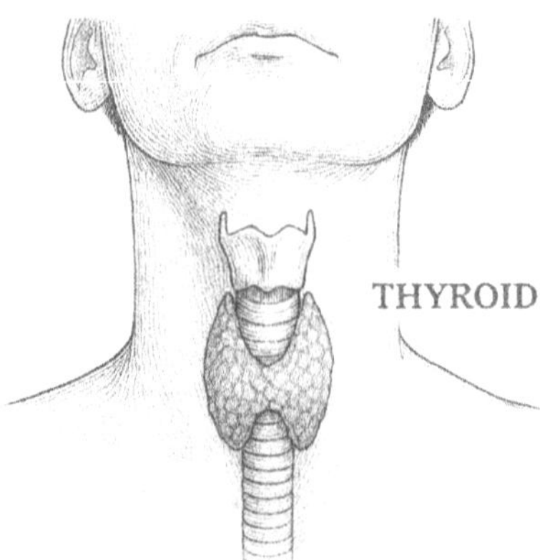

Total Gastrectomy

Step 1 – Upper midline incision and exposure
Instruments: #10 blade, Adsons with teeth, Bovie, Army Navy retractor, Richardson or Deaver retractor, suction.
Anticipation: Exposure must be wide. Prepare deep retractor early and ensure suction is immediately available due to vascular dissection.

Step 2 – Enter peritoneum and perform abdominal exploration
Instruments: Metzenbaum scissors, Debakey forceps, moist laps, Poole suction.
Anticipation: As the peritoneum is tented, anticipate fluid release. Assist with systematic exploration to rule out metastatic disease before proceeding.

Step 3 – Mobilize greater curvature of stomach
Instruments: Energy device or Bovie, Metzenbaums, Debakeys, suction.
Anticipation: Short gastric vessels bleed easily. Maintain gentle traction and keep suction close to preserve visualization.

Step 4 – Divide short gastric vessels
Instruments: Right angle clamps, clips or silk ties, energy device.
Anticipation: Preload ties and anticipate clamp tie cut rhythm. Protect spleen during division to avoid capsular injury.

Step 5 – Mobilize lesser curvature and divide gastrohepatic ligament
Instruments: Metzenbaums, Debakeys, Bovie, suction.
Anticipation: Watch for aberrant left hepatic artery. Maintain careful dissection close to the stomach.

Step 6 – Identify and divide left gastric artery and vein
Instruments: Right angle clamps, vascular clips or stapler, silk ties.
Anticipation: This is a major vascular step. Confirm proximal control before division and keep suction immediately available.

Step 7 – Divide distal esophagus
Instruments: Bowel clamp or stapler, Metzenbaums or stapler reloads.
Anticipation: Ensure adequate proximal margin. Anticipate need for esophageal mobilization to allow tension free reconstruction.

Step 8 – Divide duodenum
Instruments: Bowel clamps or stapler, Mayo scissors.
Anticipation: Confirm location distal to pylorus. Be prepared for bile spillage and maintain suction readiness.

Step 9 – Remove stomach specimen and orient for pathology
Instruments: Specimen basin, marking sutures or clips.
Anticipation: Confirm orientation requirements before specimen leaves field to avoid delays.

Step 10 – Construct Roux limb
Instruments: GIA stapler, bowel clamps, Metzenbaum scissors.
Anticipation: Anticipate multiple stapler firings. Confirm correct limb length and orientation.

Step 11 – Perform esophagojejunostomy
Instruments: Stapler or needle driver with fine sutures, atraumatic forceps.
Anticipation: This is a critical anastomosis. Maintain excellent exposure and be prepared for slow precise suturing.

Total Gastrectomy

Step 12 – Inspect anastomosis and achieve hemostasis
Instruments: Irrigation system, Poole suction, hemostatic agents.
Anticipation: Assist with visualization so the surgeon can look for leaks and bleeding. Anticipate reinforcement sutures if tissue appears fragile.

Step 13 – Place drains if indicated
Instruments: JP or Blake drains, scissors, silk or nylon sutures.
Anticipation: Prime drains early and position near anastomosis if surgeon prefers.

Step 14 – Close abdominal wall and skin
Instruments: Needle driver, #1 or #0 fascial sutures, Mayo scissors, skin closure supplies.
Anticipation: Begin closing counts early. Ensure drains are secured and functioning before final closure.

Mayo Stand Suggestion:

- #10 blade on scalpel handle
- Metzenbaum scissors
- Mayo scissors curved
- Debakey forceps
- Adsons with teeth
- Right angle clamps
- Kelly clamps
- Needle driver
- Vascular clips or silk ties
- Long Deaver or Malleable retractors

Umbilical Herniorrhaphy

Step 1 – Periumbilical incision and exposure
Instruments: #10 blade, Adsons with teeth, Bovie, Army Navy retractor, suction.
Anticipation: Incision is often curved within the umbilicus for cosmesis. Maintain careful hemostasis to preserve skin viability.

Step 2 – Dissect through subcutaneous tissue to hernia sac
Instruments: Metzenbaum scissors, Debakey forceps, Bovie.
Anticipation: Hernia sac may be adherent to skin. Use gentle dissection to avoid entering sac prematurely.

Step 3 – Identify and isolate hernia sac
Instruments: Debakeys, Metzenbaums, small retractor.
Anticipation: Keep sac intact during isolation. Anticipate need for traction to define fascial edges clearly.

Step 4 – Open hernia sac and inspect contents
Instruments: Metzenbaums, suction, moist laps.
Anticipation: Expect preperitoneal fat or bowel. Protect contents immediately and maintain moisture.

Step 5 – Reduce hernia contents into abdominal cavity
Instruments: Debakeys, Babcock forceps, moist laps.
Anticipation: Use atraumatic instruments only. Be prepared for adhesiolysis if contents are not easily reduced.

Step 6 – Excise or invert hernia sac
Instruments: Metzenbaums, Kelly clamps, absorbable ties.
Anticipation: Have ties ready for sac ligation. Maintain clear visualization of fascial defect.

Umbilical Herniorrhaphy

Step 7 – Prepare fascial edges for repair
Instruments: Debakeys, Metzenbaums.
Anticipation: Clean fascial margins improve repair strength. Expect surgeon to assess defect size for mesh consideration.

Step 8 – Perform primary fascial repair or place mesh
Instruments: Needle driver, nonabsorbable sutures, mesh if used.
Anticipation: Confirm repair method before opening mesh. Maintain proper tension to avoid ischemia or recurrence.

Step 9 – Recreate umbilicus and close subcutaneous tissue
Instruments: Needle driver, absorbable sutures, Mayo scissors.
Anticipation: Cosmetic alignment matters. Assist with accurate midline positioning of umbilicus.

Step 10 – Close skin and apply dressing
Instruments: Skin stapler or sutures, Adsonss, dressing supplies.
Anticipation: Prepare dressing early. Avoid excessive pressure over umbilicus to protect repair.

Mayo Stand Suggestion:

- #10 blade on scalpel handle
- Metzenbaum scissors
- Mayo scissors curved
- Debakey forceps
- Adsons with teeth
- Kelly clamps
- Babcock forceps
- Needle driver
- Nonabsorbable sutures
- Army Navy retractor

Ventral Incisional Herniorrhaphy

Step 1 – Incision through prior scar and exposure
Instruments: #10 blade, Adsons with teeth, Bovie, Army Navy retractor, suction.
Anticipation: Expect dense scar tissue. Control bleeding early and anticipate slow careful dissection to avoid enterotomy.

Step 2 – Dissect through subcutaneous tissue to hernia sac
Instruments: Metzenbaum scissors, Debakey forceps, Bovie.
Anticipation: Adhesions between sac and skin are common. Use blunt dissection and avoid entering the sac prematurely.

Step 3 – Identify and isolate hernia sac
Instruments: Debakeys, Metzenbaums, small retractor.
Anticipation: Maintain traction to define fascial edges clearly. Be alert for bowel adherence to sac.

Step 4 – Open hernia sac and assess contents
Instruments: Metzenbaums, suction, moist laps.
Anticipation: Protect bowel immediately if encountered. Keep contents moist and avoid traction injury.

Step 5 – Perform adhesiolysis as needed
Instruments: Metzenbaums, Debakeys, Bovie, suction.
Anticipation: Adhesiolysis increases enterotomy risk. Maintain excellent visualization and communicate closely with surgeon.

Ventral Incisional Herniorrhaphy

Step 6 – Reduce hernia contents into abdominal cavity
Instruments: Babcock forceps, Debakeys, moist laps.
Anticipation: Use atraumatic instruments only. Anticipate surgeon testing reduction before repair.

Step 7 – Excise redundant hernia sac
Instruments: Metzenbaums, Kelly clamps, absorbable ties.
Anticipation: Have ties ready for sac ligation. Preserve fascial edges for repair strength.

Step 8 – Prepare fascial defect for repair
Instruments: Debakeys, Metzenbaums.
Anticipation: Surgeon will assess defect size and tension. Confirm mesh selection if indicated.

Step 9 – Place mesh or perform primary fascial closure
Instruments: Needle driver, nonabsorbable sutures, mesh if used.
Anticipation: Confirm mesh type and orientation before opening. Maintain sterile handling and avoid mesh contact with skin.

Step 10 – Secure mesh and reinforce repair
Instruments: Needle driver, sutures, tack device if used.
Anticipation: Even tension is critical. Assist with suture management and tail control.

Step 11 – Irrigate and inspect repair
Instruments: Irrigation system, suction.
Anticipation: Remove debris and blood to evaluate repair integrity. Be ready with hemostatic agents.

Step 12 – Close subcutaneous tissue and skin
Instruments: Needle driver, absorbable sutures, Mayo scissors, skin closure supplies.
Anticipation: Drains may be placed in large repairs. Coordinate drain management and final counts.

Mayo Stand Suggestion:

- #10 blade on scalpel handle
- Metzenbaum scissors
- Mayo scissors curved
- Debakey forceps
- Adsons with teeth
- Kelly clamps
- Babcock forceps
- Needle driver
- Nonabsorbable sutures
- Small or medium retractor

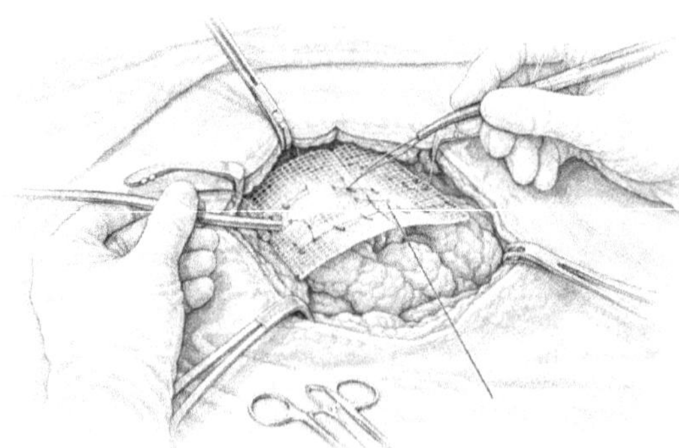

Section II: Obstetrics and Gynecological Procedures

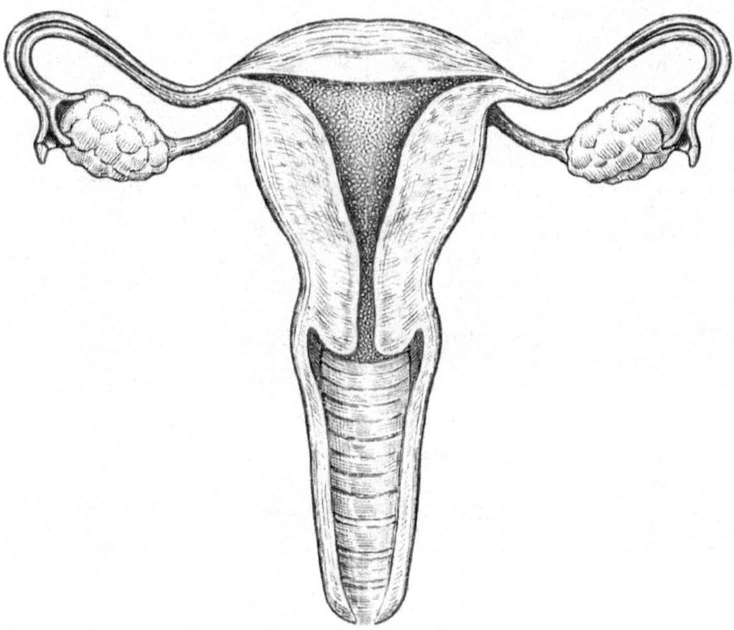

Anterior Cystocele & Posterior Rectocele Colporrhaphy

Step 1 – Patient positioning and vaginal exposure
Instruments: Allen stirrups, weighted vaginal speculum, Deaver retractor, Foley catheter.
Anticipation: Ensure bladder is drained before incision. Maintain proper positioning to prevent nerve injury and optimize vaginal exposure.

Step 2 – Vaginal mucosa infiltration
Instruments: Syringe with local anesthetic and epinephrine, fine needle.
Anticipation: Injection reduces bleeding and aids dissection. Expect tissue blanching before incision.

Step 3 – Anterior vaginal wall incision for cystocele repair
Instruments: #15 blade, Metzenbaum scissors, Adsons forceps, suction.
Anticipation: Incision is midline from urethrovesical junction toward cervix. Maintain precise suction to keep field dry.

Step 4 – Dissect bladder off vaginal mucosa
Instruments: Metzenbaum scissors, Debakey forceps, moist laps.
Anticipation: Bladder wall is thin. Use blunt dissection and gentle traction to avoid cystotomy.

Step 5 – Plicate pubocervical fascia
Instruments: Needle driver, delayed absorbable sutures, Mayo scissors.
Anticipation: Sutures restore bladder support. Maintain even tension to avoid overcorrection or urinary retention.

Step 6 – Trim excess anterior vaginal mucosa and close
Instruments: Metzenbaum scissors, needle driver, absorbable sutures.
Anticipation: Avoid narrowing vaginal canal. Assist with tissue alignment during closure.

Step 7 – Posterior vaginal wall incision for rectocele repair
Instruments: #15 blade, Metzenbaum scissors, Adsons forceps, suction.
Anticipation: Rectum lies immediately beneath mucosa. Maintain shallow dissection depth.

Step 8 – Dissect rectum from vaginal wall
Instruments: Metzenbaums, Debakeys, moist laps.
Anticipation: Gentle blunt dissection prevents rectal injury. Suction lightly to preserve tissue planes.

Step 9 – Plicate rectovaginal fascia
Instruments: Needle driver, delayed absorbable sutures.
Anticipation: This restores posterior support. Avoid sutures too deep which could penetrate rectum.

Step 10 – Perform perineorrhaphy if indicated
Instruments: Needle driver, absorbable sutures, Mayo scissors.
Anticipation: Perineal body reconstruction improves support. Confirm desired vaginal caliber with surgeon.

Step 11 – Trim excess posterior vaginal mucosa and close
Instruments: Metzenbaum scissors, needle driver, absorbable sutures.
Anticipation: Symmetry matters. Maintain smooth tissue approximation for healing and function.

Anterior Cystocele & Posterior Rectocele Colporrhaphy

Step 12 – Final inspection and vaginal packing
Instruments: Vaginal packing, lubricant, sponge forceps.
Anticipation: Packing provides hemostasis. Confirm count.

Mayo Stand Suggestion:

- #15 blade on scalpel handle
- Metzenbaum scissors
- Mayo scissors curved
- Adsons forceps
- Debakey forceps
- Needle driver
- Weighted vaginal speculum
- Deaver retractor
- Sponge forceps
- Absorbable sutures

Basic Gynecologic Laparoscopy

Step 1 – Patient positioning and preparation
Instruments: Allen stirrups, grounding pad, Foley catheter, uterine manipulator if indicated.
Anticipation: Confirm Trendelenburg capability before draping. Ensure bladder is drained and uterine manipulator is secured prior to prep.

Step 2 – Skin incision for primary port
Instruments: #11 blade, Adsons with teeth, towel clamps.
Anticipation: Incision is usually infraumbilical. Maintain midline orientation to reduce risk of vessel injury.

Step 3 – Establish pneumoperitoneum
Instruments: Veress needle or Hasson cannula, insufflation tubing.
Anticipation: Confirm needle placement with pressure readings and saline drop test if used. Watch for rising intraabdominal pressure indicating proper placement.

Step 4 – Insert primary trocar and laparoscope
Instruments: 10 mm trocar, 30 degree laparoscope, camera system.
Anticipation: Ensure camera white balance and focus before insertion. Announce entry so anesthesia can monitor patient response.

Step 5 – Perform initial pelvic survey
Instruments: Laparoscope, suction irrigation if needed.
Anticipation: Maintain steady horizon and slow camera movements. Surgeon evaluates uterus ovaries tubes and pelvic peritoneum.

Step 6 – Place accessory trocars under direct vision
Instruments: 5 mm trocars, obturators.
Anticipation: Transilluminate abdominal wall to avoid inferior epigastric vessels. Anticipate trocar repositioning for ergonomics.

Step 7 – Manipulate pelvic organs for visualization
Instruments: Atraumatic graspers, uterine manipulator.
Anticipation: Gentle traction prevents tissue injury. Coordinate uterine manipulation with camera movements.

Step 8 – Perform diagnostic or minor operative intervention
Instruments: Maryland dissector, scissors, energy device if used.
Anticipation: Be ready to escalate from diagnostic to operative laparoscopy. Keep additional instruments immediately available.

Basic Gynecologic Laparoscopy

Step 9 – Irrigate and suction pelvis if indicated
Instruments: Suction irrigation handpiece.
Anticipation: Clear blood or fluid promptly to maintain visualization. Avoid excessive suction near adnexa.

Step 10 – Final inspection and desufflation
Instruments: Laparoscope, suction.
Anticipation: Inspect port sites internally during desufflation. Ensure no bleeding before trocar removal.

Step 11 – Remove trocars and close port sites
Instruments: Needle driver, absorbable sutures, skin closure supplies.
Anticipation: Close fascia for larger ports. Confirm counts before skin closure.

Mayo Stand Suggestion:

- #11 blade on scalpel handle
- Veress needle or Hasson cannula
- 10 mm trocar
- Two 5 mm trocars
- 30 degree laparoscope
- Atraumatic graspers
- Maryland dissector
- Laparoscopic scissors
- Suction irrigation handpiece
- Needle driver

Cervical Cerclage

Step 1 – Patient positioning and vaginal exposure
Instruments: Allen stirrups, weighted vaginal speculum or Sims retractors, Foley catheter.
Anticipation: Ensure bladder is emptied to improve visualization and reduce injury risk. Proper positioning is critical for cervical access.

Step 2 – Cervical visualization and traction
Instruments: Single tooth tenaculum or ring forceps.
Anticipation: Apply gentle traction to avoid cervical laceration. Maintain steady exposure throughout the procedure.

Step 3 – Vaginal mucosal incision near cervix
Instruments: #15 blade, Metzenbaum scissors, Adsons forceps.
Anticipation: Incision is placed high on the cervix. Maintain shallow depth to avoid bladder injury anteriorly.

Step 4 – Bladder dissection and mobilization
Instruments: Metzenbaum scissors, Debakey forceps, moist laps.
Anticipation: Bladder is dissected off cervix anteriorly. Use blunt dissection and gentle traction to prevent cystotomy.

Step 5 – Create submucosal tunnel around cervix
Instruments: Right angle clamp or blunt dissector.
Anticipation: Maintain correct plane to allow tape passage without entering cervical canal.

Step 6 – Pass cerclage tape around cervix
Instruments: Mersilene tape or nonabsorbable suture, clamp or needle driver.
Anticipation: Confirm tape lies evenly without twisting. Avoid excessive tension which may compromise cervical blood supply.

Cervical Cerclage

Step 7 – Secure cerclage knot posteriorly
Instruments: Needle driver, scissors.
Anticipation: Posterior knot placement reduces irritation. Confirm cervical canal remains patent.

Step 8 – Reapproximate vaginal mucosa over cerclage
Instruments: Needle driver, absorbable sutures, Mayo scissors.
Anticipation: Ensure complete coverage of tape to reduce infection risk.

Step 9 – Final inspection and hemostasis
Instruments: Suction, sponge forceps.
Anticipation: Confirm no bleeding or bladder injury before completing procedure.

Step 10 – Vaginal packing if indicated
Instruments: Vaginal packing, lubricant.
Anticipation: Communicate packing removal timing to recovery staff.

Mayo Stand Suggestion:

- Weighted vaginal speculum
- Graves or Pederson speculum
- Single tooth tenaculum or ring forceps
- Metzenbaum scissors
- Right angle clamp or blunt dissector
- Needle driver
- Mayo scissors curved
- Mersilene tape or nonabsorbable suture
- Sponge forceps
- Vaginal packing

Cesarean Section

Step 1 – Patient positioning and preparation
Instruments: Foley catheter, grounding pad, Allen stirrups if used, abdominal prep supplies.
Anticipation: Ensure left uterine displacement to prevent supine hypotension. Confirm fetal monitoring and antibiotic timing before incision.

Step 2 – Skin incision
Instruments: #10 blade, Adsons with teeth, Bovie, Army Navy retractor.
Anticipation: Incision is usually Pfannenstiel. Maintain meticulous hemostasis as dissection proceeds through subcutaneous tissue.

Step 3 – Dissect through subcutaneous tissue and fascia
Instruments: Bovie, Metzenbaum scissors, Mayo scissors, Debakey forceps.
Anticipation: Expect brisk bleeding from subcutaneous vessels. Prepare to widen exposure quickly with retractor.

Step 4 – Open rectus fascia and separate muscles
Instruments: Mayo scissors, Debakeys, Army Navy retractor.
Anticipation: Rectus muscles are separated bluntly. Maintain midline orientation to reduce bleeding.

Step 5 – Enter peritoneum
Instruments: Metzenbaum scissors, Debakey forceps, suction.
Anticipation: As the peritoneum is tented, anticipate fluid release. Protect underlying bowel and bladder.

Cesarean Section

Step 6 – Expose lower uterine segment
Instruments: Bladder blade, Deaver retractors, moist laps.
Anticipation: Ensure bladder is reflected inferiorly. Proper retraction prevents bladder injury.

Step 7 – Incise uterus
Instruments: #10 blade, bandage scissors or Metzenbaums.
Anticipation: Incision is controlled and shallow initially. Be prepared for amniotic fluid release.

Step 8 – Deliver infant
Instruments: Hands, suction bulb, cord clamps.
Anticipation: Coordinate with anesthesia and pediatrics. Have bulb suction ready immediately upon delivery.

Step 9 – Clamp and cut umbilical cord
Instruments: Two cord clamps, scissors.
Anticipation: Timing may vary for delayed cord clamping. Confirm surgeon preference.

Step 10 – Deliver placenta and inspect uterus
Instruments: Ring forceps, sponge forceps, suction.
Anticipation: Watch for retained placental tissue. Anticipate uterine atony and readiness for uterotonic medications.

Step 11 – Close uterine incision
Instruments: Needle driver, absorbable sutures, Mayo scissors.
Anticipation: Maintain clear field for multilayer closure. Assist with suture management and tension control.

Step 12 – Irrigate and close abdominal layers
Instruments: Irrigation system, suction, needle driver, sutures.
Anticipation: Confirm hemostasis before closure. Closure proceeds uterus fascia subcutaneous tissue and skin.

Step 13 – Skin closure and dressing
Instruments: Skin stapler or sutures, Adsonss, dressing supplies.
Anticipation: Prepare dressing early. Final counts must be correct before patient transfer.

Mayo Stand Suggestion:

- #10 blade on scalpel handle
- Metzenbaum scissors
- Mayo scissors curved
- Debakey forceps
- Adsons with teeth
- Army Navy retractor
- Bladder blade
- Ring forceps
- Needle driver
- Cord clamps

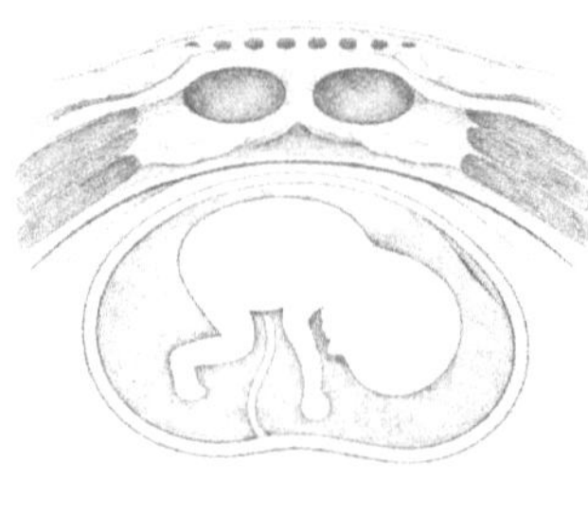

Dilation and Curettage

Step 1 – Patient positioning and vaginal preparation
Instruments: Allen stirrups, vaginal prep supplies, Foley catheter if ordered.
Anticipation: Confirm bladder is emptied to reduce uterine perforation risk. Proper lithotomy positioning is essential for cervical alignment.

Step 2 – Vaginal exposure and cervical visualization
Instruments: Weighted vaginal speculum or Sims retractors, sponge forceps.
Anticipation: Maintain steady exposure. Poor visualization increases risk of cervical injury.

Step 3 – Grasp cervix for stabilization
Instruments: Single tooth tenaculum or ring forceps.
Anticipation: Apply controlled traction only. Excess force can cause cervical laceration.

Step 4 – Sound the uterus
Instruments: Uterine sound.
Anticipation: Note uterine depth and direction. This guides dilation and curettage technique and helps prevent perforation.

Step 5 – Dilate cervix
Instruments: Cervical dilators graduated sizes.
Anticipation: Dilate gradually and sequentially. Anticipate resistance in nulliparous or postmenopausal patients.

Step 6 – Perform curettage of uterine lining
Instruments: Sharp curette or suction curette, suction tubing if used.
Anticipation: Use gentle even strokes. Excessive force increases perforation and bleeding risk.

Step 7 – Inspect tissue and achieve hemostasis
Instruments: Sponge forceps, suction.
Anticipation: Watch for excessive bleeding or inadequate tissue removal. Be alert for signs of uterine atony.

Step 8 – Remove instruments and reassess cervix
Instruments: Sponge forceps, suction.
Anticipation: Inspect cervix for bleeding or lacerations before completing the procedure.

Step 9 – Specimen handling
Instruments: Specimen container with formalin.
Anticipation: Ensure specimen is properly labeled and communicated to circulator immediately.

Step 10 – Vaginal packing if indicated
Instruments: Vaginal packing, lubricant.
Anticipation: Communicate packing presence and removal timing to recovery staff.

Mayo Stand Suggestion:

- Weighted vaginal speculum
- Graves or Sims retractor
- Single tooth tenaculum
- Uterine sound
- Cervical dilators
- Sharp curette
- Suction curette
- Sponge forceps
- Ring forceps
- Specimen container

Endometrial Ablation

Step 1 – Patient positioning and preparation
Instruments: Allen stirrups, grounding pad if required, vaginal prep supplies.
Anticipation: Confirm pregnancy test is negative and patient selection criteria are met. Ensure bladder is emptied before starting.

Step 2 – Vaginal exposure and cervical stabilization
Instruments: Weighted vaginal speculum, Deaver retractor, single tooth tenaculum.
Anticipation: Maintain steady cervical traction. Poor stabilization increases risk of uterine perforation during device insertion.

Step 3 – Sound the uterus
Instruments: Uterine sound.
Anticipation: Measure uterine depth and note direction. Accurate sounding is critical for correct device sizing and safe ablation.

Step 4 – Dilate cervix as needed
Instruments: Cervical dilators.
Anticipation: Dilate only to manufacturer requirements. Excessive dilation increases fluid leakage and reduces treatment effectiveness.

Step 5 – Perform diagnostic hysteroscopy if indicated
Instruments: Hysteroscope, light source, distension media tubing.
Anticipation: Inspect cavity for polyps fibroids or perforation before ablation. Maintain clear visualization with controlled fluid inflow.

Step 6 – Insert endometrial ablation device
Instruments: Endometrial ablation device specific to system used.
Anticipation: Confirm correct orientation and depth. Device must contact entire endometrial surface evenly.

Step 7 – Activate ablation cycle
Instruments: Ablation generator control unit.
Anticipation: Monitor time and parameters closely. Communicate immediately if alarms or abnormal readings occur.

Step 8 – Complete ablation and remove device
Instruments: Device handle, sponge forceps.
Anticipation: Remove slowly to avoid cervical trauma. Inspect device for integrity after removal.

Step 9 – Assess uterus and cervix for bleeding
Instruments: Sponge forceps, suction.
Anticipation: Watch for unexpected bleeding which may indicate perforation or inadequate coagulation.

Step 10 – Specimen handling if curettage performed
Instruments: Specimen container.
Anticipation: Label specimens clearly and communicate findings to circulator.

Step 11 – Vaginal packing if indicated
Instruments: Vaginal packing, lubricant.
Anticipation: Communicate packing presence and removal timing to recovery staff.

Endometrial Ablation

Mayo Stand Suggestion:

- Weighted vaginal speculum
- Graves or Sims retractors
- Single tooth tenaculum
- Uterine sound
- Cervical dilators
- Hysteroscope
- Endometrial ablation device
- Sponge forceps
- Suction tubing
- Specimen container

Hysteroscopy

Step 1 – Patient positioning and vaginal preparation
Instruments: Allen stirrups, vaginal prep supplies, grounding pad if operative hysteroscopy planned.
Anticipation: Confirm bladder is emptied. Proper lithotomy positioning is critical for straight cervical access.

Step 2 – Vaginal exposure and cervical visualization
Instruments: Weighted vaginal speculum, Deaver retractor, sponge forceps.
Anticipation: Maintain steady exposure. Poor visualization increases risk of cervical trauma during scope insertion.

Step 3 – Grasp cervix for stabilization
Instruments: Single tooth tenaculum or ring forceps.
Anticipation: Apply gentle traction only. Excess force can cause cervical laceration or patient discomfort.

Step 4 – Sound the uterus
Instruments: Uterine sound.
Anticipation: Note uterine depth and direction. This guides safe hysteroscope insertion and helps prevent perforation.

Step 5 – Dilate cervix if required
Instruments: Cervical dilators.
Anticipation: Dilate only as much as necessary for the hysteroscope size. Over dilation increases fluid leakage.

Step 6 – Insert hysteroscope and initiate distension
Instruments: Hysteroscope, light source, camera, distension media tubing.
Anticipation: Start distension before advancing the scope. Maintain continuous visualization during insertion.

Step 7 – Inspect uterine cavity systematically
Instruments: Hysteroscope, camera controls.
Anticipation: Surgeon evaluates fundus tubal ostia and endometrium. Keep camera steady and adjust light to avoid glare.

Step 8 – Perform operative intervention if indicated
Instruments: Operative hysteroscope instruments such as scissors graspers or resectoscope.
Anticipation: Be ready to transition quickly from diagnostic to operative. Monitor fluid deficit closely throughout the procedure.

Hysteroscopy

Step 9 – Manage distension media and suction
Instruments: Fluid management system suction tubing.
Anticipation: Communicate fluid intake and output regularly. Excess fluid absorption can lead to serious complications.

Step 10 – Final cavity inspection and scope removal
Instruments: Hysteroscope, suction.
Anticipation: Inspect for bleeding or perforation before withdrawal. Remove scope slowly to avoid cervical trauma.

Step 11 – Specimen handling if tissue removed
Instruments: Specimen container.
Anticipation: Confirm correct labeling and communicate specimen details to circulator immediately.

Step 12 – Vaginal packing if indicated
Instruments: Vaginal packing, lubricant.
Anticipation: Communicate packing presence and removal timing to recovery staff.

Mayo Stand Suggestion:

- Weighted vaginal speculum
- Graves or Pederson speculum
- Single tooth tenaculum
- Uterine sound
- Cervical dilators
- Hysteroscope
- Light source and camera head
- Operative hysteroscopy instruments
- Sponge forceps
- Specimen container

Labiaplasty

Step 1 – Patient positioning and preparation
Instruments: Allen stirrups, grounding pad if electrosurgery used, vaginal prep supplies.
Anticipation: Ensure proper lithotomy positioning with padding to prevent nerve injury. Confirm procedure type and extent since techniques vary.

Step 2 – Surgical marking of labial tissue
Instruments: Skin marker, sterile gauze.
Anticipation: Surgeon often marks before infiltration. Confirm symmetry and planned excision lines before proceeding.

Step 3 – Local anesthetic infiltration
Instruments: Syringe with local anesthetic and epinephrine, fine needle.
Anticipation: Injection minimizes bleeding and improves visualization. Expect tissue blanching before incision.

Step 4 – Labial incision and tissue excision
Instruments: #15 blade, Metzenbaum scissors, Adsons forceps with teeth, suction.
Anticipation: Incisions are precise and superficial. Maintain excellent suction control to keep field dry and avoid obscuring margins.

Step 5 – Hemostasis of labial tissue
Instruments: Bipolar forceps or Bovie with fine tip, suction.
Anticipation: Labial tissue is highly vascular. Anticipate frequent coagulation and keep suction immediately available.

Labiaplasty

Step 6 – Symmetry check and tissue contouring
Instruments: Metzenbaum scissors, Adsons forceps.
Anticipation: Surgeon may pause to compare sides. Be prepared for small additional excisions to achieve symmetry.

Step 7 – Deep tissue closure if required
Instruments: Needle driver, fine absorbable sutures, Mayo scissors.
Anticipation: Sutures are delicate and closely spaced. Manage suture tails carefully to maintain clean visualization.

Step 8 – Skin closure
Instruments: Needle driver, fine absorbable sutures, Adsons forceps.
Anticipation: Closure is cosmetic. Assist with precise edge alignment to reduce scarring.

Step 9 – Final inspection and hemostasis
Instruments: Suction, sponge forceps.
Anticipation: Even minor bleeding can cause postoperative hematoma. Ensure field is completely dry before dressing.

Step 10 – Apply dressing and padding
Instruments: Nonadherent dressing, gauze, perineal pad.
Anticipation: Dressing should protect without compression. Communicate postoperative care instructions to recovery staff.

Mayo Stand Suggestion:

- #15 blade on scalpel handle
- Metzenbaum scissors
- Mayo scissors curved
- Adsons forceps with teeth
- Needle driver
- Bipolar forceps or fine tip cautery
- Sponge forceps
- 2 Mosquito Hemostats
- 2 Kelly Hemostats
- Skin marker

Laparoscopic Hysterectomy

Step 1 – Patient positioning and preparation
Instruments: Allen stirrups, Foley catheter, uterine manipulator, grounding pad.
Anticipation: Confirm uterine manipulator placement and secure positioning. Ensure Trendelenburg is achievable before draping.

Step 2 – Establish pneumoperitoneum
Instruments: #11 blade, Veress needle or Hasson cannula, insufflation tubing.
Anticipation: Maintain midline orientation and confirm pressure readings. Be alert for failed entry requiring alternate access.

Step 3 – Insert primary trocar and laparoscope
Instruments: 10 to 12 mm trocar, 30 degree laparoscope, camera system.
Anticipation: White balance and focus camera before insertion. Announce entry so anesthesia can monitor response.

Step 4 – Place accessory trocars under direct vision
Instruments: Two or three 5 mm trocars.
Anticipation: Transilluminate abdominal wall to avoid inferior epigastric vessels. Adjust placement for surgeon ergonomics.

Step 5 – Perform pelvic survey and expose uterus
Instruments: Laparoscope, atraumatic graspers.
Anticipation: Coordinate uterine manipulation with camera movements. Maintain a stable horizon.

Step 6 – Divide round ligaments
Instruments: Energy device or bipolar, atraumatic grasper.
Anticipation: Expect bilateral division early. Keep suction ready for small bleeders.

Step 7 – Open broad ligament and identify ureters
Instruments: Maryland dissector, energy device, suction.
Anticipation: Ureter identification is critical. Maintain clear visualization and gentle traction.

Step 8 – Control uterine vessels
Instruments: Energy device or vascular clips, Maryland dissector.
Anticipation: This is a key bleeding risk step. Keep suction close and avoid blind activation of energy.

Step 9 – Dissect bladder flap
Instruments: Maryland dissector, energy device, suction.
Anticipation: Maintain correct tissue plane to prevent cystotomy. Expect frequent small bleeders.

Step 10 – Colpotomy
Instruments: Hook cautery or energy device, uterine manipulator cup.
Anticipation: Communicate with vaginal team if present. Expect smoke and maintain clear visualization.

Step 11 – Remove uterus vaginally or via containment
Instruments: Sponge forceps, specimen bag if used.
Anticipation: Open specimen container early. Anticipate morcellation if uterus is enlarged.

Step 12 – Close vaginal cuff
Instruments: Laparoscopic needle driver, absorbable sutures.
Anticipation: Prepare multiple sutures early. Maintain exposure and manage suture tails carefully.

Step 13 – Irrigate pelvis and inspect hemostasis
Instruments: Suction irrigation handpiece.
Anticipation: Inspect cuff angles and pedicles closely. Offer hemostatic agents if oozing persists.

Step 14 – Desufflate and remove trocars
Instruments: Laparoscope, suction.
Anticipation: Watch cuff and pedicles during desufflation. Confirm no bleeding before trocar removal.

Step 15 – Close port sites and apply dressings
Instruments: Needle driver, absorbable sutures, skin closure supplies.
Anticipation: Close fascia for larger ports. Complete counts before skin closure.

Mayo Stand Suggestion:

- #11 blade on scalpel handle
- Veress needle or Hasson cannula
- 10 to 12 mm trocar
- Two 5 mm trocars
- Maryland dissector
- Atraumatic graspers
- Energy device handpiece
- Laparoscopic scissors
- Laparoscopic needle driver
- Suction irrigation handpiece

Laparoscopic Resection of Unruptured Tubal Pregnancy

Step 1 – Patient positioning and preparation
Instruments: Allen stirrups, Foley catheter, uterine manipulator if used, grounding pad.
Anticipation: Confirm pregnancy location and laterality. Ensure Trendelenburg positioning is achievable before draping.

Step 2 – Establish pneumoperitoneum
Instruments: #11 blade, Veress needle or Hasson cannula, insufflation tubing.
Anticipation: Maintain midline orientation. Watch pressure readings closely to confirm safe entry.

Step 3 – Insert primary trocar and laparoscope
Instruments: 10 to 12 mm trocar, 30 degree laparoscope, camera system.
Anticipation: White balance and focus camera prior to insertion. Announce entry to anesthesia.

Step 4 – Place accessory trocars under direct vision
Instruments: Two or three 5 mm trocars.
Anticipation: Avoid inferior epigastric vessels by transillumination. Placement should allow comfortable access to adnexa.

Step 5 – Perform pelvic survey and identify ectopic pregnancy
Instruments: Laparoscope, atraumatic graspers, suction irrigation.
Anticipation: Confirm tubal pregnancy is unruptured. Clear small amounts of blood to maintain visualization.

Step 6 – Stabilize fallopian tube
Instruments: Atraumatic grasper.
Anticipation: Handle tube gently to prevent rupture. Maintain steady traction without compressing the gestational sac.

Step 7 – Perform salpingostomy or salpingectomy
Instruments: Energy device or bipolar, Maryland dissector, laparoscopic scissors.
Anticipation: Be prepared for brisk bleeding. Keep suction immediately available and anticipate rapid instrument exchanges.

Step 8 – Remove ectopic tissue
Instruments: Atraumatic graspers, specimen bag.
Anticipation: Remove tissue carefully to prevent spillage. Open specimen bag before extraction.

Step 9 – Achieve hemostasis of tubal site
Instruments: Bipolar energy, suction irrigation.
Anticipation: Inspect closely for continued bleeding. Avoid excessive coagulation which can damage remaining tube.

Step 10 – Irrigate pelvis and inspect contralateral tube
Instruments: Suction irrigation handpiece.
Anticipation: Confirm hemostasis and evaluate opposite adnexa for pathology.

Step 11 – Desufflate and remove trocars
Instruments: Laparoscope, suction.
Anticipation: Watch operative site during desufflation. Remove trocars under direct vision.

Laparoscopic Resection of Unruptured Tubal Pregnancy

Step 12 – Close port sites and apply dressings
Instruments: Needle driver, absorbable sutures, skin closure supplies.
Anticipation: Close fascia for larger ports. Confirm counts before skin closure.

Mayo Stand Suggestion:

- #11 blade on scalpel handle
- Veress needle or Hasson cannula
- 10 to 12 mm trocar
- Two 5 mm trocars
- Maryland dissector
- Atraumatic graspers
- Energy device handpiece
- Laparoscopic scissors
- Suction irrigation handpiece

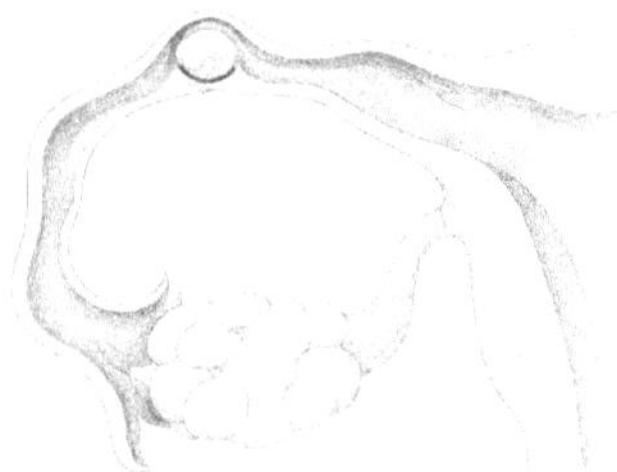

Marsupialization of Bartholin's Gland Cyst

Step 1 – Patient positioning and preparation
Instruments: Allen stirrups, perineal prep supplies, grounding pad if electrosurgery used.
Anticipation: Ensure proper lithotomy positioning with padding. Confirm laterality of the cyst before prep and drape.

Step 2 – Vaginal and vulvar exposure
Instruments: Graves or Pederson speculum if needed, Sims retractors, sponge forceps.
Anticipation: Exposure is usually external. Speculum use is minimal and only if vaginal visualization is required.

Step 3 – Local anesthetic infiltration
Instruments: Syringe with local anesthetic and epinephrine, fine needle.
Anticipation: Injection reduces pain and bleeding. Expect tissue blanching prior to incision.

Step 4 – Incision into cyst wall
Instruments: #15 blade, Metzenbaum scissors, suction.
Anticipation: Incision is made at the mucocutaneous junction. Be ready for purulent drainage and immediate suctioning.

Step 5 – Drain cyst contents and obtain culture if ordered
Instruments: Suction tip, culture swab, specimen container.
Anticipation: Maintain control of drainage to prevent contamination. Prepare culture materials before incision if ordered.

Step 6 – Break up loculations and irrigate cyst cavity
Instruments: Hemostat, suction irrigation.
Anticipation: Gentle exploration prevents missed pockets. Avoid aggressive probing that could damage surrounding tissue.

Step 7 – Marsupialize cyst wall to skin edges
Instruments: Needle driver, absorbable sutures, Mayo scissors.
Anticipation: Sutures are placed circumferentially. Assist with precise suture spacing to keep cyst open for drainage.

Marsupialization of Bartholin's Gland Cyst

Step 8 – Achieve hemostasis and inspect site
Instruments: Bipolar cautery if needed, suction.
Anticipation: Even small bleeders can cause postoperative hematoma. Ensure field is dry before dressing.

Step 9 – Place packing if indicated
Instruments: Vaginal packing or gauze strip, lubricant.
Anticipation: Communicate packing presence and removal timing clearly to recovery staff.

Step 10 – Apply dressing and perineal pad
Instruments: Nonadherent dressing, gauze, perineal pad.
Anticipation: Dressing should protect without pressure. Confirm postoperative instructions regarding sitz baths.

Mayo Stand Suggestion:

- #15 blade on scalpel handle
- Metzenbaum scissors
- Mayo scissors curved
- Adsons forceps
- 2 Mosquito Hemostats
- 2 Kelly Hemostats
- Sponge forceps

Myomectomy Abdominal Approach

Step 1 – Lower abdominal incision and exposure
Instruments: #10 blade, Adsons with teeth, monopolar pencil if incision begins immediately, suction tip if needed.
Anticipation: Incision is usually Pfannenstiel or lower midline. Expect brisk bleeding in subcutaneous tissue and fascia.

Step 2 – Dissect through fascia and enter peritoneum
Instruments: Metzenbaum scissors, Mayo scissors, Debakey forceps.
Anticipation: Maintain midline orientation. As the peritoneum is tented, be ready for fluid release and protect bowel.

Step 3 – Pack bowel and expose uterus
Instruments: Moist laps , Debakey forceps.
Anticipation: Uterus may be enlarged and vascular. Exposure shifts quickly so keep the field organized and dry.

Step 4 – Identify fibroid location and plan incision
Instruments: Debakey forceps, marking pen if used.
Anticipation: Surgeon confirms size depth and number of fibroids. Be prepared for multiple uterine incisions.

Step 5 – Inject vasoconstrictive agent into myometrium if ordered
Instruments: Syringe with vasopressin solution, fine needle.
Anticipation: Confirm correct dilution verbally. Watch anesthesia closely for hemodynamic changes.

Step 6 – Incise uterine serosa over fibroid
Instruments: #10 blade or monopolar pencil, Metzenbaum scissors.
Anticipation: Bleeding can be immediate. Suction must stay close without obscuring the incision.

Myomectomy Abdominal Approach

Step 7 – Enucleate fibroid from myometrium
Instruments: Tenaculum or myoma screw, Debakey forceps, Metzenbaums.
Anticipation: Expect strong traction and countertraction. Fibroid may release suddenly so maintain controlled handling.

Step 8 – Inspect fibroid bed for additional nodules
Instruments: Debakey forceps, suction.
Anticipation: Surgeon may palpate deeply for satellite fibroids. Be ready for repeat enucleation.

Step 9 – Remove fibroid specimen from field
Instruments: Specimen basin.
Anticipation: Prepare basin early. Confirm specimen orientation and count if multiple fibroids removed.

Step 10 – Achieve hemostasis of myometrial bed
Instruments: Monopolar pencil if needed, suction.
Anticipation: Bleeding control is critical before closure. Hemostatic agents are back table add ons if requested.

Step 11 – Irrigate uterus and pelvis
Instruments: Irrigation system, suction.
Anticipation: Clear pooled blood to reassess hemostasis and identify additional bleeding sites.

Step 12 – Uterine closure
Instruments: Suture, Mayo Scissors, and Forceps
Anticipation: This is the transition point where needle driver and sutures come to the field. Assist with layered closure awareness.

Step 13 – Abdominal closure
Instruments: Suture, Mayo Scissors, and Forceps
Anticipation: Begin closing counts early. Ensure uterine repair is complete before fascial closure.

Mayo Stand Suggestion:

- #10 blade on scalpel handle
- Metzenbaum scissors
- Mayo scissors
- Adsons forceps with teeth
- Debakey forceps
- Tenaculum or myoma screw

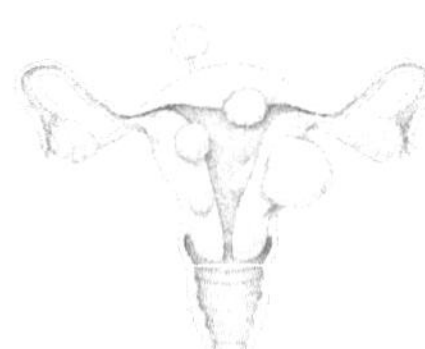

Oophorectomy

Step 1 – Patient positioning and preparation
Instruments: Allen stirrups, Foley catheter, uterine manipulator if used, grounding pad.
Anticipation: Confirm laterality and indication. Ensure Trendelenburg positioning is achievable and the bladder is drained.

Step 2 – Establish pneumoperitoneum
Instruments: #11 blade, Veress needle or Hasson cannula, insufflation tubing.
Anticipation: Confirm entry with pressure readings. Be prepared for alternate entry if prior surgery suggests adhesions.

Oophorectomy

Step 3 – Insert primary trocar and laparoscope
Instruments: 10 to 12 mm trocar, 30 degree laparoscope, camera system.
Anticipation: White balance and focus camera before insertion. Announce entry for anesthesia awareness.

Step 4 – Place accessory trocars under direct vision
Instruments: Two 5 mm trocars.
Anticipation: Transilluminate to avoid inferior epigastric vessels. Ensure ports allow safe approach to infundibulopelvic ligament.

Step 5 – Perform pelvic survey and identify ureter
Instruments: Atraumatic graspers, suction irrigation if needed.
Anticipation: Ureter identification is essential before energy use near the pelvic sidewall. Maintain a clear dry field.

Step 6 – Elevate adnexa and tension infundibulopelvic ligament
Instruments: Atraumatic grasper, Maryland dissector.
Anticipation: Apply traction and countertraction to open the avascular plane. Avoid crushing ovarian tissue if malignancy is suspected.

Step 7 – Seal and divide infundibulopelvic ligament
Instruments: Energy device handpiece, Maryland dissector, laparoscopic scissors if needed.
Anticipation: This is the key bleeding risk step. Keep suction ready but do not obscure the field. Confirm ureter is away from the seal line.

Step 8 – Divide utero ovarian ligament and fallopian tube if needed
Instruments: Energy device, atraumatic grasper.
Anticipation: Be prepared to convert to salpingo oophorectomy depending on indication. Maintain orientation to avoid uterine or tubal injury.

Step 9 – Free remaining attachments and inspect pedicles
Instruments: Suction irrigation, atraumatic grasper.
Anticipation: Inspect for bleeding at the pelvic sidewall pedicle. Expect brief irrigation and reassessment before retrieval.

Step 10 – Remove ovary from abdomen
Instruments: Specimen retrieval bag brought up when requested.
Anticipation: Bag is an add on, not on initial Mayo. For large ovaries, anticipate controlled decompression only if surgeon directs and pathology permits.

Step 11 – Desufflate and remove trocars
Instruments: Laparoscope, suction.
Anticipation: Watch pedicles during desufflation. Remove trocars under visualization to confirm hemostasis.

Step 12 – Close port sites and dressings
Instruments: Suture, Mayo Scissors, and Forceps
Anticipation: Fascia closure is required for larger ports. Needle driver and sutures come up only at closure.

Oophorectomy

Mayo Stand Suggestion:

- #11 blade on scalpel handle
- Veress needle or Hasson cannula
- 10 to 12 mm trocar
- Two 5 mm trocars
- Maryland dissector
- Atraumatic grasper
- Energy device handpiece
- Laparoscopic scissors
- Suction irrigation handpiece

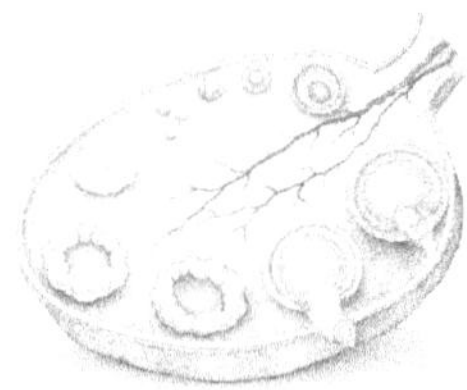

Pelvic Exenteration

Pelvic Exenteration
Step 1 – Midline abdominal incision and wide exposure
Instruments: #10 blade, Adsons with teeth, suction
Anticipation: Incision is long and exposure is critical. Expect early bleeding from scar tissue and prior radiation changes.

Step 2 – Enter peritoneum and perform abdominal exploration
Instruments: Metzenbaum scissors, Debakey forceps.
Anticipation: Surgeon confirms resectability before committing. Be prepared to pause if disease is unresectable.

Step 3 – Mobilize bowel and pack abdomen
Instruments: Moist laps from back table, Debakey forceps.
Anticipation: Bowel is often friable from radiation. Maintain constant moisture and gentle handling.

Step 4 – Identify and protect ureters
Instruments: Debakey forceps, vessel loops if requested.
Anticipation: Ureter identification is critical early. Anticipate stents or marking loops to remain in place throughout the case.

Step 5 – Control major pelvic vessels
Instruments: Right angle clamps, Debakey forceps, suction.
Anticipation: Vascular control precedes organ removal. Expect clamp cut tie rhythm but closure instruments remain until requested.

Step 6 – Resection of involved pelvic organs
Instruments: Metzenbaum scissors, monopolar pencil, suction.
Anticipation: Organs removed may include bladder rectum uterus or vagina. Expect frequent suction and specimen handoff.

Step 7 – Manage pelvic floor and perineal dissection
Instruments: Metzenbaum scissors, Debakey forceps, suction.
Anticipation: This phase often overlaps with perineal team. Communicate clearly and maintain orientation of specimens.

Step 8 – Inspect pelvic cavity and achieve hemostasis
Instruments: Suction irrigation.
Anticipation: Bleeding control is ongoing. Hemostatic agents are added from back table when requested.

Pelvic Exenteration

Step 9 – Urinary or fecal diversion preparation
Instruments: Bowel clamps and staplers brought up when requested.
Anticipation: Diversions are planned preoperatively but executed later. Do not preload Mayo with diversion supplies.

Step 10 – Irrigation and final inspection
Instruments: Irrigation, suction.
Anticipation: Surgeon reassesses all pedicles and raw surfaces before reconstruction or closure.

Step 11 – Reconstruction and diversion creation
Instruments: Added from back table when requested.
Anticipation: This is a major transition point. Mayo stand contents change significantly here.

Step 12 – Abdominal and perineal closure
Instruments: Brought up from back table when closure begins.
Anticipation: Closure may be staged. Begin closing counts early and confirm drain placement before final closure.

Mayo Stand Suggestion:

- #10 blade on scalpel handle
- Metzenbaum scissors
- Mayo scissors
- Adsons forceps with teeth
- Debakey forceps
- Right angle clamp

Radical Hysterectomy (Wertheim Procedure)

Step 1 – Midline abdominal incision and exposure
Instruments: #10 blade, Adsons with teeth, Bovie if incision begins immediately, suction tip if needed.
Anticipation: Wide exposure is required. Expect adhesions and friable tissue from prior radiation or biopsy.

Step 2 – Enter peritoneum and explore abdomen
Instruments: Metzenbaum scissors, Debakey forceps.
Anticipation: Surgeon confirms operability before proceeding. Be prepared to pause if metastatic disease is found.

Step 3 – Pack bowel and expose pelvis
Instruments: Moist laps from back table, Debakey forceps.
Anticipation: Maintain bowel moisture and clear pelvic visualization. Exposure will be adjusted frequently.

Step 4 – Identify and mobilize ureters
Instruments: Debakey forceps, right angle clamp, suction.
Anticipation: Ureter identification is critical and ongoing. Vessel loops may be placed and remain throughout the case.

Step 5 – Control uterine vessels at origin
Instruments: Right angle clamps, Debakey forceps, Bovie.
Anticipation: This is a high bleeding risk step. Maintain suction readiness and clear clamp cut sequence awareness.

Radical Hysterectomy (Wertheim Procedure)

Step 6 – Divide cardinal and uterosacral ligaments
Instruments: Metzenbaum scissors, right angle clamps, Bovie.
Anticipation: Deep pelvic dissection requires excellent visualization. Avoid tension on ureters during division.

Step 7 – Dissect bladder and rectum from vagina
Instruments: Metzenbaum scissors, Debakey forceps, suction.
Anticipation: Bladder and rectum are at high risk for injury. Maintain correct planes and gentle traction.

Step 8 – Perform colpotomy and remove specimen
Instruments: Bovie, sponge forceps.
Anticipation: Specimen is large and complex. Open specimen basin early and confirm orientation for pathology.

Step 9 – Inspect pelvis and achieve hemostasis
Instruments: Suction irrigation, Bovie.
Anticipation: Expect prolonged hemostasis checks. Hemostatic agents are added from back table when requested.

Step 10 – Pelvic lymph node dissection if indicated
Instruments: Metzenbaum scissors, Debakey forceps, suction.
Anticipation: Node dissection increases bleeding risk. Maintain a clean dry field and careful specimen handling.

Step 11 – Irrigate pelvis and reassess ureters
Instruments: Irrigation system, suction.
Anticipation: Confirm ureteral integrity and hemostasis before closure phase begins.

Step 12 – Vaginal cuff and abdominal closure
Instruments: Suture, Mayo Scissors, and Forceps
Anticipation: This is the transition point where needle drivers and sutures come to the Mayo.

Mayo Stand Suggestion:

- #10 blade on scalpel handle
- Metzenbaum scissors
- Mayo scissors
- Adsons forceps with teeth
- Debakey forceps
- Right angle clamp

Robot Assisted Hysterectomy

Step 1 – Patient positioning and preparation
Instruments: Allen stirrups, Foley catheter, uterine manipulator, grounding pad.
Anticipation: Positioning is critical for long operative time. Pad pressure points and confirm steep Trendelenburg capability before draping.

Step 2 – Establish pneumoperitoneum
Instruments: #11 blade, Veress needle or Hasson cannula, insufflation tubing.
Anticipation: Maintain midline entry and confirm insufflation pressures. Prior abdominal surgery may require alternate entry.

Robot Assisted Hysterectomy

Step 3 – Insert camera port and laparoscope
Instruments: 8 to 12 mm robotic camera trocar, laparoscope.
Anticipation: Camera must be perfectly centered and focused before docking. Poor placement complicates the entire case.

Step 4 – Place robotic and assistant trocars
Instruments: Robotic trocars, assistant port trocar.
Anticipation: Spacing is critical to prevent robotic arm collisions. Confirm port placement before docking.

Step 5 – Dock robotic system
Instruments: Robotic arms and instruments.
Anticipation: Maintain sterile field while docking. Communicate clearly during arm positioning.

Step 6 – Perform pelvic survey and expose uterus
Instruments: Robotic graspers, camera control.
Anticipation: Coordinate uterine manipulation with robotic movements to optimize visualization.

Step 7 – Divide round ligaments
Instruments: Robotic energy instrument, grasper.
Anticipation: Expect bilateral division early. Keep suction ready via assistant port.

Step 8 – Open broad ligament and identify ureters
Instruments: Robotic Maryland dissector
Anticipation: Ureter identification is essential and continuous. Loss of visualization requires immediate correction.

Step 9 – Control uterine vessels
Instruments: Robotic energy device, grasper.
Anticipation: High bleeding risk. Assistant must be ready with suction and clip applier if needed.

Step 10 – Dissect bladder flap
Instruments: Robotic dissector
Anticipation: Maintain correct tissue plane to avoid cystotomy. Expect slow controlled dissection.

Step 11 – Perform colpotomy
Instruments: Robotic energy device, uterine manipulator cup.
Anticipation: Communicate with anesthesia and vaginal team. Smoke evacuation is critical.

Step 12 – Remove uterus vaginally or via containment
Instruments: Sponge forceps, specimen bag brought up when requested.
Anticipation: Bag is an add on only. Open specimen container early.

Step 13 – Close vaginal cuff robotically
Instruments: Robotic needle driver and sutures brought up when requested.
Anticipation: Transition to closure phase. Ensure sutures are correct type and length before docking needle drivers.

Step 14 – Undock robot and inspect abdomen
Instruments: Laparoscope, suction irrigation.
Anticipation: Inspect pedicles after undocking to confirm hemostasis.

Robot Assisted Hysterectomy

Step 15 – Desufflate and close port sites
Instruments: Suture, Mayo Scissors, and Forceps
Anticipation: Close fascia for larger ports. Complete final counts before skin closure.

Mayo Stand Suggestion:

- #11 blade on scalpel handle
- Veress needle or Hasson cannula
- Robotic camera trocar
- Two or three robotic trocars
- Assistant port trocar
- Laparoscopic suction irrigation handpiece

Vulvectomy

Step 1 – Patient positioning and preparation
Instruments: Allen stirrups, perineal prep supplies, grounding pad.
Anticipation: Positioning must protect nerves and allow wide perineal access. Confirm lesion location and laterality before prep and drape.

Step 2 – Mark excision margins
Instruments: Skin marker, sterile gauze.
Anticipation: Margins are planned for complete excision while preserving function. Confirm planned margin width with surgeon before incision.

Step 3 – Local anesthetic infiltration if used
Instruments: Syringe with local anesthetic and epinephrine, fine needle.
Anticipation: Tissue blanching indicates vasoconstriction. Communicate with anesthesia if large volumes are injected.

Step 4 – Incise skin and begin vulvar excision
Instruments: #15 blade, Adsons with teeth, Metzenbaum scissors, suction
Anticipation: Vulvar tissue is vascular. Keep the field dry and maintain precise traction to avoid tearing skin edges.

Step 5 – Continue dissection to remove lesion with adequate depth
Instruments: Bovie, Metzenbaum scissors, Adsons with teeth.
Anticipation: Maintain anatomic awareness of urethra clitoris and vaginal introitus. Avoid excessive thermal spread near sensitive structures.

Step 6 – Achieve hemostasis and reassess margins
Instruments: Bovie, suction.
Anticipation: Hemostasis must be meticulous to prevent hematoma. Surgeon may request additional margin excision based on gross appearance.

Step 7 – Remove specimen and orient for pathology
Instruments: Specimen basin, marking suture or clip if requested.
Anticipation: Confirm orientation requirements before passing off specimen. Communicate laterality and margin designation clearly.

Step 8 – Irrigate and final hemostasis check
Instruments: Irrigation system, suction.
Anticipation: Even small bleeders can expand postoperatively. Ensure field is fully dry prior to closure.

Vulvectomy Continued

Step 9 – Closure
Instruments: Suture, Mayo Scissors, and Forceps
Anticipation: This is when needle driver and sutures come to the Mayo. Closure may require layered repair and careful alignment.

Step 10 – Dressing and padding
Instruments: Nonadherent dressing, gauze, perineal pad.
Anticipation: Dressing should protect without compression. Communicate postoperative instructions about wound care and bleeding monitoring.

Mayo Stand Suggestion:

- #15 blade on scalpel handle
- Metzenbaum scissors
- Mayo scissors
- 2 Mosquito Hemostats
- Skin Marker
- Adsons with teeth

Total Abdominal Hysterectomy

Step 1 – Lower abdominal incision and exposure
Instruments: #10 blade, Adsons with teeth, Bovie, suction tip if needed.
Anticipation: Incision is usually Pfannenstiel or midline. Expect bleeding from subcutaneous tissue and fascia early.

Step 2 – Dissect through fascia and enter peritoneum
Instruments: Metzenbaum scissors, Mayo scissors, Debakey forceps.
Anticipation: Maintain midline orientation. As the peritoneum is tented, be prepared for fluid release and protect bowel.

Step 3 – Pack bowel and expose uterus
Instruments: Moist laps from back table, Debakey forceps.
Anticipation: Exposure must be maintained throughout. Anticipate frequent retractors adjustments by the assistant.

Step 4 – Clamp and divide round ligaments
Instruments: Kelly or Crile clamps, Metzenbaum scissors, Bovie.
Anticipation: Expect bilateral clamp cut sequence. Maintain rhythm and keep suction ready.

Step 5 – Develop bladder flap
Instruments: Metzenbaum scissors, Debakey forceps, Bovie, suction.
Anticipation: Correct tissue plane prevents cystotomy. Bleeding can obscure the field quickly.

Step 6 – Clamp uterine vessels
Instruments: Heaney or curved clamps, Metzenbaum scissors, Bovie.
Anticipation: This is a major bleeding risk step. Be ready with clamps immediately.

Step 7 – Divide cardinal and uterosacral ligaments
Instruments: Heaney or curved clamps, Metzenbaum scissors, Bovie.
Anticipation: Maintain ureter awareness. Deep pelvic visualization is critical.

Step 8 – Perform colpotomy and remove uterus
Instruments: Bovie, sponge forceps.
Anticipation: Specimen removal is imminent. Open specimen basin early and confirm orientation.

Total Abdominal Hysterectomy Continued

Step 9 – Inspect pedicles and achieve hemostasis
Instruments: Suction irrigation, Bovie.
Anticipation: Bleeding control here prevents postoperative hemorrhage. Expect additional clamps or sutures.

Step 10 – Close vaginal cuff
Instruments: Suture, Mayo Scissors, and Forceps
Anticipation: Transition to closure phase. Needle driver and sutures come to the Mayo now.

Step 11 – Irrigate pelvis and final inspection
Instruments: Irrigation system, suction.
Anticipation: Confirm ureteral integrity and hemostasis before abdominal closure.

Step 12 – Abdominal wall closure
Instruments: Suture, Mayo Scissors, and Forceps
Anticipation: Begin closing counts early and confirm drains if placed.

Mayo Stand Suggestion:

- #10 blade on scalpel handle
- Metzenbaum scissors
- **Adsons** forceps with teeth
- **Debakey** forceps
- 2 Mosquito hemostats
- 1 Kelly or Crile clamp
- 1 Heaney clamp
- Mayo scissors

Total Salpingectomy

Step 1 – Patient positioning and preparation
Instruments: Allen stirrups, Foley catheter, uterine manipulator if used, grounding pad.
Anticipation: Confirm laterality or bilateral intent. Ensure Trendelenburg positioning is achievable and bladder is drained.

Step 2 – Establish abdominal access
Instruments: #11 blade, Veress needle or Hasson cannula, insufflation tubing.
Anticipation: Confirm proper insufflation pressures. Prior surgery may require alternate entry technique.

Step 3 – Insert primary trocar and laparoscope
Instruments: 10 to 12 mm trocar, 30 degree laparoscope.
Anticipation: White balance and focus camera before insertion. Announce entry to anesthesia.

Step 4 – Place accessory trocars under direct vision
Instruments: Two 5 mm trocars.
Anticipation: Avoid inferior epigastric vessels by transillumination. Port placement should allow safe access to adnexa.

Step 5 – Perform pelvic survey and identify ureter
Instruments: Atraumatic graspers, suction irrigation if needed.
Anticipation: Identify ureter before any energy use near the pelvic sidewall. Maintain a dry field.

Step 6 – Elevate fallopian tube and apply traction
Instruments: Atraumatic grasper.
Anticipation: Gentle traction opens the avascular plane between tube and ovary. Avoid crushing tubal tissue.

Total Salpingectomy Continued

Step 7 – Seal and divide mesosalpinx
Instruments: Energy device handpiece, Maryland dissector, laparoscopic scissors if needed.
Anticipation: Bleeding can occur along the mesosalpinx. Keep suction ready and advance in controlled segments.

Step 8 – Divide tubal attachment at uterine cornua
Instruments: Energy device, Maryland dissector.
Anticipation: Stay close to the tube to avoid uterine vessel injury. Confirm complete separation before moving on.

Step 9 – Inspect pedicle and achieve hemostasis
Instruments: Suction irrigation.
Anticipation: Inspect entire length of mesosalpinx. Small bleeders should be addressed before retrieval.

Step 10 – Remove fallopian tube from abdomen
Instruments: Specimen retrieval bag brought up when requested.
Anticipation: Bag is an add on only. Open specimen basin early if vaginal extraction is planned.

Step 11 – Desufflate and remove trocars
Instruments: Laparoscope, suction.
Anticipation: Observe pedicles during desufflation. Remove trocars under direct vision.

Step 12 – Close port sites and apply dressings
Instruments: Suture, Mayo Scissors, and Forceps
Anticipation: Fascia closure is required for larger ports. Needle driver and sutures come up only at closure.

Mayo Stand Suggestion:

- #11 blade on scalpel handle
- Veress needle or Hasson cannula
- 10 to 12 mm trocar
- Two 5 mm trocars
- Maryland dissector
- Atraumatic grasper
- Energy device handpiece
- Laparoscopic scissors
- Suction irrigation handpiece

Tubal Sterilization

Step 1 – Patient positioning and preparation
Instruments: Allen stirrups, Foley catheter, uterine manipulator if used, grounding pad.
Anticipation: Confirm sterilization method planned clip band cautery or partial salpingectomy. Ensure Trendelenburg positioning and bladder drainage.

Step 2 – Establish pneumoperitoneum
Instruments: #11 blade, Veress needle or Hasson cannula, insufflation tubing.
Anticipation: Confirm proper entry with pressure readings. Prior abdominal surgery may require alternate entry technique.

Step 3 – Insert primary trocar and laparoscope
Instruments: 10 mm trocar, 30 degree laparoscope.
Anticipation: White balance and focus camera before insertion. Announce entry to anesthesia.

Tubal Sterilization Continued

Step 4 – Place accessory trocar
Instruments: One or two 5 mm trocars.
Anticipation: Place ports to allow comfortable access to both adnexa without crossing instruments.

Step 5 – Perform pelvic survey and identify tubes
Instruments: Atraumatic graspers, suction irrigation if needed.
Anticipation: Identify uterus tubes and ovaries. Confirm no unexpected pathology before proceeding.

Step 6 – Elevate fallopian tube
Instruments: Atraumatic grasper.
Anticipation: Gentle traction isolates the tube. Avoid grasping the mesosalpinx near vessels.

Step 7 – Apply sterilization method
Instruments: Clip applicator banding device or Bovie depending on method.
Anticipation: Confirm correct tube and location before application. Surgeon may verbally confirm laterality before division.

Step 8 – Inspect for hemostasis and tubal separation
Instruments: Suction irrigation.
Anticipation: Assist with visualization so the surgeon can look for bleeding or incomplete occlusion. Address immediately before moving to the opposite side.

Step 9 – Repeat on contralateral side
Instruments: Same as above.
Anticipation: Maintain consistent technique bilaterally. Reconfirm anatomy to avoid wrong structure error.

Step 10 – Desufflate and remove trocars
Instruments: Laparoscope, suction.
Anticipation: Observe pedicles during desufflation. Remove trocars under direct vision.

Step 11 – Close port sites and apply dressings
Instruments: Closing suture, Mayo Scissors, and Dressings
Anticipation: Fascia closure for larger ports. Needle driver and sutures come up only at closure.

Mayo Stand Suggestion:

- #11 blade on scalpel handle
- Veress needle or Hasson cannula
- 10 mm trocar
- One or two 5 mm trocars
- Atraumatic grasper
- Maryland dissector
- Bovie handpiece
- 2 Mosquito hemostats
- 1 Kelly or Crile clamp
- Clip Applicator

Tuboplasty

Step 1 – Patient positioning and preparation
Instruments: Allen stirrups, Foley catheter, uterine manipulator if used, grounding pad.
Anticipation: Confirm laterality and type of tubal pathology. Ensure Trendelenburg positioning and bladder drainage before draping.

Step 2 – Establish pneumoperitoneum
Instruments: #11 blade, Veress needle or Hasson cannula, insufflation tubing.
Anticipation: Confirm proper insufflation pressures. Prior pelvic surgery increases adhesion risk and may alter entry technique.

Step 3 – Insert primary trocar and laparoscope
Instruments: 10 to 12 mm trocar, 30 degree laparoscope.
Anticipation: White balance and focus camera before insertion. Announce entry so anesthesia can monitor patient response.

Step 4 – Place accessory trocars under direct vision
Instruments: Two or three 5 mm trocars.
Anticipation: Port placement must allow fine instrument control. Avoid inferior epigastric vessels and allow ergonomic access to adnexa.

Step 5 – Perform pelvic survey and identify ureters
Instruments: Atraumatic graspers, suction irrigation handpiece.
Anticipation: Ureter identification is critical before any tubal reconstruction. Maintain a clear dry field.

Step 6 – Isolate fallopian tube and assess damage
Instruments: Atraumatic grasper, Maryland dissector.
Anticipation: Surgeon determines feasibility of repair. Excessive manipulation can compromise tubal viability.

Step 7 – Excise scarred or occluded tubal segment
Instruments: Laparoscopic scissors, Bovie, Maryland dissector.
Anticipation: Bleeding can occur along mesosalpinx. Control small bleeders promptly to maintain visualization.

Step 8 – Reapproximate tubal ends or open fimbrial end
Instruments: Laparoscopic needle driver and fine sutures brought up when requested.
Anticipation: This marks transition to microsurgical precision. Ensure correct suture type and needle size are ready before handoff.

Step 9 – Inspect repair and ensure tubal patency
Instruments: Suction irrigation handpiece.
Anticipation: Surgeon may inject dye via uterine manipulator. Watch for leakage or bleeding at repair site.

Step 10 – Achieve final hemostasis
Instruments: Bovie, suction irrigation handpiece.
Anticipation: Hemostasis must be meticulous to protect tubal function. Avoid excessive thermal spread.

Step 11 – Desufflate and remove trocars
Instruments: Laparoscope, suction.
Anticipation: Observe repair during desufflation. Remove trocars under direct vision.

Tuboplasty Continued

Step 12 – Close port sites and apply dressings
Instruments: Suture, Mayo Scissors, and Forceps
Anticipation: Fascia closure for larger ports. Needle driver and sutures come up only at closure.

Mayo Stand Suggestion:

- #11 blade on scalpel handle
- Veress needle or Hasson cannula
- 10 to 12 mm trocar
- Two or three 5 mm trocars
- Atraumatic grasper
- Laparoscopic scissors
- Bovie handpiece
- 2 Mosquito hemostats
- 1 Kelly or Crile clamp
- Maryland dissector

Vaginal Hysterectomy

Step 1 – Patient positioning and vaginal preparation
Instruments: Allen stirrups, Foley catheter, vaginal prep supplies, grounding pad.
Anticipation: Lithotomy positioning must allow wide vaginal access without nerve compression. Ensure bladder is fully drained.

Step 2 – Vaginal exposure and cervical visualization
Instruments: Weighted vaginal speculum or Graves speculum, Sims retractors, sponge forceps.
Anticipation: Stable exposure is essential. Adjust retractor early to avoid repeated repositioning later.

Step 3 – Grasp cervix for traction
Instruments: Single tooth tenaculum or double tooth tenaculum.
Anticipation: Apply firm but controlled traction. Cervical tearing complicates the entire case.

Step 4 – Circumferential cervical incision
Instruments: #15 blade, Bovie, Metzenbaum scissors, suction tip if needed.
Anticipation: Bleeding begins early. Be ready with clamps immediately rather than relying only on Bovie.

Step 5 – Develop vesicovaginal space and reflect bladder
Instruments: Metzenbaum scissors, Debakey forceps, Bovie, suction.
Anticipation: Correct plane protects the bladder. Loss of plane increases cystotomy risk.

Step 6 – Enter posterior cul de sac
Instruments: Metzenbaum scissors, sponge forceps.
Anticipation: Posterior entry is usually easier. Be prepared for peritoneal fluid release.

Step 7 – Clamp and divide uterosacral ligaments
Instruments: Heaney or curved clamps, Metzenbaum scissors, Bovie.
Anticipation: Maintain awareness of ureters laterally. Clamp placement must be deliberate and secure.

Step 8 – Clamp and divide cardinal ligaments
Instruments: Heaney clamps, Metzenbaum scissors, Bovie.
Anticipation: This is a major support structure. Expect firm resistance and bleeding if clamp placement is off.

Step 9 – Clamp uterine vessels
Instruments: Heaney clamps, Metzenbaum scissors, Bovie.
Anticipation: High bleeding risk step. Anticipate immediate clamp placement before division.

Vaginal Hysterectomy Continued

Step 11 – Inspect pedicles and achieve hemostasis
Instruments: Suction, Bovie.
Anticipation: Bleeding control here prevents postoperative hemorrhage. Expect additional clamps or sutures.

Step 12 – Close vaginal cuff
Instruments: Brought up from back table when requested.
Anticipation: Needle driver and sutures come to the Mayo now. Assist with organized suture management.

Step 13 – Vaginal packing if indicated
Instruments: Vaginal packing, lubricant.
Ant

Mayo Stand Suggestion:

- #15 blade on scalpel handle
- Metzenbaum scissors
- Mayo scissors
- Adsons forceps with teeth
- Debakey forceps
- 2 Mosquito hemostats
- 1 Kelly or Crile clamp
- 2 Heaney clamps

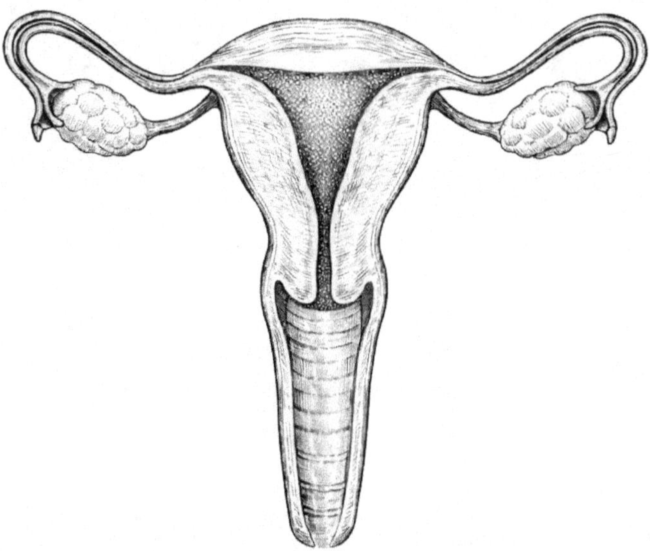

Section III:
Ophthalmic Procedures

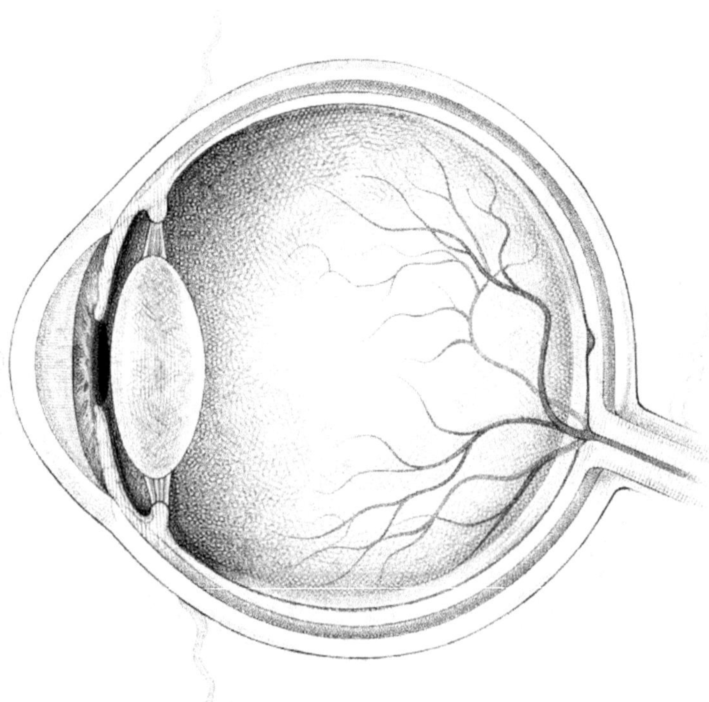

Dacryocystorhinostomy

Step 1 – Patient positioning and preparation
Instruments: Donut, eye prep supplies, nasal prep supplies, grounding pad if Bovie used.
Anticipation: Head is slightly elevated. Confirm laterality carefully. Nasal packing with vasoconstrictor may be placed to reduce bleeding.

Step 2 – Skin marking and local infiltration
Instruments: Skin marker, syringe with local anesthetic and epinephrine, fine needle.
Anticipation: Mark incision just medial to the medial canthus. Epinephrine minimizes bleeding in a highly vascular area.

Step 3 – Skin incision and dissection to lacrimal sac
Instruments: #15 blade, fine Adsons forceps, Westcott scissors, Bovie on low setting, suction tip.
Anticipation: Dissection is delicate and shallow. Avoid injury to medial canthal structures and angular vessels.

Step 4 – Expose lacrimal sac fossa
Instruments: Periosteal elevator, fine retractor, suction.
Anticipation: Bone exposure must be clean. Maintain gentle retraction to avoid orbital injury.

Step 5 – Create bony ostium
Instruments: Kerrison rongeur or bone punch, suction.
Anticipation: Have suction in hand before rongeur use. Pass Kerrison in correct orientation and be ready to clear blood immediately without obscuring the field.

Step 6 – Incise lacrimal sac and nasal mucosa
Instruments: Westcott scissors, fine forceps.
Anticipation: Identify sac lumen clearly before incision. Maintain orientation to avoid false passage.

Step 7 – Create mucosal flaps and anastomose
Instruments: Needle driver and fine sutures brought up from back table when requested.
Anticipation: This is the transition to closure level work. Bring fine needle driver and sutures only when surgeon commits to flap anastomosis.

Step 8 – Place silicone stent if indicated
Instruments: Silicone lacrimal stent.
Anticipation: Stent placement may be fiddly. Maintain patience and avoid tension that could dislodge flaps.

Step 9 – Achieve hemostasis and irrigate
Instruments: Bovie on low setting, suction.
Anticipation: Hemostasis must be meticulous to prevent postoperative hematoma or epistaxis.

Step 10 – Close skin incision
Instruments: Suture, Mayo Scissors, and Forceps
Anticipation: Fine skin closure is cosmetic. Assist with precise edge alignment.

Step 11 – Apply dressing and nasal packing
Instruments: Eye pad, nasal packing if used.
Anticipation: Communicate packing presence and removal timing clearly.

Dacryocystorhinostomy

Mayo Stand Suggestion:

- #15 blade on scalpel handle
- Westcott scissors
- Fine Adsons forceps
- Periosteal elevator
- Kerrison rongeur or bone punch
- 2 Mosquito hemostats
- 1 small curved hemostat
- Fine skin retractor
- Lacrimal Stent
- Needle Driver

Enucleation

Step 1 – Patient positioning and eye preparation
Instruments: Headrest or donut, ophthalmic prep supplies, eyelid speculum, grounding pad if Bovie used.
Anticipation: Confirm laterality verbally with the team. Head must be stable since small movements affect orbital control.

Step 2 – Eyelid retraction and exposure
Instruments: Barraquer or Lieberman eyelid speculum.
Anticipation: Maintain consistent exposure without excessive pressure on the globe.

Step 3 – Conjunctival peritomy
Instruments: Westcott scissors, fine toothed forceps, Bovie on low setting, suction tip if needed.
Anticipation: Circumferential incision allows access to extraocular muscles. Keep the field dry to maintain visualization.

Step 4 – Isolate and secure rectus muscles
Instruments: Muscle hook, fine hemostats, 4 0 silk ties brought up when requested.
Anticipation: Each muscle is isolated individually. Maintain control of sutures to prevent muscle retraction into the orbit.

Step 5 – Transect extraocular muscles
Instruments: Westcott scissors, fine hemostats, Bovie if needed.
Anticipation: Cut only after the muscle is secured. Maintain orientation to avoid losing muscle ends.

Step 6 – Identify and clamp optic nerve
Instruments: Long curved hemostat or enucleation clamp, suction.
Anticipation: Anticipate enucleation clamp before nerve exposure. Keep clamp ready and suction immediately available before transection.

Step 7 – Transect optic nerve and remove globe
Instruments: Enucleation scissors, specimen basin.
Anticipation: Globe removal is immediate after nerve division. Be prepared for sudden bleeding and pass globe off promptly.

Step 8 – Inspect orbit and achieve hemostasis
Instruments: Bovie on low setting, suction.
Anticipation: Bleeding control is essential to prevent postoperative hematoma. Expect oozing from muscle beds and optic nerve stump.

Enucleation

Step 9 – Place orbital implant if indicated
Instruments: Orbital implant brought up when requested.
Anticipation: Implant size and type are surgeon specific. Handle gently to avoid contamination.

Step 10 – Close Tenons capsule and conjunctiva
Instruments: Suture, Mayo Scissors, and Forceps
Anticipation: This is the transition to closure. Fine needle driver and sutures are now brought to the Mayo.

Step 11 – Apply conformer and dressing
Instruments: Ocular conformer, antibiotic ointment, eye pad and shield.
Anticipation: Confirm conformer placement before dressing. Communicate dressing care clearly to recovery staff.

Mayo Stand Suggestion:

- Eyelid speculum
- Westcott scissors
- Fine toothed forceps
- Muscle hook
- Enucleation scissors
- 2 fine mosquito hemostats
- 1 long curved hemostat or enucleation clamp

Extracapsular Cataract Extraction

Step 1 – Patient positioning and sterile eye preparation
Instruments: Headrest or donut, ophthalmic prep supplies, sterile drape with adhesive aperture, lid speculum.
Anticipation: Head must be stable and centered. Confirm laterality and lens plan before draping.

Step 2 – Place lid speculum and assess exposure
Instruments: Barraquer lid speculum.
Anticipation: Avoid excessive lid tension. A stable speculum prevents corneal drying and movement.

Step 3 – Create conjunctival peritomy if planned
Instruments: Westcott scissors, fine toothed forceps, cellulose spears.
Anticipation: Some surgeons use a limbal based flap. Maintain moisture with balanced salt solution.

Step 4 – Control bleeding at limbus if present
Instruments: Wet field cautery if used, Weck Cel sponges.
Anticipation: Hemostasis must be gentle. Excess cautery can damage scleral tissue.

Step 5 – Create scleral tunnel or limbal incision
Instruments: Crescent blade, keratome, fixation forceps.
Anticipation: Anticipate immediate viscoelastic request once chamber is entered. Have syringe uncapped and ready

Step 6 – Enter anterior chamber and instill viscoelastic
Instruments: Viscoelastic cannula and syringe, Weck Cel sponges.
Anticipation: Maintain chamber stability. Keep the wound controlled to prevent iris prolapse.

Step 7 – Perform capsulotomy
Instruments: Cystotome or capsulorhexis forceps, Utrata forceps if used.
Anticipation: Capsular tear control is key. Keep eye stable and pass instruments gently to avoid sudden chamber collapse.

Extracapsular Cataract Extraction

Step 8 – Hydrodissection and nucleus delivery
Instruments: Hydrodissection cannula with syringe, lens loop or vectis, irrigating solution.
Anticipation: Be ready with Weck Cel at wound edge to control fluid egress and prevent iris prolapse.

Step 9 – Remove cortical material
Instruments: Simcoe irrigation aspiration cannula or manual aspiration system.
Anticipation: Cortical cleanup must be systematic. Protect posterior capsule and maintain chamber depth.

Step 10 – Insert intraocular lens
Instruments: Lens injector or lens forceps, viscoelastic.
Anticipation: Confirm correct lens power and type before opening. Maintain a controlled chamber during insertion.

Step 11 – Remove viscoelastic and reform chamber
Instruments: Irrigation aspiration cannula, balanced salt solution.
Anticipation: Residual viscoelastic can raise intraocular pressure. Ensure chamber is stable at conclusion.

Step 12 – Close wound and conjunctiva if required
Instruments: Suture, Mayo Scissors, and Forceps
Anticipation: Sutures and needle driver come up only when surgeon commits to closure. Prepare for watertight wound check.

Step 13 – Apply antibiotic and dressing
Instruments: Antibiotic drops or ointment, eye pad and shield.
Anticipation: Confirm wound integrity before dressing. Communicate shield instructions to recovery staff.

Mayo Stand Suggestion:

- Barraquer lid speculum
- Westcott scissors
- Fine toothed forceps
- Fixation forceps
- Crescent blade
- Keratome
- Cystotome or capsulorhexis forceps
- Weck Cel sponges
- Viscoelastic syringe with cannula
- Simcoe irrigation aspiration cannula

Iridectomy

Step 1 – Patient positioning and sterile eye preparation
Instruments: Headrest or donut, ophthalmic prep supplies, sterile drape with adhesive aperture, lid speculum.
Anticipation: Head must be stable and centered. Confirm laterality and planned iridectomy location before draping.

Step 2 – Place lid speculum and assess exposure
Instruments: Barraquer lid speculum.
Anticipation: Avoid excessive lid tension. Corneal drying increases risk of epithelial injury.

Step 3 – Create corneal or limbal incision
Instruments: Keratome or micro blade, fixation forceps, Weck Cel sponges.
Anticipation: Incision must be controlled and self sealing. Anticipate viscoelastic immediately after entry.

Iridectomy

Step 4 – Enter anterior chamber and instill viscoelastic
Instruments: Viscoelastic syringe with cannula.
Anticipation: Chamber stability is critical. Maintain gentle injection to avoid iris prolapse.

Step 5 – Grasp iris tissue
Instruments: Iris forceps.
Anticipation: Use minimal traction. Excess pull increases bleeding and pupil distortion.

Step 6 – Excise iris tissue
Instruments: Vannas scissors or DeWecker scissors.
Anticipation: Have Vannas scissors oriented and ready once iris is grasped. Be prepared for immediate irrigation if bleeding occurs.

Step 7 – Control bleeding
Instruments: Irrigation cannula, Weck Cel sponges.
Anticipation: Minor bleeding is common. Gentle irrigation usually clears blood without cautery.

Step 8 – Remove viscoelastic and reform chamber
Instruments: Irrigation aspiration cannula, balanced salt solution.
Anticipation: Residual viscoelastic may increase intraocular pressure. Ensure chamber stability before closure.

Step 9 – Close incision if required
Instruments: Suture, Mayo Scissors, and Forceps
Anticipation: Needle driver and fine sutures come to the Mayo only if wound is not self sealing.

Step 10 – Apply medication and dressing
Instruments: Antibiotic drops or ointment, eye pad and shield.
Anticipation: Confirm patency of iridectomy before dressing.

Mayo Stand Suggestion:

- Barraquer lid speculum
- Westcott scissors
- Fine toothed forceps
- Fixation forceps
- Crescent blade
- Keratome
- Cystotome or capsulorhexis forceps
- Weck Cel sponges
- Viscoelastic syringe with cannula
- Simcoe irrigation aspiration cannula

Keratoplasty Corneal Transplant

Step 1 – Patient positioning and sterile eye preparation
Instruments: Headrest or donut, ophthalmic prep supplies, sterile drape with adhesive aperture, lid speculum.
Anticipation: Confirm laterality and donor tissue details before draping. Keep cornea continuously moist with balanced salt solution.

Step 2 – Place lid speculum and stabilize globe
Instruments: Barraquer lid speculum, fixation forceps.
Anticipation: Globe must be stable for trephination. Avoid excessive pressure that can distort the cornea.

Keratoplasty Corneal Transplant

Step 3 – Mark and center the graft
Instruments: Calipers, marking pen if used, fixation forceps.
Anticipation: Centering is critical for visual outcome. Confirm intended graft size before trephine touches the cornea.

Step 4 – Trephine host cornea
Instruments: Corneal trephine, Weck Cel sponges.
Anticipation: Depth control prevents injury to iris and lens. Expect an anterior chamber opening once full thickness is reached.

Step 5 – Enter anterior chamber and maintain chamber stability
Instruments: Viscoelastic syringe with cannula, balanced salt solution syringe, Weck Cel sponges.
Anticipation: Chamber can shallow quickly and iris can prolapse. Anticipate viscoelastic immediately to protect intraocular structures.

Step 6 – Excise host corneal button
Instruments: Corneal scissors, corneal forceps.
Anticipation: Ensure donor tissue is open and positioned on the field before host button removal. Do not allow open sky time without donor immediately available.

Step 7 – Prepare donor corneal button
Instruments: Donor corneal punch, donor block, fine forceps.
Anticipation: Confirm donor size matches plan. Ensure donor is oriented correctly and handled gently to protect endothelium.

Step 8 – Place donor button on host bed
Instruments: Corneal forceps, Weck Cel sponges, balanced salt solution.
Anticipation: Prevent endothelial touch and desiccation. Expect micro adjustments for centration.

Step 9 – Initial fixation of graft
Instruments: Suture, Mayo Scissors, and Forceps
Anticipation: This is the cue to bring needle driver and 10-0 nylon to the Mayo. Confirm suture count and needle orientation before handoff.

Step 10 – Complete suturing and adjust tension
Instruments: Suture, Mayo Scissors, and Forceps
Anticipation: Surgeon may use interrupted or continuous sutures. Expect frequent rotation of the eye and suture tail management.

Step 11 – Reform anterior chamber and check wound integrity
Instruments: Balanced salt solution syringe, Weck Cel sponges.
Anticipation: Confirm watertight seal and proper chamber depth. Watch for leakage at suture bites and iris prolapse.

Step 12 – Apply medication and dressing
Instruments: Antibiotic drops or ointment, eye pad and shield.
Anticipation: Confirm graft is centered and surface is protected before dressing.

Mayo Stand Suggestion:

- Barraquer lid speculum
- Fixation forceps
- Calipers
- Corneal trephine
- Corneal scissors
- Corneal forceps
- Weck Cel sponges
- Viscoelastic syringe with cannula
- Balanced salt solution syringe
- Donor corneal punch and donor block

Repair of Traumatic Eyelid Laceration

Step 1 – Patient positioning and eye protection
Instruments: Headrest or donut, ophthalmic prep supplies, corneal shield if globe intact, grounding pad if Bovie used.
Anticipation: First priority is globe protection. Confirm whether the laceration involves lid margin canaliculus or tarsal plate.

Step 2 – Eyelid exposure and assessment
Instruments: Barraquer or Lieberman eyelid speculum, fine skin retractor.
Anticipation: Full assessment determines complexity. Canalicular involvement changes the entire repair plan.

Step 3 – Irrigate wound and remove debris
Instruments: Saline syringe with cannula, suction tip, Weck Cel sponges.
Anticipation: Debridement must be conservative. Preserve as much tissue as possible for reconstruction.

Step 4 – Local anesthetic infiltration if used
Instruments: Syringe with local anesthetic and epinephrine, fine needle.
Anticipation: Tissue blanching reduces bleeding. Avoid distortion of wound edges with over injection.

Step 5 – Achieve hemostasis
Instruments: Bovie on low setting, fine mosquito hemostats.
Anticipation: Bleeding control is critical before alignment. Excess cautery risks tissue necrosis.

Step 6 – Align eyelid margin and tarsal plate
Instruments: Fine toothed forceps, skin hooks if needed.
Anticipation: Hold tissue steady with fine forceps and avoid traction on skin edges. Anticipate deep layer sutures before skin closure.

Step 7 – Repair deep structures
Instruments: Suture, Mayo Scissors, and Forceps
Anticipation: This is the transition to suturing. Fine needle driver and sutures are now brought to the Mayo.

Step 8 – Close skin
Instruments: Suture, Mayo Scissors, and Forceps
Anticipation: Skin closure should be tension free. Assist with precise edge eversion.

Step 9 – Apply ointment and dressing
Instruments: Antibiotic ointment, eye pad and shield.
Anticipation: Confirm globe integrity before dressing. Communicate wound care and follow up instructions.

Mayo Stand Suggestion:

- Barraquer or Lieberman eyelid speculum
- Fine skin retractor
- Westcott scissors
- Fine toothed forceps
- 2 fine mosquito hemostats
- Bovie handpiece
- Saline syringe with cannula
- Weck Cel sponges

Scleral Buckle

Step 1 – Patient positioning and eye preparation
Instruments: Headrest or donut, ophthalmic prep supplies, sterile drape with adhesive aperture, grounding pad if Bovie used.
Anticipation: Confirm laterality and retinal break location. Head stability is critical for precise scleral work.

Step 2 – Place lid speculum and expose globe
Instruments: Barraquer lid speculum.
Anticipation: Maintain corneal moisture throughout the case.

Step 3 – Perform conjunctival peritomy
Instruments: Westcott scissors, fine toothed forceps, Bovie on low setting, Weck Cel sponges.
Anticipation: Wide exposure allows access to all quadrants. Gentle cautery minimizes conjunctival scarring.

Step 4 – Isolate rectus muscles
Instruments: Muscle hook, fine mosquito hemostats, 2 0 silk ties brought up when requested.
Anticipation: Each muscle is isolated and tagged. Maintain suture control to prevent muscle loss into the orbit.

Step 5 – Identify retinal breaks and mark sclera
Instruments: Indirect ophthalmoscope used by surgeon, marking pen.
Anticipation: Accurate localization determines buckle placement. Remain still during retinal examination.

Step 6 – Apply cryotherapy to retinal breaks
Instruments: Cryoprobe and console.
Anticipation: Confirm cryoprobe is connected and functioning before application. Keep probe tip clean and immediately available

Step 7 – Place scleral buckle element
Instruments: Buckle element band or sponge, scleral depressor, fine forceps.
Anticipation: Confirm correct buckle size and orientation before placement.

Step 8 – Secure buckle to sclera
Instruments: Suture, Mayo Scissors, and Forceps
Anticipation: Suturing phase begins here. Needle driver and sutures are now placed on the Mayo.

Step 9 – Adjust buckle tension and reassess retina
Instruments: Scleral depressor.
Anticipation: Surgeon may re examine retina. Buckle height and position may need adjustment.

Step 10 – Drain subretinal fluid if indicated
Instruments: Fine needle or blade, suction.
Anticipation: This step carries hemorrhage risk. Be prepared with suction and gentle pressure.

Step 11 – Close conjunctiva
Instruments: Suture, Mayo Scissors, and Forceps
Anticipation: Ensure buckle is fully covered to prevent exposure.

Step 12 – Apply medication and dressing
Instruments: Antibiotic ointment, eye pad and shield.
Anticipation: Confirm retinal reattachment and buckle stability before dressing.

Scleral Buckle

Mayo Stand Suggestion:

- Barraquer lid speculum
- Westcott scissors
- Fine toothed forceps
- Muscle hook
- 2 fine mosquito hemostats
- Scleral depressor
- Buckle element band or sponge
- Cryoprobe
- Weck Cel sponges

Strabismus Correction Recession and Resection

Step 1 – Patient positioning and eye preparation
Instruments: Headrest or donut, ophthalmic prep supplies, sterile drape with adhesive aperture, grounding pad if Bovie used.
Anticipation: Confirm operative eye and specific muscle plan. Head must be stable since muscle orientation is critical.

Step 2 – Place lid speculum and expose globe
Instruments: Barraquer lid speculum.
Anticipation: Ensure even lid retraction without excessive pressure. Keep cornea moist.

Step 3 – Perform conjunctival incision
Instruments: Westcott scissors, fine toothed forceps, Weck Cel sponges, Bovie on low setting if needed.
Anticipation: Anticipate gentle cautery for small bleeders.

Step 4 – Isolate target extraocular muscle
Instruments: Muscle hook, fine mosquito hemostats.
Anticipation: Have muscle hook ready before conjunctival dissection is complete. Maintain control of muscle once hooked to prevent slippage.

Step 5 – Clear intermuscular septum and expose muscle insertion
Instruments: Westcott scissors, fine forceps.
Anticipation: Dissection is delicate. Keep field dry with Weck Cel to maintain visualization.

Step 6 – Secure muscle with suture
Instruments: Suture, Mayo Scissors, and Forceps
Anticipation: This is the transition to suturing. Bring needle driver and preloaded muscle sutures only when surgeon commits to muscle fixation.

Step 7 – Perform muscle recession or resection
Instruments: Westcott scissors, muscle hook.
Anticipation: Anticipate immediate cut after suture placement. Be ready to manage muscle ends and prevent retraction.

Step 8 – Reattach muscle at new position
Instruments: Needle driver and sutures already on field.
Anticipation: Maintain organization of suture ends. Prevent tangling and inadvertent needle loss.

Step 9 – Inspect muscle tension and alignment
Instruments: Muscle hook
Anticipation: Surgeon may adjust placement. Be prepared to reposition hook quickly without excess manipulation.

Strabismus Correction Recession and Resection

Step 10 – Close conjunctiva
Instruments: Suture, Mayo Scissors, and Forceps
Anticipation: Assist with smooth tissue handling and maintain moisture to prevent tearing.

Step 11 – Apply medication and dressing
Instruments: Antibiotic drops or ointment, eye pad and shield.
Anticipation: Confirm muscle stability and hemostasis before dressing.

Mayo Stand Suggestion:

- Barraquer lid speculum
- Westcott scissors
- Fine toothed forceps
- Muscle hook
- 2 fine mosquito hemostats
- Weck Cel sponges
- Saline syringe for irrigation
- Muscle Sutures
- Needle Driver

Surgical Repair of Chalazion

Step 1 – Patient positioning and eye preparation
Instruments: Headrest or donut, ophthalmic prep supplies, sterile drape with adhesive aperture.
Anticipation: Confirm correct eyelid and lesion location before prep. Head stability is important even for short cases.

Step 2 – Place lid speculum or eyelid retraction
Instruments: Barraquer lid speculum or eyelid retractors.
Anticipation: Ensure adequate exposure without excessive pressure on the globe.

Step 3 – Evert eyelid and apply chalazion clamp
Instruments: Chalazion clamp
Anticipation: Have clamp opened and oriented correctly before the surgeon asks. Confirm clamp tightness to provide hemostasis.

Step 4 – Incise conjunctival surface over chalazion
Instruments: #11 blade or Westcott scissors, fine toothed forceps.
Anticipation: Incision is usually from the conjunctival side. Be ready to manage thick contents immediately.

Step 5 – Curette chalazion contents
Instruments: Chalazion curette
Anticipation: Anticipate repeated passes of the curette. Keep the field clear and pass curette without delay.

Step 6 – Scrape chalazion capsule
Instruments: Chalazion curette.
Anticipation: Thorough capsule disruption reduces recurrence. Expect firm scraping and maintain clamp stability.

Step 7 – Achieve hemostasis
Instruments: Pressure with clamp, Weck Cel sponges, Bovie on low setting if needed.
Anticipation: Most bleeding is controlled by clamp pressure. Use Bovie sparingly to avoid lid damage.

Surgical Repair of Chalazion

Step 8 – Release clamp and inspect site
Instruments: Weck Cel sponges.
Anticipation: Expect brief bleeding after clamp release. Be ready with gentle pressure immediately.

Step 9 – Apply antibiotic ointment and dressing
Instruments: Antibiotic ointment, eye pad.
Anticipation: Confirm lesion cavity is adequately treated before dressing. Communicate postoperative care instructions.

Mayo Stand Suggestion:

- Barraquer lid speculum or eyelid retractors
- Chalazion clamp
- #11 blade or Westcott scissors
- Fine toothed forceps
- Chalazion curette
- 2 fine mosquito hemostats
- Weck Cel sponges

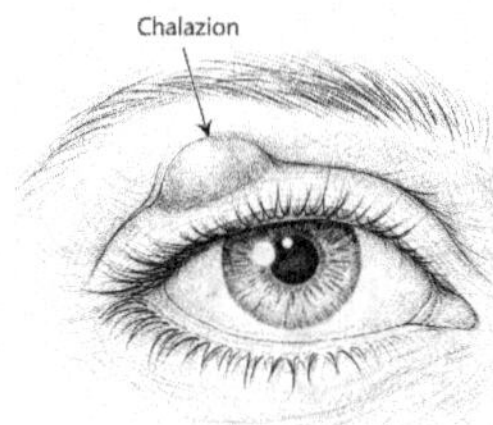

Surgical Repair of Entropion

Step 1 – Patient positioning and eye preparation
Instruments: Headrest or donut, ophthalmic prep supplies, sterile drape with adhesive aperture.
Anticipation: Confirm eyelid and laterality before prep. Head stability is important for precise lid work.

Step 2 – Eyelid exposure and stabilization
Instruments: Barraquer lid speculum or eyelid retractors.
Anticipation: Ensure adequate exposure without excessive pressure on the globe. Keep cornea protected and moist.

Step 3 – Mark incision and infiltrate local anesthetic
Instruments: Skin marker, syringe with local anesthetic and epinephrine, fine needle.
Anticipation: Tissue blanching reduces bleeding. Avoid over injection that distorts lid anatomy.

Step 4 – Skin incision along lower eyelid
Instruments: #15 blade, fine toothed forceps, Westcott scissors.
Anticipation: Incision is shallow and precise. Anticipate small bleeders and have hemostats ready.

Step 5 – Dissect to expose lower lid retractor
Instruments: Westcott scissors, fine forceps, 2 fine mosquito hemostats, Bovie on low setting if needed.
Anticipation: Dissection is delicate. Use clamps for small bleeders rather than relying on cautery.

Step 6 – Tighten or reattach lower lid retractor
Instruments: Suture, Mayo Scissors, and Forceps
Anticipation: This marks transition to suturing. Bring needle driver and sutures only when surgeon commits to repair.

Step 7 – Assess lid position and stability
Instruments: Lid retractors, fine forceps.
Anticipation: Surgeon may adjust tension. Be ready to assist with gentle traction and repositioning.

Surgical Repair of Entropion

Step 8 – Close skin incision
Instruments: Suture, Mayo Scissors, and Forceps
Anticipation: Skin closure requires precise edge alignment. Assist with controlled suture handling.

Step 9 – Apply ointment and dressing
Instruments: Antibiotic ointment, eye pad.
Anticipation: Confirm lid position and globe protection before dressing.

Mayo Stand Suggestion:

- Barraquer lid speculum or eyelid retractors
- #15 blade on scalpel handle
- Westcott scissors
- Fine toothed forceps
- 2 fine mosquito hemostats
- Weck Cel sponges

Vitrectomy

Step 1 – Patient positioning and eye preparation
Instruments: Headrest or donut, ophthalmic prep supplies, sterile drape with adhesive aperture, grounding pad if Bovie used.
Anticipation: Confirm laterality and surgical plan. Head must be completely stable. Ensure microscope and foot pedals are positioned before draping.

Step 2 – Place lid speculum and protect cornea
Instruments: Barraquer lid speculum.
Anticipation: Ensure even lid retraction without pressure on the globe. Maintain corneal lubrication throughout the case.

Step 3 – Mark sclerotomy sites
Instruments: Calipers, marking pen if used.
Anticipation: Accurate port spacing prevents instrument collision. Be ready to adjust microscope focus as globe orientation changes.

Step 4 – Create pars plana sclerotomies
Instruments: Micro blade or trocar cannula system, fine toothed forceps.
Anticipation: Have infusion cannula ready before vitreous instruments are inserted. Confirm infusion placement before flow is initiated.

Step 5 – Insert infusion cannula and confirm flow
Instruments: Infusion cannula, balanced salt solution tubing.
Anticipation: Do not allow infusion to start until surgeon confirms correct placement. Incorrect flow can collapse the globe.

Step 6 – Insert vitrector and illumination probe
Instruments: Vitrector handpiece, light pipe.
Anticipation: Anticipate coordinated hand movements. Keep cords organized to prevent drag on the eye.

Step 7 – Perform core vitrectomy
Instruments: Vitrector, light pipe.
Anticipation: Monitor tubing and foot pedal cords continuously. Be prepared to adjust microscope or reposition lines.

Vitrectomy

Step 8 – Address pathology
Instruments: Forceps, scissors, laser probe, suction depending on case.
Anticipation: Instruments change quickly. Anticipate next tool based on pathology discussed during time out.

Step 9 – Fluid air or gas exchange if indicated
Instruments: Air or gas tubing, syringe if needed.
Anticipation: Confirm correct gas concentration verbally before opening. Gas errors are critical safety events.

Step 10 – Inspect retina and achieve hemostasis
Instruments: Light pipe, suction, laser probe if used.
Anticipation: Final inspection requires a quiet stable field. Avoid unnecessary movement.

Step 11 – Remove instruments and close sclerotomies
Instruments: Suture, Mayo Scissors, and Forceps
Anticipation: This is the transition to closure. Needle driver and fine sutures come to the Mayo only if sclerotomies require closure.

Step 12 – Apply medication and dressing
Instruments: Antibiotic ointment, eye pad and shield.
Anticipation: Confirm globe integrity and intraocular pressure before dressing.

Mayo Stand Suggestion:

- Barraquer lid speculum
- Calipers
- Micro blade or trocar cannula system
- Fine toothed forceps
- Vitrector handpiece
- Light pipe
- Infusion cannula
- Weck Cel sponges
- Balanced salt solution tubing

VITRECTOMY

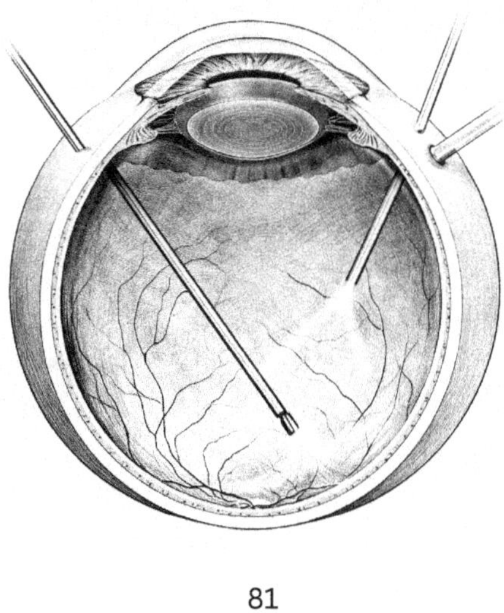

Section IV:

Otorhinolaryngologic Procedures

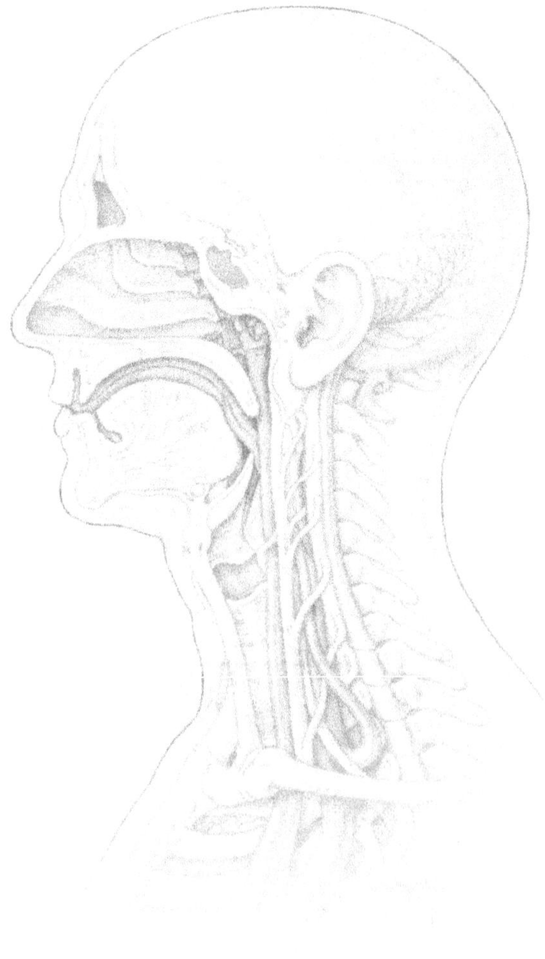

Caldwell Luc Procedure

Step 1 – Patient positioning and oral cavity preparation
Instruments: Headrest, oral prep supplies, throat pack, grounding pad if Bovie used.
Anticipation: Confirm laterality and dentition status. Place and document throat pack before incision.

Step 2 – Local anesthetic infiltration
Instruments: Syringe with local anesthetic and epinephrine, dental needle.
Anticipation: Tissue blanching reduces bleeding. Have suction ready for oral pooling.

Step 3 – Gingivobuccal incision above canine fossa
Instruments: #15 blade, Adsons with teeth, suction tip.
Anticipation: Oral mucosa bleeds readily. Anticipate immediate suction and small clamps.

Step 4 – Elevate mucoperiosteal flap
Instruments: Periosteal elevator, Adsons with teeth, suction.
Anticipation: Maintain steady retraction without tearing mucosa. Keep flap moist.

Step 5 – Create bony window into maxillary sinus
Instruments: Osteotome and mallet or burr with drill, Kerrison rongeur.
Anticipation: Have suction and irrigation ready before bone work begins. Protect soft tissue from rotating instruments.

Step 6 – Enlarge sinus opening and remove pathology
Instruments: Kerrison rongeur, sinus curettes, suction.
Anticipation: Expect frequent instrument exchanges. Keep curettes organized by size and shape.

Step 7 – Irrigate maxillary sinus
Instruments: Irrigation syringe or bulb, suction.
Anticipation: Control fluid runoff to prevent aspiration. Monitor throat pack saturation.

Step 8 – Create inferior meatal antrostomy if indicated
Instruments: Nasal speculum, Kerrison rongeur, suction.
Anticipation: Be ready to transition between oral and nasal fields without contamination.

Step 9 – Achieve hemostasis
Instruments: Bovie on low setting, suction, hemostats.
Anticipation: Oral bleeding can be brisk. Use clamps before cautery when possible.

Step 10 – Close gingivobuccal incision
Instruments: Suture, Mayo Scissors, and Forceps
Anticipation: This is the closure transition. Bring needle driver and absorbable sutures only when surgeon commits to closure.

Step 11 – Remove throat pack and final oral inspection
Instruments: Sponge forceps, suction.
Anticipation: Throat pack removal must be verbalized and documented before extubation.

Mayo Stand Suggestion:

- #15 blade on scalpel handle
- Adsons forceps with teeth
- Periosteal elevator
- Kerrison rongeur
- Sinus curettes
- 2 mosquito hemostats
- 1 Kelly clamp
- Osteotome and mallet
- Nasal Speculum
- Needle Driver and Absorbable Surture

Choanal Atresia Repair

Step 1 – Patient positioning and airway preparation
Instruments: Headrest, shoulder roll if infant, nasal prep supplies, throat pack if used, grounding pad if Bovie used.
Anticipation: This is an airway critical case. Confirm secured airway before draping and clearly communicate throat pack placement.

Step 2 – Nasal decongestion and local infiltration
Instruments: Cottonoids with vasoconstrictor, syringe with local anesthetic and epinephrine.
Anticipation: Pass cottonoids in sequence and track removal. Vasoconstriction improves visualization and reduces bleeding.

Step 3 – Insert nasal endoscope and assess atresia
Instruments: Rigid nasal endoscope, camera system, suction.
Anticipation: Ensure camera is white balanced and focused before insertion. Keep suction immediately available.

Step 4 – Remove membranous or bony atresia plate
Instruments: Microdebrider or drill with burr, curettes, suction.
Anticipation: Protect endoscope lens from debris. Anticipate frequent suction and irrigation during bone removal.

Step 5 – Enlarge choanal opening
Instruments: Kerrison rongeur, curettes, suction.
Anticipation: Have multiple instrument sizes ready. Maintain clear visualization to avoid skull base injury.

Step 6 – Smooth edges and confirm patency
Instruments: Microdebrider or curette, suction.
Anticipation: Be ready to reposition endoscope frequently. Avoid allowing blood to pool and obscure landmarks.

Step 7 – Place stent if indicated
Instruments: Choanal stent or endotracheal tube segment.
Anticipation: Do not open stent until surgeon confirms placement plan. Secure stent carefully to prevent migration.

Step 8 – Achieve hemostasis
Instruments: Bovie on low setting, suction.
Anticipation: Use cautery sparingly near delicate nasal structures. Suction must be continuous but gentle.

Step 9 – Remove throat pack and final airway check
Instruments: Sponge forceps, suction.
Anticipation: Throat pack removal must be verbalized and confirmed before extubation.

Mayo Stand Suggestion:

- Rigid nasal endoscope
- Endoscope camera and light cord
- Suction tip
- Cottonoids with vasoconstrictor
- Curettes
- Kerrison rongeur
- 2 mosquito hemostats
- Microdebrider
- Stent Materials
- Needle Driver

Cochlear Implant

Step 1 – Patient positioning and head stabilization
Instruments: Headrest or donut, head strap or tape, grounding pad if Bovie used.
Anticipation: Head must be completely immobile. Confirm operative ear and ensure microscope and drill foot pedals are positioned before prep.

Step 2 – Ear preparation and sterile draping
Instruments: Ear prep supplies, sterile drape with ear aperture, microscope drape.
Anticipation: Drape microscope early to avoid breaking sterility once the case starts.

Step 3 – Postauricular skin incision
Instruments: #15 blade, Adsons with teeth, suction tip.
Anticipation: Anticipate immediate suction. Ear incisions bleed more than expected.

Step 4 – Elevate periosteal flap and expose mastoid cortex
Instruments: Periosteal elevator, Adsons with teeth, 2 mosquito hemostats, Bovie on low setting.
Anticipation: Control small bleeders with clamps first. Avoid excessive cautery near skin flaps.

Step 5 – Perform cortical mastoidectomy
Instruments: High speed drill with cutting and diamond burrs, suction irrigation.
Anticipation: Have correct burrs opened and organized by size. Manage irrigation and suction continuously to maintain visualization.

Step 6 – Identify facial recess landmarks
Instruments: Drill with diamond burr, suction irrigation.
Anticipation: Maintain a dry field. Avoid moving microscope or cords during delicate drilling.

Step 7 – Create cochleostomy or expose round window
Instruments: Fine diamond burr, suction irrigation.
Anticipation: Burr size often changes quickly. Anticipate exchange without delay.

Step 8 – Prepare implant receiver bed
Instruments: Drill with cutting burr, suction irrigation.
Anticipation: Have implant template ready but unopened. Do not open implant until surgeon confirms readiness.

Step 9 – Insert cochlear implant electrode array
Instruments: Cochlear implant system brought up when requested.
Anticipation: This is a sterile critical moment. Open implant only when surgeon and audiology confirm readiness.

Step 10 – Secure implant and test function
Instruments: Implant accessories, testing cables handled by audiology.
Anticipation: Protect implant cables and maintain a dry field during testing.

Step 11 – Achieve hemostasis and irrigate
Instruments: Suction irrigation, Bovie on low setting if needed.
Anticipation: Bleeding control prevents postoperative hematoma and implant displacement.

Step 12 – Layered closure
Instruments: Suture, Mayo Scissors, and Forceps
Anticipation: Needle driver and sutures come to the Mayo only when surgeon commits to closure.

Cochlear Implant

Step 13 – Apply mastoid dressing
Instruments: Mastoid dressing supplies.
Anticipation: Ensure dressing pressure is adequate without compromising circulation.

Mayo Stand Suggestion:

- #15 blade on scalpel handle
- Adsons forceps with teeth
- Periosteal elevator
- 2 mosquito hemostats
- Drill and burrs
- Cochlear implant system
- Needle Driver and sutures

Functional Endoscopic Sinus Surgery (FESS)

Step 1 – Patient positioning and airway preparation
Instruments: Headrest, shoulder roll if needed, nasal prep supplies, throat pack if used, grounding pad if Bovie used.
Anticipation: This is an airway and bleeding sensitive case. Confirm secured airway and document throat pack placement before draping.

Step 2 – Nasal decongestion and local infiltration
Instruments: Cottonoids with vasoconstrictor, syringe with local anesthetic and epinephrine.
Anticipation: Track cottonoid count carefully. Replace soaked pledgets promptly to maintain visualization.

Step 3 – Insert nasal endoscope and perform initial survey
Instruments: Rigid nasal endoscope, camera and light source, suction.
Anticipation: Ensure camera is white balanced and focused. Keep suction immediately available to prevent lens obscuration.

Step 4 – Uncinectomy and middle meatal access
Instruments: Backbiting forceps, sickle knife, suction.
Anticipation: Anticipate rapid instrument exchange. Hand backbiters oriented correctly to avoid mucosal tearing.

Step 5 – Maxillary antrostomy
Instruments: Kerrison rongeur, curettes, suction.
Anticipation: Maintain constant suction to keep landmarks visible. Avoid allowing blood to pool in the maxillary sinus.

Step 6 – Anterior ethmoidectomy
Instruments: Blakesley forceps, microdebrider, suction irrigation.
Anticipation: Instruments alternate quickly. Anticipate next tool based on surgeon sequence to avoid delays.

Step 7 – Posterior ethmoid and sphenoid access if indicated
Instruments: Straight and angled Blakesley forceps, suction irrigation.
Anticipation: Maintain orientation of angled instruments. Do not pass sharp instruments without direct visualization

Step 8 – Hemostasis and cavity inspection
Instruments: Bovie on low setting, suction, cottonoids.
Anticipation: Use cautery sparingly. Anticipate placement of hemostatic cottonoids and track removal.

Functional Endoscopic Sinus Surgery (FESS)

Step 9 – Nasal packing or splints if used
Instruments: Nasal packing materials or splints.
Anticipation: Do not open packing until surgeon commits. Confirm type and laterality before placement.

Step 10 – Remove throat pack and final airway check
Instruments: Sponge forceps, suction.
Anticipation: Throat pack removal must be verbalized and confirmed before extubation.

Mayo Stand Suggestion:

- Rigid nasal endoscope
- Endoscope camera and light cord
- Suction tip
- Cottonoids with vasoconstrictor
- Sickle knife
- Backbiting forceps
- Blakesley forceps
- 2 mosquito hemostats
- Microdebrider system
- Nasal packing or splints

Laryngectomy

tep 1 – Patient positioning and airway confirmation
Instruments: Headrest, shoulder roll, tracheostomy tray available, grounding pad.
Anticipation: This is an airway critical case. Confirm secured airway and backup tracheostomy equipment before prep and drape.

Step 2 – Neck preparation and draping
Instruments: Neck prep supplies, sterile drapes, towel clips.
Anticipation: Prep must extend widely for possible neck dissection or stoma creation.

Step 3 – Cervical skin incision and flap elevation
Instruments: #10 blade, Adsons with teeth, Bovie, suction.
Anticipation: Anticipate brisk bleeding from platysma and subcutaneous tissue. Keep suction and clamps immediately available.

Step 4 – Expose laryngeal framework
Instruments: Metzenbaum scissors, Debakey forceps, 2 mosquito hemostats, 1 Kelly clamp.
Anticipation: Maintain organized clamp placement. Anticipate frequent clamp cut rhythm during muscle division.

Step 5 – Identify and protect major vessels and nerves
Instruments: Right angle clamp, Debakey forceps, suction.
Anticipation: Be ready with vessel loops when requested. Do not clutter the field with unused ties.

Step 6 – Divide pharyngeal musculature and mobilize larynx
Instruments: Bovie, Metzenbaum scissors, clamps.
Anticipation: Expect heavy clamp usage. Follow the surgeon's rhythm and keep clamps oriented consistently.

Step 7 – Transect trachea and create permanent stoma
Instruments: #10 blade, Bovie, tracheal hook if used, suction.
Anticipation: This is a critical airway transition. Have tracheostomy tube open and ready before tracheal division.

Laryngectomy

Step 8 – Remove laryngeal specimen
Instruments: Specimen basin.
Anticipation: Open specimen container early. Confirm orientation and labeling for pathology.

Step 9 – Pharyngeal closure
Instruments: Suture, Mayo Scissors, and Forceps
Anticipation: Transition to closure phase. Bring needle driver and sutures only when surgeon commits to closure.

Step 10 – Test pharyngeal closure integrity
Instruments: Saline syringe, suction.
Anticipation: Be prepared to suction immediately during leak testing.

Step 11 – Hemostasis and drain placement
Instruments: Suction, Bovie, drains brought up when requested.
Anticipation: Confirm drain type and exit site before placement.

Step 12 – Layered neck closure
Instruments: Suture, Mayo Scissors, and Forceps
Anticipation: Begin closing counts early. Confirm stoma patency before final skin closure.

Mayo Stand Suggestion:

- #10 blade on scalpel handle
- Metzenbaum scissors
- Mayo scissors
- Adsons forceps with teeth
- Debakey forceps
- Right angle clamp
- Tracheostomy tube
- Drains
- Vessel loops

Mastoidectomy

Step 1 – Patient positioning and head stabilization
Instruments: Headrest or donut, head strap or tape, grounding pad placed off field.
Anticipation: Head must be immobile for microscope and drill work. Confirm microscope position and foot pedals before prep.

Step 2 – Ear preparation and sterile draping
Instruments: Ear prep supplies, sterile ear drape, microscope drape.
Anticipation: Drape microscope early. Avoid breaking sterility once drilling begins.

Step 3 – Postauricular skin incision
Instruments: #15 blade, Adsons with teeth.
Anticipation: Be ready to hand off suction and Bovie from the back table as bleeding begins, but do not stage them on the Mayo.

Step 4 – Elevate periosteal flap and expose mastoid cortex
Instruments: Periosteal elevator, Adsons with teeth.
Anticipation: Maintain flap exposure without excessive traction. Anticipate frequent instrument switching during exposure.

Step 5 – Transition to drilling phase
Instruments: None added to Mayo. Drill system managed from back table.
Anticipation: Confirm correct burr sequence is open and ready. Manage irrigation and suction actively from the back table.

Mastoidectomy

Step 6 – Cortical mastoidectomy drilling
Instruments: Drill and burrs handled .
Anticipation: Anticipate burr changes quickly. Pass burrs safely without contaminating microscope field.

Step 7 – Identify anatomic landmarks
Instruments: Otologic curettes, suction.
Anticipation: Be ready to pass curettes immediately when drilling pauses. Maintain clear instrument organization to avoid delays.

Step 8 – Disease removal and cavity refinement
Instruments: Otologic curettes, picks.
Anticipation: Anticipate frequent switching between curettes and drill. Keep fine hand instruments dry and visible on Mayo.

Step 9 – Inspect cavity and prepare for reconstruction if needed
Instruments: Otologic mirrors or picks if used.
Anticipation: Surgeon may pause drilling. Be ready to hand fine instruments promptly without clutter.

Step 10 – Hemostasis and irrigation
Instruments: Managed from back table.
Anticipation: Assist with suction and irrigation without placing tubing onto the Mayo.

Step 11 – Closure preparation
Instruments: None added to Mayo yet.
Anticipation: This is the cue to prepare closure instruments on the back table only when surgeon commits.

Step 12 – Layered closure and dressing
Instruments: Brought to field from back table when requested.
Anticipation: Maintain count awareness and prepare mastoid dressing supplies.

Mayo Stand Suggestion:

- Periosteal elevator
- Otologic curettes
- Otologic picks
- ·Tenotomy scissors if used
- #15 Blade on Scalpel
- Metzenbaum Scissors
- Adsons forceps with teeth

Myringotomy

Step 1 – Patient positioning and microscope setup
Instruments: Headrest or donut, microscope drape, ear prep supplies.
Anticipation: Confirm operative ear and microscope focus before prep. Once the microscope is in use, instrument flow must be smooth to avoid repositioning delays.

Step 2 – Place ear speculum and visualize tympanic membrane
Instruments: Ear speculum.
Anticipation: Have correct speculum size ready before surgeon asks. A size change mid step disrupts microscope alignment.

Myringotomy

Step 3 – Incise tympanic membrane
Instruments: Myringotomy blade (Beaver myringotomy knife such as #64 or #67).
Anticipation: Blade must be on the Mayo and oriented correctly. Hand it immediately once membrane is centered in view.

Step 4 – Aspirate middle ear fluid
Instruments: Suction managed off the Mayo.
Anticipation: Be ready to immediately hand suction from the back table after incision. Do not place suction tubing on the Mayo.

Step 5 – Insert ventilation tube if indicated
Instruments: Ventilation tube, tube inserter, alligator forceps.
Anticipation: Have tube opened and loaded only after incision is complete. Confirm tube type before opening.

Step 6 – Adjust tube position
Instruments: Rosen needle or pick.
Anticipation: Anticipate fine adjustments. Keep pick immediately accessible without cluttering the field.

Step 7 – Apply medication if ordered
Instruments: Drops or ointment.
Anticipation: Medication is applied after tube placement. Confirm correct drug and side before handoff.

Step 8 – Remove speculum and conclude procedure
Instruments: None additional.
Anticipation: Maintain microscope position until surgeon confirms completion.

Mayo Stand Suggestion:

- Myringotomy blade (Beaver #64 or #67)
- Ear speculum
- Alligator forceps
- Ventilation tube inserter
- Rosen needle or pick

Parotidectomy

Step 1 – Patient positioning and nerve monitoring setup
Instruments: Headrest, shoulder roll, facial nerve monitor leads placed by anesthesia or neuromonitoring team.
Anticipation: Confirm nerve monitor is functioning before prep. Protect monitor leads and cables throughout positioning and draping.

Step 2 – Skin preparation and wide draping
Instruments: Neck and facial prep supplies, sterile drapes.
Anticipation: Prep must extend from temporal region to clavicle. Anticipate need for wide exposure if neck dissection becomes necessary.

Step 3 – Preauricular and cervical skin incision
Instruments: Scalpel handle with #10 or #15 blade, Adsons with teeth.
Anticipation: Incision is long and curved. Be ready to exchange blades if requested but do not preload extras.

Parotidectomy

Step 4 – Elevate skin flaps
Instruments: Metzenbaum scissors, Adsons with teeth.
Anticipation: Maintain gentle traction on skin edges. Anticipate frequent instrument switching during flap elevation.

Step 5 – Identify parotid landmarks
Instruments: Fine forceps, blunt dissectors.
Anticipation: Surgeon will slow down here. Keep field organized and avoid unnecessary instrument clutter.

Step 6 – Identify and protect facial nerve trunk
Instruments: Nerve stimulator probe managed fine dissectors.
Anticipation: Do not pass instruments abruptly. Anticipate pauses while nerve is stimulated and confirmed.

Step 7 – Dissect parotid tissue from facial nerve branches
Instruments: Metzenbaum scissors, fine forceps.
Anticipation: This phase is repetitive and delicate. Keep frequently used instruments immediately accessible and clean.

Step 8 – Control small vessels as encountered
Instruments: Hemostats or ties passed from back table as requested.
Anticipation: Do not stage clamps on the Mayo. Be ready to pass them quickly when bleeding occurs.

Step 9 – Remove parotid specimen
Instruments: Specimen basin.
Anticipation: Open specimen container early and confirm orientation and labeling requirements

Step 10 – Inspect field and prepare for closure
Instruments: None added to Mayo yet.
Anticipation: This is the cue to prepare closure instruments on the back table only when surgeon commits.

Step 11 – Drain placement if indicated
Instruments: Drain passed from back table when requested.
Anticipation: Confirm drain type and exit site before placement.

Step 12 – Layered closure and dressing
Instruments: Brought from back table when requested.
Anticipation: Maintain count awareness and protect facial nerve monitor leads during closure.

Mayo Stand Suggestion:

- Scalpel handle with #10 or #15 blade
- Adsons forceps with teeth
- Metzenbaum scissors
- Fine forceps or blunt dissector
- Nerve Stimulator
- Drains
- 2 Mosquito Hemostats

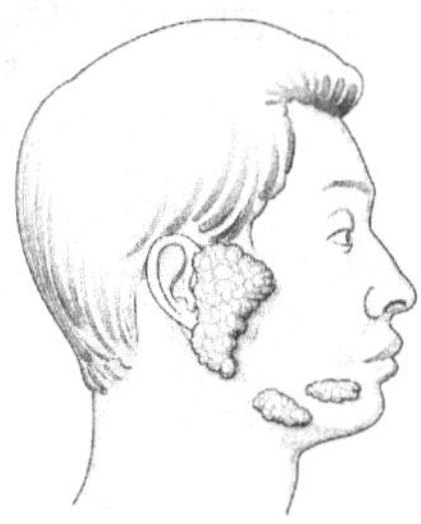

Polypectomy

Step 1 – Patient positioning and nasal preparation
Instruments: Headrest, nasal prep supplies, throat pack if used.
Anticipation: Confirm laterality and extent of disease. Track throat pack placement if used.

Step 2 – Nasal decongestion
Instruments: Cottonoids with vasoconstrictor.
Anticipation: Count cottonoids carefully. Replace promptly to maintain visualization.

Step 3 – Insert nasal endoscope and assess polyps
Instruments: Rigid nasal endoscope managed .
Anticipation: Ensure camera is focused and white balanced before insertion. Keep Mayo clear for hand instruments.

Step 4 – Grasp and remove polyp tissue
Instruments: Blakesley forceps.
Anticipation: Polyps are slippery. Pass forceps oriented correctly to avoid repeated repositioning.

Step 5 – Control bleeding as encountered
Instruments: Mosquito hemostats passed from Mayo, packing materials from back table.
Anticipation: Anticipate clamp use for small bleeders. Do not reach for cautery unless requested.

Step 6 – Continue polyp removal and cavity inspection
Instruments: Blakesley forceps, angled forceps if needed.
Anticipation: Instrument exchanges are frequent. Maintain clean orientation of forceps on Mayo.

Step 7 – Irrigation and final inspection
Instruments: Managed from back table.
Anticipation: Be ready to assist without adding tubing to the Mayo.

Step 8 – Nasal packing if indicated
Instruments: Packing materials.
Anticipation: Do not open packing until surgeon commits. Confirm side and type.

Step 9 – Remove throat pack and conclude procedure
Instruments: Sponge forceps.
Anticipation: Throat pack removal must be verbalized and confirmed.

Mayo Stand Suggestion:

- Blakesley forceps
- Angled Blakesley forceps (if used)
- 2 mosquito hemostats
- Cottonoid forceps

Radical Neck Dissection with Mandibulectomy

Step 1 – Patient positioning and airway planning
Instruments: Headrest, shoulder roll, tracheostomy tray available, grounding pad placed off field.
Anticipation: Airway is critical. Confirm secured airway and availability of tracheostomy equipment before prep and drape.

Step 2 – Wide neck and facial preparation and draping
Instruments: Neck and facial prep supplies, sterile drapes.
Anticipation: Prep widely to allow extension. Anticipate need for simultaneous oral and neck access.

Radical Neck Dissection with Mandibulectomy

Step 3 – Cervical skin incision and flap elevation
Instruments: Scalpel handle with #10 blade, Adsons with teeth, Metzenbaum scissors.
Anticipation: This is a long incision with brisk bleeding. Be ready to pass clamps from the Mayo as vessels are encountered.

Step 4 – Identify and ligate major vessels
Instruments: 2 mosquito hemostats, right angle clamp passed from Mayo if surgeon routinely uses one.
Anticipation: Follow clamp cut tie rhythm closely. Keep ties prepared on the back table.

Step 5 – Dissect cervical lymph node levels
Instruments: Metzenbaum scissors, Debakey forceps, 2 mosquito hemostats.
Anticipation: This phase is repetitive. Keep frequently used instruments clean and immediately accessible.

Step 6 – Identify and protect cranial nerves
Instruments: Fine forceps, nerve hooks passed from back table if requested.
Anticipation: Minimize instrument clutter. Pass instruments deliberately and avoid sudden movements.

Step 7 – Mandibular exposure and osteotomy preparation
Instruments: Periosteal elevator, retractor passed from back table.
Anticipation: Power equipment is coming next. Confirm saw and plates are available but unopened until requested.

Step 8 – Mandibulectomy osteotomy and specimen removal
Instruments: Power saw handled , specimen basin.
Anticipation: Open specimen container early. Confirm orientation and margin labeling requirements.

Step 9 – Hemostasis and field inspection
Instruments: Mosquito hemostats, ties passed as requested.
Anticipation: Bleeding control is ongoing. Anticipate repeated clamp usage without staging extras.

Step 10 – Reconstruction planning and transition
Instruments: Plates and screws passed from back table when requested.
Anticipation: Do not open reconstruction hardware until surgeon commits to reconstruction plan.

Step 11 – Drain placement
Instruments: Drains passed from back table.
Anticipation: Confirm number and exit sites before placement.

Step 12 – Layered closure
Instruments: Brought from back table when requested.
Anticipation: Begin closing counts early. Maintain awareness of airway and drain patency.

Mayo Stand Suggestion:

- Scalpel handle with #10 blade
- Adsons forceps with teeth
- Metzenbaum scissors
- Debakey forceps
- 2 mosquito hemostats
- Periosteal elevator

SMR Septoplasty

Step 1 – Patient positioning and nasal preparation
Instruments: Headrest, nasal prep supplies, throat pack if used.
Anticipation: Confirm laterality and degree of deviation. Track throat pack placement if used.

Step 2 – Nasal decongestion and local infiltration
Instruments: Cottonoids with vasoconstrictor, syringe with local anesthetic and epinephrine.
Anticipation: Replace pledgets as they saturate. Careful cottonoid counts are essential.

Step 3 – Insert nasal speculum and expose septum
Instruments: Cottle or Killian nasal speculum.
Anticipation: Have multiple speculum sizes available. Avoid changing speculum mid step if possible.

Step 4 – Septal incision
Instruments: Scalpel handle with #15 blade.
Anticipation: Blade should be ready and oriented. Be prepared to pass suction from back table immediately after incision.

Step 5 – Elevate mucoperichondrial flaps
Instruments: Freer elevator, Cottle elevator.
Anticipation: Gentle elevation is key. Anticipate switching elevators quickly to maintain clean planes.

Step 6 – Resect deviated cartilage and bone
Instruments: Takahashi forceps, Jansen Middleton forceps, 2 mosquito hemostats.
Anticipation: Resection occurs in stages. Keep forceps organized and ready for repeated passes.

Step 7 – Preserve structural support
Instruments: Freer elevator.
Anticipation: Be aware when surgeon pauses to assess septal support. Do not rush instrument exchanges.

Step 8 – Reposition septal flaps
Instruments: Freer elevator.
Anticipation: Maintain gentle handling to avoid flap tears.

Step 9 – Achieve hemostasis and packing placement if indicated
Instruments: Packing materials passed from back table.
Anticipation: Do not open packing until surgeon confirms need and type.

Step 10 – Remove throat pack and final airway check
Instruments: Sponge forceps.
Anticipation: Throat pack removal must be verbalized and confirmed.

Mayo Stand Suggestion:

- Scalpel handle with #15 blade
- Cottle or Killian nasal speculum
- Freer elevator
- Cottle elevator
- Takahashi forceps
- Jansen Middleton forceps
- 2 mosquito hemostats

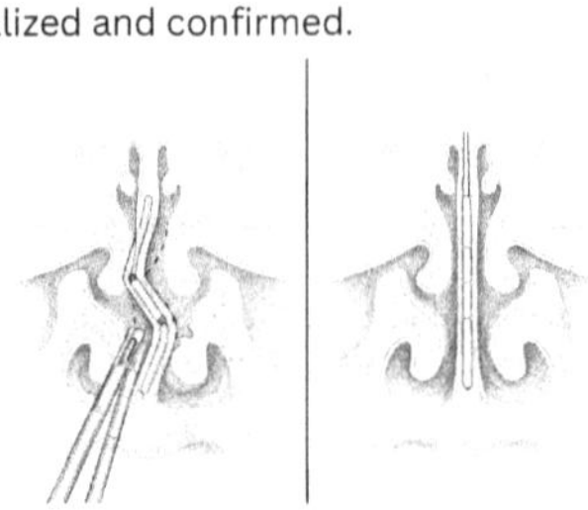

Stapedectomy

Step 1 – Patient positioning and microscope setup
Instruments: Headrest or donut, microscope drape, ear prep supplies.
Anticipation: Confirm operative ear and microscope focus before prep. Once the microscope is positioned, avoid unnecessary instrument movement.

Step 2 – Place ear speculum and expose tympanic membrane
Instruments: Ear speculum.
Anticipation: Have multiple speculum sizes available. A change after microscope alignment disrupts workflow.

Step 3 – Elevate tympanomeatal flap
Instruments: Rosen knife, fine suction.
Anticipation: Hand Rosen knife smoothly and deliberately. Be ready to pass suction immediately after flap elevation.

Step 4 – Expose ossicular chain
Instruments: Fine picks, micro hooks.
Anticipation: Surgeon will pause to assess ossicular mobility. Keep fine instruments organized and visible.

Step 5 – Disarticulate incudostapedial joint
Instruments: Joint knife or micro scissors.
Anticipation: This is a precise moment. Hand the correct instrument immediately once requested.

Step 6 – Remove stapes superstructure
Instruments: Micro forceps.
Anticipation: Maintain a steady, quiet field. Avoid passing unnecessary instruments during removal.

Step 7 – Create fenestra in footplate
Instruments: Micro perforator or laser probe.
Anticipation: Confirm laser or perforator readiness before footplate work begins.

Step 8 – Measure and place prosthesis
Instruments: Measuring rod, stapes prosthesis.
Anticipation: Do not open prosthesis until surgeon confirms measurement. Open only the selected size.

Step 9 – Crimp prosthesis to incus
Instruments: Crimping forceps.
Anticipation: Hand crimper precisely and avoid instrument crowding near ossicles.

Step 10 – Reposition tympanomeatal flap
Instruments: Rosen needle or pick.
Anticipation: Gentle handling prevents flap tears. Keep picks immediately available.

Step 11 – Pack middle ear if indicated
Instruments: Gelfoam passed from back table.
Anticipation: Confirm packing amount before opening. Excess packing can affect hearing outcomes.

Stapedectomy

Step 12 – Remove speculum and conclude procedure
Instruments: None additional.
Anticipation: Maintain microscope position until surgeon confirms completion

Mayo Stand Suggestion:

- Ear speculum
- Rosen knife
- Fine picks and micro hooks
- Joint knife or micro scissors
- Micro forceps
- Crimping forceps
- Measuring rod

Tonsillectomy and Adenoidectomy

Step 1 – Patient positioning and airway protection
Instruments: Shoulder roll, headrest, mouth gag system available, throat pack if used.
Anticipation: Airway awareness is critical. Confirm throat pack placement and ensure mouth gag system is assembled before draping.

Step 2 – Place mouth gag and expose oropharynx
Instruments: Crowe Davis or McIvor mouth gag with tongue blade.
Anticipation: Have multiple blade sizes available. Secure gag to prevent movement during surgery.

Step 3 – Assess tonsils and adenoid tissue
Instruments: Headlight or microscope if used.
Anticipation: Surgeon may adjust gag position. Be ready to assist without disturbing airway.

Step 4 – Dissect tonsil from tonsillar fossa
Instruments: Tonsil dissector, Fisher knife, 2 mosquito hemostats.
Anticipation: Follow clamp cut rhythm closely. Anticipate repeated use of dissector and clamps.

Step 5 – Control tonsillar vessels
Instruments: Mosquito hemostats, ties passed from back table.
Anticipation: Bleeding can be brisk. Pass clamps immediately when bleeding is seen.

Step 6 – Remove tonsil specimen
Instruments: Tonsil sponge forceps.
Anticipation: Open specimen container early and confirm labeling if required.

Step 7 – Perform adenoidectomy
Instruments: Adenoid curette, mirror if used.
Anticipation: Be ready to hand curette promptly. Visualization can be limited.

Step 8 – Control adenoid bed bleeding
Instruments: Packing passed from back table.
Anticipation: Do not over pack. Track packing removal carefully.

Step 9 – Inspect surgical sites
Instruments: Headlight or mirror.
Anticipation: Surgeon may reassess multiple times. Maintain quiet organized field.

Step 10 – Remove throat pack and release gag
Instruments: Sponge forceps.
Anticipation: Throat pack removal must be verbalized and confirmed before extubation.

Tonsillectomy and Adenoidectomy

Mayo Stand Suggestion:

- Tonsil dissector
- Fisher knife
- Tonsil sponge forceps
- Tonsil dissector
- Fisher knife
- Tonsil Schnidt

Tracheotomy

Step 1 – Patient positioning and airway confirmation
Instruments: Shoulder roll, headrest, endotracheal tube secured, tracheostomy tray available.
Anticipation: Airway awareness is constant. Confirm tube position and ensure tracheostomy tube of correct size is opened and ready before incision.

Step 2 – Neck preparation and draping
Instruments: Neck prep supplies, sterile drapes.
Anticipation: Prep widely from mandible to upper chest in case the incision must be extended.

Step 3 – Skin incision over trachea
Instruments: Scalpel handle with #10 blade, Adsons with teeth.
Anticipation: Incision is midline. Be ready to pass clamps from the Mayo as small vessels are encountered.

Step 4 – Blunt dissection through strap muscles
Instruments: Metzenbaum scissors, 2 mosquito hemostats.
Anticipation: Follow clamp spread rhythm closely. Maintain midline orientation.

Step 5 – Identify thyroid isthmus
Instruments: Right angle clamp passed from Mayo if surgeon uses one, mosquito hemostats.
Anticipation: Isthmus management varies. Be ready to pass clamps or ties without staging extras.

Step 6 – Expose tracheal rings
Instruments: Tracheal hook, Army Navy retractors passed from back table if needed.
Anticipation: Do not clutter Mayo with retractor. Hand tracheal hook promptly when requested.

Step 7 – Create tracheal opening
Instruments: Scalpel handle with #11 blade.
Anticipation: Confirm tracheostomy tube is open and assembled before tracheal incision.

Step 8 – Insert tracheostomy tube
Instruments: Tracheostomy tube with obturator.
Anticipation: Coordinate with anesthesia. Do not release tube until ventilation is confirm**ed.**

Step 9 – Secure tube and assess ventilation
Instruments: Ties or sutures passed from back table.
Anticipation: Be ready with ties immediately after insertion to prevent dislodgement.

Step 10 – Apply dressing and confirm airway
Instruments: Tracheostomy dressing supplies.
Anticipation: Confirm tube position, cuff inflation, and securement before final draping is removed.

Tracheotomy

Mayo Stand Suggestion:

- Scalpel handle with #10 blade
- Scalpel handle with #11 blade
- Adsons forceps with teeth
- Metzenbaum scissors
- 2 mosquito hemostats
- Tracheal hook

Turbinectomy

Step 1 – Patient positioning and nasal preparation
Instruments: Headrest, nasal prep supplies, throat pack if used.
Anticipation: Confirm laterality and extent of turbinate reduction. Track throat pack placement if used.

Step 2 – Nasal decongestion and local infiltration
Instruments: Cottonoids with vasoconstrictor, syringe with local anesthetic and epinephrine.
Anticipation: Replace cottonoids as they saturate. Maintain accurate cottonoid counts.

Step 3 – Insert nasal speculum and expose turbinate
Instruments: Nasal speculum.
Anticipation: Have appropriate speculum size ready to avoid repeated adjustments.

Step 4 – Incise turbinate mucosa
Instruments: Scalpel handle with #15 blade.
Anticipation: Blade must be immediately available. Anticipate suction handoff from back table once incision is made.

Step 5 – Reduce or resect turbinate tissue
Instruments: Turbinectomy scissors or turbinate forceps, 2 mosquito hemostats.
Anticipation: Tissue removal occurs incrementally. Keep forceps and clamps organized and ready for repeated passes.

Step 6 – Control bleeding
Instruments: Mosquito hemostats, packing passed from back table.
Anticipation: Bleeding is expected. Pass clamps promptly and avoid over packing.

Step 7 – Inspect nasal airway
Instruments: Nasal speculum.
Anticipation: Surgeon may reassess airway multiple times. Maintain clear Mayo layout.

Step 8 – Place nasal packing if indicated
Instruments: Packing materials.
Anticipation: Do not open packing until surgeon confirms need and type.

Step 9 – Remove throat pack and conclude procedure
Instruments: Sponge forceps.
Anticipation: Throat pack removal must be verbalized and confirmed before extubation.

Mayo Stand Suggestion:

- Scalpel handle with #15 blade
- Nasal speculum
- Turbinectomy scissors or turbinate forceps
- 2 mosquito hemostats

Tympanoplasty

Step 1 – Patient positioning and microscope setup
Instruments: Headrest or donut, microscope drape, ear prep supplies.
Anticipation: Confirm operative ear and microscope focus before prep. Once microscope is positioned, avoid unnecessary movement.

Step 2 – Place ear speculum and visualize tympanic membrane
Instruments: Ear speculum.
Anticipation: Have multiple speculum sizes available. Changing sizes after microscope alignment disrupts workflow.

Step 3 – Harvest graft material
Instruments: Scalpel handle with #15 blade, Adsons with teeth, Metzenbaum scissors.
Anticipation: Graft is often harvested early. Keep graft moist immediately after harvest and protect it from drying.

Step 4 – Elevate tympanomeatal flap
Instruments: Rosen knife, round knife.
Anticipation: Hand knives deliberately. Be ready to pass suction from the back table as the flap elevates.

Step 5 – Inspect middle ear and ossicles
Instruments: Fine picks, micro hooks.
Anticipation: Surgeon may pause to assess mobility. Keep fine instruments organized and immediately accessible.

Step 6 – Prepare tympanic membrane remnant
Instruments: Micro scissors, picks.
Anticipation: Anticipate frequent instrument exchanges. Maintain a clean, uncluttered Mayo.

Step 7 – Place graft
Instruments: Fine forceps.
Anticipation: This is a precision step. Have graft ready and oriented before surgeon asks for it.

Step 8 – Reposition tympanomeatal flap
Instruments: Rosen needle or pick.
Anticipation: Gentle handling prevents flap tears. Keep pick immediately available.

Step 9 – Pack middle ear and canal if indicated
Instruments: Gelfoam passed from back table.
Anticipation: Do not open packing until surgeon confirms amount and location.

Step 10 – Final inspection and conclude procedure
Instruments: Ear speculum.
Anticipation: Maintain microscope position until surgeon confirms completion.

Mayo Stand Suggestion:

- Ear speculum
- Scalpel handle with #15 blade
- Adsons forceps with teeth
- Metzenbaum scissors
- Rosen knife
- Round knife
- Fine picks or micro hooks
- Fine forceps
- 2 mosquito hemostats

Uvulopalatopharyngoplasty UPPP

Step 1 – Patient positioning and airway protection
Instruments: Shoulder roll, headrest, mouth gag system available, throat pack if used.
Anticipation: Airway is critical. Confirm throat pack placement and ensure gag system is assembled before draping.

Step 2 – Place mouth gag and expose oropharynx
Instruments: Crowe Davis or McIvor mouth gag with tongue blade.
Anticipation: Have correct blade size ready. Secure gag to prevent movement during resection.

Step 3 – Assess tonsils and soft palate anatomy
Instruments: Headlight or microscope if used.
Anticipation: Surgeon may adjust gag position. Be ready to assist without disturbing airway or pack.

Step 4 – Incise mucosa of soft palate and uvula
Instruments: Scalpel handle with #15 blade, Adsons with teeth.
Anticipation: Incision is precise. Be ready to pass clamps promptly if bleeding is encountered.

Step 5 – Resect uvula and redundant soft palate tissue
Instruments: Metzenbaum scissors, 2 mosquito hemostats.
Anticipation: Follow clamp cut rhythm closely. Anticipate repeated clamp use for bleeding control.

Step 6 – Contour palatal edges
Instruments: Metzenbaum scissors, fine forceps.
Anticipation: Tissue handling must be gentle. Keep scissors clean and immediately available.

Step 7 – Inspect surgical field and achieve hemostasis
Instruments: Mosquito hemostats, packing passed from back table.
Anticipation: Bleeding can be brisk. Anticipate clamp placement without overpacking.

Step 8 – Reapproximate palatal mucosa
Instruments: Brought from back table when requested.
Anticipation: This marks transition to closure. Bring needle driver and sutures only when surgeon commits.

Step 9 – Final airway inspection
Instruments: Mouth gag remains in place.
Anticipation: Surgeon may reassess multiple times. Maintain a quiet, organized field.

Step 10 – Remove throat pack and release gag
Instruments: Sponge forceps.
Anticipation: Throat pack removal must be verbalized and confirmed before extubation.

Mayo Stand Suggestion:

- Scalpel handle with #15 blade
- Adsons forceps with teeth
- Metzenbaum scissors
- 2 mosquito hemostats

Section V:

Oral and Maxillofacial Procedures

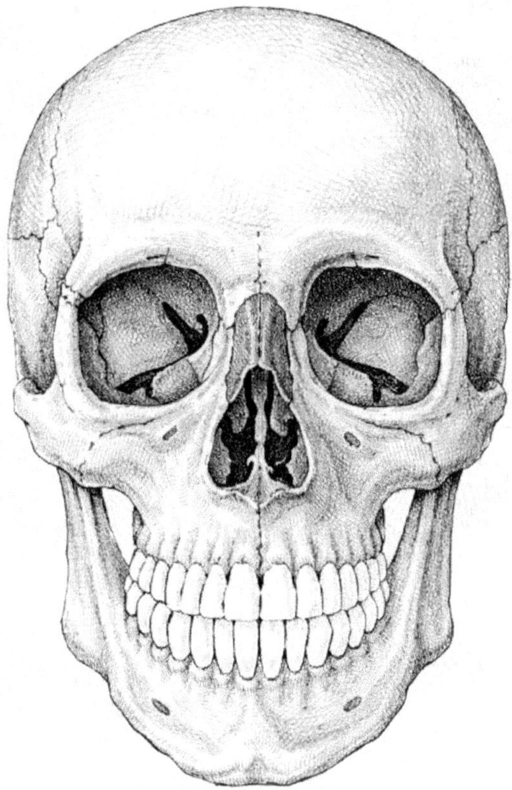

Application of Arch Bars

Step 1 – Patient positioning and airway planning
Instruments: Headrest, shoulder roll if needed, throat pack if used.
Anticipation: This is an airway sensitive case. Confirm secured airway and throat pack placement before draping.

Step 2 – Oral cavity preparation and exposure
Instruments: Mouth prop or bite block, cheek retractor.
Anticipation: Ensure adequate exposure of both arches. Maintain moisture control without placing suction on the Mayo.

Step 3 – Select and size arch bars
Instruments: Arch bars.
Anticipation: Have both maxillary and mandibular arch bars available. Do not open additional bars unless requested.

Step 4 – Place arch bar along dental arch
Instruments: Wire twisters, wire cutters.
Anticipation: Anticipate repetitive wire placement. Keep wire ends organized to prevent sharps injury.

Step 5 – Secure arch bar with circumdental wires
Instruments: Precut stainless steel wires, needle drivers or wire drivers, 2 mosquito hemostats.
Anticipation: Pass wires smoothly and track sharp ends carefully. Anticipate clamp use to control wire tails.

Step 6 – Continue fixation tooth by tooth
Instruments: Wire twisters, wire cutters, mosquito hemostats.
Anticipation: This is repetitive work. Maintain consistent instrument orientation to prevent delays.

Step 7 – Apply intermaxillary fixation if indicated
Instruments: Elastics or fixation wires.
Anticipation: Do not apply elastics until surgeon confirms occlusion. Have scissors ready for emergency release.

Step 8 – Trim and tuck wire ends
Instruments: Wire cutters, mosquito hemostats.
Anticipation: Ensure all wire ends are tucked to prevent mucosal injury.

Step 9 – Final occlusion check
Instruments: None additional.
Anticipation: Surgeon may make adjustments. Keep wire tools immediately available.

Step 10 – Remove throat pack and conclude procedure
Instruments: Sponge forceps.
Anticipation: Throat pack removal must be verbalized and confirmed before extubation.

Mayo Stand Suggestion:

- Arch bars
- Wire twisters
- Wire cutters
- Needle driver or wire driver
- Precut stainless steel wires
- 2 mosquito hemostats

Le Fort I Fracture Repair

Step 1 – Patient positioning and airway planning
Instruments: Headrest, shoulder roll if needed, throat pack if used.
Anticipation: This is an airway sensitive case. Confirm secured airway and throat pack placement before draping.

Step 2 – Oral cavity preparation and exposure
Instruments: Mouth prop or bite block, cheek retractor.
Anticipation: Ensure wide exposure of maxillary vestibule. Maintain moisture control without placing suction on the Mayo.

Step 3 – Maxillary vestibular incision
Instruments: Scalpel handle with #15 blade, Adsons with teeth.
Anticipation: Incision is long and mucosal bleeding is expected. Be ready to pass clamps from the Mayo when bleeding is encountered.

Step 4 – Elevate mucoperiosteal flap
Instruments: Periosteal elevator, 2 mosquito hemostats.
Anticipation: Maintain steady flap retraction. Anticipate clamp use for small bleeders along the maxilla.

Step 5 – Identify fracture line and mobilize maxilla
Instruments: Periosteal elevator, Rowe disimpaction forceps passed from back table if needed.
Anticipation: Surgeon may request disimpaction instruments suddenly. Have them ready but unopened until requested.

Step 6 – Establish occlusion and apply intermaxillary fixation
Instruments: Arch bars or IMF screws if used, wire twisters, wire cutters.
Anticipation: Occlusion must be confirmed before fixation. Keep wire tools organized and immediately accessible.

Step 7 – Reduce fracture and confirm alignment
Instruments: Bone holding forceps passed from back table.
Anticipation: Do not open fixation hardware until occlusion is confirmed.

Step 8 – Plate and screw fixation of maxilla
Instruments: Plates and screws passed from back table when requested.
Anticipation: Open only selected plate sizes. Keep screws controlled to prevent loss.

Step 9 – Irrigate and inspect fixation
Instruments: Managed from back table.
Anticipation: Assist with irrigation and inspection without adding tubing to the Mayo.

Step 10 – Remove intermaxillary fixation if temporary
Instruments: Wire cutters.
Anticipation: Be ready to cut fixation promptly once surgeon confirms stability.

Step 11 – Close vestibular incision
Instruments: Brought from back table when requested.
Anticipation: Closure instruments come to Mayo only when surgeon commits.

Step 12 – Remove throat pack and final airway check
Instruments: Sponge forceps.
Anticipation: Throat pack removal must be verbalized and confirmed before extubation.

Le Fort I Fracture Repair

Mayo Stand Suggestion:

- Scalpel handle with #15 blade
- Adsons forceps with teeth
- Periosteal elevator
- 2 mosquito hemostats
- Wire twisters
- Wire cutters

Le Fort II and III Fracture Repair

Step 1 – Patient positioning and airway planning
Instruments: Headrest, shoulder roll if needed, throat pack if used.
Anticipation: These are high risk airway cases. Confirm secured airway and throat pack placement before draping. Anticipate possible tracheostomy backup.

Step 2 – Wide facial and oral preparation and draping
Instruments: Facial and oral prep supplies, sterile drapes.
Anticipation: Prep must allow access to oral cavity, nasal region, and orbits. Do not limit exposure.

Step 3 – Establish occlusion and apply intermaxillary fixation
Instruments: Arch bars or IMF screws, wire twisters, wire cutters.
Anticipation: Occlusion is set early and controls reduction. Keep wire tools organized and immediately accessible.

Step 4 – Intraoral vestibular incision
Instruments: Scalpel handle with #15 blade, Adsons with teeth.
Anticipation: Bleeding is expected. Be ready to pass mosquito hemostats promptly.

Step 5 – Elevate mucoperiosteal flaps
Instruments: Periosteal elevator, 2 mosquito hemostats.
Anticipation: Maintain steady retraction and clamp small bleeders quickly.

Step 6 – Access midface fracture sites
Instruments: Periosteal elevator, malar retractor passed from back table.
Anticipation: Exposure expands quickly. Do not crowd the Mayo with large retractor.

Step 7 – Reduce midface fractures
Instruments: Bone holding forceps passed from back table.
Anticipation: Reduction may occur in stages. Keep fixation sequence in mind.

Step 8 – Plate and screw fixation of midface and orbital rims
Instruments: Plates and screws passed from back table when requested.
Anticipation: Open only requested hardware. Maintain strict screw control.

Step 9 – Orbital floor assessment and repair if indicated
Instruments: Orbital implant passed from back table.
Anticipation: Implant handling must be delicate. Do not open until surgeon confirms need and size.

Step 10 – Verify occlusion and facial symmetry
Instruments: Wire cutters.
Anticipation: Be ready to adjust IMF quickly if occlusion is altered during fixation.

Step 11 – Remove temporary intermaxillary fixation if indicated
Instruments: Wire cutters.
Anticipation: Do not remove fixation until surgeon confirms stability.

Le Fort II and III Fracture Repair

Step 12 – Close incisions
Instruments: Brought from back table when requested.
Anticipation: Closure phase begins only after all fixation is verified.

Step 13 – Remove throat pack and final airway check
Instruments: Sponge forceps.
Anticipation: Throat pack removal must be verbalized and confirmed before extubation.

Mayo Stand Suggestion:

- Scalpel handle with #15 blade
- Adsons forceps with teeth
- Periosteal elevator
- 2 mosquito hemostats
- Wire twisters
- Wire cutters

Orbital Floor Fracture Repair

Step 1 – Patient positioning and eye protection
Instruments: Headrest, eye shield for nonoperative eye, corneal protector.
Anticipation: Confirm operative side and that the nonoperative eye is protected before prep.

Step 2 – Facial preparation and draping
Instruments: Facial prep supplies, sterile drapes.
Anticipation: Prep widely to include eyelid, cheek, and nose. Avoid pooling prep solution near eyes.

Step 3 – Access incision
Instruments: Scalpel handle with #15 blade, Adsons with teeth.
Anticipation: Incision is precise and cosmetic. Be ready to pass mosquito hemostats promptly for small bleeders.

Step 4 – Elevate soft tissue flap
Instruments: Fine scissors, periosteal elevator, 2 mosquito hemostats.
Anticipation: Tissue planes are delicate. Maintain gentle traction and clear instrument orientation.

Step 5 – Expose orbital floor fracture
Instruments: Periosteal elevator, Malleable retractors passed from back table.
Anticipation: retractors placement is critical. Do not stage large retractor on the Mayo.

Step 6 – Free entrapped orbital contents
Instruments: Periosteal elevator, fine forceps.
Anticipation: This is a delicate step. Hand instruments slowly and deliberately.

Step 7 – Size and prepare orbital implant
Instruments: Orbital implant passed from back table when requested.
Anticipation: Do not open implant until surgeon confirms size and need.

Step 8 – Place orbital floor implant
Instruments: Implant positioning forceps.
Anticipation: Implant must be handled gently and kept clean. Maintain a clutter free Mayo

Step 9 – Confirm globe position and mobility
Instruments: None additional.
Anticipation: Surgeon may pause to assess eye movement. Maintain still field and readiness.

Orbital Floor Fracture Repair

Step 10 – Achieve hemostasis and irrigate
Instruments: Managed from back table.
Anticipation: Assist with irrigation and suction without adding tubing to the Mayo.

Step 11 – Close incision
Instruments: Brought from back table when requested.
Anticipation: Closure instruments come forward only after implant placement is finalized.

Step 12 – Apply dressing and eye protection
Instruments: Eye pad, dressing supplies.
Anticipation: Ensure dressing does not apply pressure to the globe.

Mayo Stand Suggestion:

- Scalpel handle with #15 blade
- Adsons forceps with teeth
- Fine scissors
- Periosteal elevator
- 2 mosquito hemostats
- Fine forceps

Plate and Screw Fixation of Mandibular Fracture

Step 1 – Patient positioning and airway planning
Instruments: Headrest, shoulder roll if needed, throat pack if used.
Anticipation: Mandibular fractures are airway sensitive. Confirm secured airway and throat pack placement before draping.

Step 2 – Oral and facial preparation and draping
Instruments: Oral and facial prep supplies, sterile drapes.
Anticipation: Prep must allow access to mandible and oral cavity. Do not limit exposure.

Step 3 – Establish occlusion and apply temporary intermaxillary fixation
Instruments: Arch bars or IMF screws, wire twisters, wire cutters.
Anticipation: Occlusion guides fracture reduction. Keep wire tools immediately available.

Step 4 – Incision over fracture site
Instruments: Scalpel handle with #15 blade, Adsons with teeth.
Anticipation: Bleeding is expected. Be ready to pass mosquito hemostats promptly.

Step 5 – Elevate periosteum and expose fracture
Instruments: Periosteal elevator, 2 mosquito hemostats.
Anticipation: Maintain exposure and control small bleeders quickly.

Step 6 – Reduce mandibular fracture
Instruments: Bone holding forceps passed from back table.
Anticipation: Reduction may require repositioning. Keep fixation sequence in mind.

Step 7 – Select plate and drill screw holes
Instruments: Plates, screws, and drill passed from back table when requested.
Anticipation: Open only requested hardware. Maintain strict screw control.

Step 8 – Secure plate with screws
Instruments: Screwdriver passed from back table.
Anticipation: Hand screws deliberately to prevent loss.

Plate and Screw Fixation of Mandibular Fracture

Step 9 – Verify occlusion and stability
Instruments: Wire cutters.
Anticipation: Be ready to adjust IMF promptly if occlusion shifts.

Step 10 – Remove temporary intermaxillary fixation if indicated
Instruments: Wire cutters.
Anticipation: Do not remove fixation until surgeon confirms stability.

Step 11 – Irrigate and inspect fixation
Instruments: Managed from back table.
Anticipation: Assist without placing suction on the Mayo.

Step 12 – Close incision
Instruments: Brought from back table when requested.
Anticipation: Closure instruments come forward only after fixation is finalized.

Step 13 – Remove throat pack and final airway check
Instruments: Sponge forceps.
Anticipation: Throat pack removal must be verbalized and confirmed before extubation.

Mayo Stand Suggestion:

- Scalpel handle with #15 blade
- Adsons forceps with teeth
- Periosteal elevator
- 2 mosquito hemostats
- Wire twisters
- Wire cutters

Tooth Extraction Odontectomy

Step 1 – Patient positioning and airway planning
Instruments: Headrest, shoulder roll if needed, throat pack if used.
Anticipation: Oral cases are airway sensitive. Confirm secured airway and throat pack placement before draping.

Step 2 – Oral cavity preparation and exposure
Instruments: Mouth prop or bite block, cheek retractor.
Anticipation: Ensure adequate exposure of operative quadrant. Maintain moisture control without placing suction on the Mayo.

Step 3 – Incision of gingival tissue
Instruments: Scalpel handle with #15 blade, Adsons with teeth.
Anticipation: Incision is small but bleeding is expected. Be ready to pass mosquito hemostats promptly.

Step 4 – Elevate mucoperiosteal flap
Instruments: Periosteal elevator, 2 mosquito hemostats.
Anticipation: Maintain flap integrity. Control small bleeders early to keep field visible.

Step 5 – Remove bone overlying tooth if needed
Instruments: Bone rongeur or chisel passed from back table.
Anticipation: Surgeon may request bone removal unexpectedly. Have instruments available but unopened until requested.

Step 6 – Section tooth if indicated
Instruments: Sectioning instruments passed from back table.
Anticipation: Anticipate multiple stages of sectioning. Keep elevator and forceps ready for immediate use.

Step 7 – Luxate and extract tooth
Instruments: Dental elevators, extraction forceps.
Anticipation: Follow extraction sequence closely. Hand forceps oriented correctly to avoid repeated repositioning.

Step 8 – Inspect socket and remove debris
Instruments: Curette.
Anticipation: Be ready to hand curette promptly. Socket inspection is brief but important.

Step 9 – Control bleeding
Instruments: Mosquito hemostats, packing passed from back table.
Anticipation: Bleeding control is immediate. Do not over pack the socket.

Step 10 – Irrigate extraction site
Instruments: Managed from back table.
Anticipation: Assist with irrigation and suction without placing tubing on the Mayo.

Step 11 – Close flap if indicated
Instruments: Brought from back table when requested.
Anticipation: Closure instruments come to Mayo only when surgeon commits to closure.

Step 12 – Remove throat pack and final airway check
Instruments: Sponge forceps.
Anticipation: Throat pack removal must be verbalized and confirmed before extubation.

Mayo Stand Suggestion:

- Scalpel handle with #15 blade
- Adsons forceps with teeth
- Periosteal elevator
- Dental elevators
- Extraction forceps
- 2 mosquito hemostats

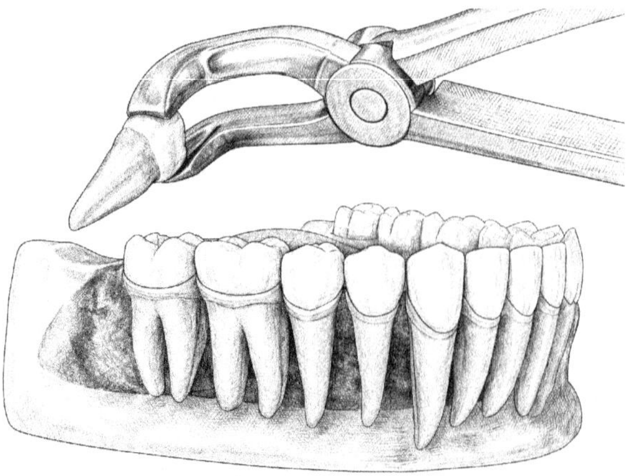

Section VI:

Plastic and Reconstructive Procedures

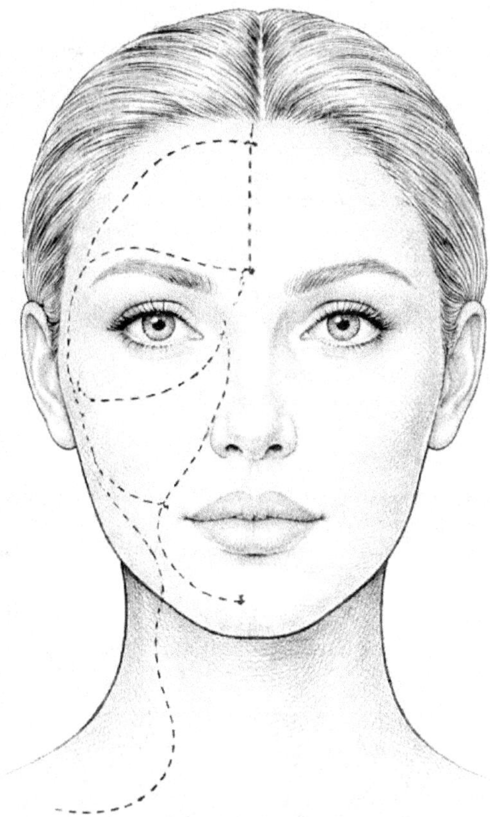

Abdominoplasty

Step 1 – Patient positioning and marking verification
Instruments: Headrest, positioning aids, skin marker (markings typically done preop).
Anticipation: Confirm surgical markings are visible before prep. Position patient to allow full abdominal exposure from costal margins to pubis.

Step 2 – Abdominal preparation and wide draping
Instruments: Abdominal prep supplies, sterile drapes.
Anticipation: Prep widely to accommodate flap elevation and possible drain exit sites.

Step 3 – Lower abdominal incision
Instruments: Scalpel handle with #10 blade, Adsons forceps with teeth.
Anticipation: Incision is long with brisk bleeding. Be ready to pass mosquito hemostats promptly.

Step 4 – Elevate abdominal skin flap
Instruments: Metzenbaum scissors, 2 mosquito hemostats, Adsons with teeth.
Anticipation: Follow clamp cut rhythm closely. Maintain organized clamp placement to avoid clutter.

Step 5 – Dissect to xiphoid and costal margins
Instruments: Metzenbaum scissors, long scissors if requested.
Anticipation: Dissection is extensive. Anticipate repeated instrument exchanges and keep scissors clean.

Step 6 – Identify and preserve umbilicus
Instruments: Metzenbaum scissors, fine forceps.
Anticipation: Umbilical stalk must be protected.

Step 7 – Rectus muscle plication if indicated
Instruments: Brought from back table when requested.
Anticipation: This marks transition to suturing. Bring needle driver and heavy sutures only when surgeon commits.

Step 8 – Excise excess abdominal skin and fat
Instruments: Scalpel handle with #10 blade, scissors.
Anticipation: Large specimen removal is imminent. Open specimen container early.

Step 9 – Achieve hemostasis and irrigate
Instruments: Managed from back table.
Anticipation: Assist with irrigation and clamp control without placing suction on the Mayo.

Step 10 – Place drains if indicated
Instruments: Drains passed from back table.
Anticipation: Confirm number and exit sites before placement.

Step 11 – Recreate umbilical opening
Instruments: Scalpel handle with #15 blade, Adsons with teeth.
Anticipation: Incision is small and cosmetic. Be ready to hand blade promptly.

Step 12 – Layered closure
Instruments: Brought from back table when requested.
Anticipation: Begin closing counts early. Closure instruments come forward only after surgeon commits.

Abdominoplasty

Step 13 – Apply dressing and abdominal binder
Instruments: Dressing supplies, binder.
Anticipation: Ensure drains are secured and not kinked before binder placement.

Mayo Stand Suggestion:

- Scalpel handle with #10 blade
- Scalpel handle with #15 blade
- Adsons forceps with teeth
- Metzenbaum scissors
- 2 mosquito hemostats

Ablation of Radial Thumb and Collateral Ligament

Step 1 – Patient positioning and extremity setup
Instruments: Hand table, arm board, tourniquet placed but not inflated, padding.
Anticipation: Confirm correct digit and side. Ensure tourniquet tubing is routed away from sterile field.

Step 2 – Prep and sterile draping of extremity
Instruments: Extremity prep supplies, sterile towels and drapes.
Anticipation: Prep must include entire hand and forearm. Maintain visibility of all digits for comparison.

Step 3 – Tourniquet inflation if used
Instruments: Tourniquet controlled by anesthesia.
Anticipation: Confirm time is noted. Bloodless field improves visualization for ligament reconstruction.

Step 4 – Skin incision over radial thumb
Instruments: Scalpel handle with #15 blade, Adsons forceps with teeth.
Anticipation: Incision is small but precise. Be ready to pass mosquito hemostats for small bleeders.

Step 5 – Identify and protect neurovascular structures
Instruments: Fine forceps, 2 mosquito hemostats.
Anticipation: This is delicate dissection. Pass instruments slowly and deliberately.

Step 6 – Excise supernumerary thumb
Instruments: Metzenbaum scissors, periosteal elevator if bone involved.
Anticipation: Specimen is small. Open specimen cup early to avoid delays.

Step 7 – Prepare collateral ligament reconstruction
Instruments: Fine forceps, small scissors.
Anticipation: Surgeon may pause to assess alignment. Maintain a quiet organized Mayo.

Step 8 – Reattach collateral ligament to remaining thumb
Instruments: Brought from back table when requested.
Anticipation: This is transition to suturing. Bring needle driver and fine sutures only when surgeon commits.

Step 9 – Assess thumb stability and alignment
Instruments: None additional.
Anticipation: Surgeon may test range of motion. Keep instruments available but unobtrusive.

Ablation of Radial Thumb and Collateral Ligament

Step 10 – Achieve hemostasis and irrigate
Instruments: Managed from back table.
Anticipation: Assist without placing suction on the Mayo.

Step 11 – Skin closure
Instruments: Brought from back table when requested.
Anticipation: Closure instruments come forward only after reconstruction is complete.

Step 12 – Apply dressing and splint if indicated
Instruments: Dressing and splint supplies.
Anticipation: Ensure thumb is positioned correctly before splint application.

Mayo Stand Suggestion:

- Scalpel handle with #15 blade
- Adsons forceps with teeth
- Metzenbaum scissors
- Fine forceps
- 2 mosquito hemostats

Augmentation Mammoplasty

Step 1 – Patient positioning and marking verification
Instruments: Headrest, arm boards, positioning aids.
Anticipation: Confirm surgical markings and implant plan (type, size, pocket location) before prep. Arms should be positioned symmetrically to avoid distortion.

Step 2 – Chest preparation and sterile draping
Instruments: Chest prep supplies, sterile drapes.
Anticipation: Prep widely to include possible drain sites or pocket extension. Keep markings visible if surgeon prefers.

Step 3 – Skin incision
Instruments: Scalpel handle with #15 blade, Adsons forceps with teeth.
Anticipation: Incision is precise and cosmetic. Be ready to pass mosquito hemostats promptly for small bleeders.

Step 4 – Dissection to implant pocket
Instruments: Metzenbaum scissors, 2 mosquito hemostats.
Anticipation: Dissection proceeds in layers. Follow clamp cut rhythm closely and keep scissors clean.

Step 5 – Create implant pocket
Instruments: Metzenbaum scissors, blunt dissectors.
Anticipation: Pocket creation may switch between sharp and blunt dissection. Anticipate instrument changes without clutter.

Step 6 – Achieve hemostasis and irrigate pocket
Instruments: Managed from back table.
Anticipation: Hemostasis must be complete before implant insertion. Assist with irrigation without placing suction on the Mayo.

Step 7 – Trial sizer placement if used
Instruments: Sizers passed from back table when requested.
Anticipation: Do not open multiple sizers. Maintain strict implant handling discipline.

Augmentation Mammoplasty

Step 8 – Prepare and insert implant
Instruments: Implant passed from back table when requested.
Anticipation: This is a sterile critical moment. Open implant only when surgeon confirms readiness.

Step 9 – Confirm implant position and symmetry
Instruments: None additional.
Anticipation: Surgeon may sit patient up. Be ready to assist with repositioning safely.

Step 10 – Close deep layers
Instruments: Brought from back table when requested.
Anticipation: Transition to suturing phase. Bring needle driver and sutures only after surgeon commits.

Step 11 – Skin closure
Instruments: Brought from back table when requested.
Anticipation: Cosmetic closure requires quiet, organized field.

Step 12 – Apply dressings and support garment
Instruments: Dressing supplies, surgical bra or binder.
Anticipation: Ensure implants are stable and incisions are protected before garment placement.

Mayo Stand Suggestion:

- Scalpel handle with #15 blade
- Adsons forceps with teeth
- Metzenbaum scissors
- Rake retractors
- Blunt dissector
- 2 mosquito hemostats
- Army Navy
- Senn retractors

Blepharoplasty

Step 1 – Patient positioning and eye protection
Instruments: Headrest, eye shield for nonoperative eye, corneal protectors if used.
Anticipation: Confirm operative eyelid(s) and markings before prep. Ensure eyes are protected before draping.

Step 2 – Facial preparation and sterile draping
Instruments: Facial prep supplies, sterile drapes.
Anticipation: Avoid prep solution pooling near eyes. Maintain clear access to eyelids and brows.

Step 3 – Markings verification
Instruments: Skin marker.
Anticipation: Surgeon may re confirm markings after draping. Keep marker accessible.

Step 4 – Eyelid incision
Instruments: Scalpel handle with #15 blade, Adsons forceps with teeth.
Anticipation: Incision is cosmetic and precise. Be ready to pass mosquito hemostats promptly for small bleeders.

Step 5 – Elevate skin and muscle flap
Instruments: Fine scissors, 2 mosquito hemostats, fine forceps.
Anticipation: Tissue is delicate. Maintain gentle traction and keep scissors clean.

Step 6 – Expose and excise excess fat if indicated
Instruments: Fine scissors, fine forceps.
Anticipation: Fat pads are fragile. Handle gently and anticipate clamp placement for bleeding control.

Blepharoplasty

Step 7 – Achieve hemostasis
Instruments: Mosquito hemostats passed as needed.
Anticipation: Avoid excessive clamping. Keep field dry and clear.

Step 8 – Assess symmetry and contour
Instruments: None additional.
Anticipation: Surgeon may pause and re check eyelid height. Maintain quiet organized field.

Step 9 – Close incision
Instruments: Brought from back table when requested.
Anticipation: Transition to closure phase. Bring needle driver and fine sutures only when surgeon commits.

Step 10 – Apply ointment and dressing if used
Instruments: Ointment, eye pads if used.
Anticipation: Ensure no pressure is placed on the globe.

Mayo Stand Suggestion:

- Scalpel handle with #15 blade
- Adsons forceps with teeth
- Fine scissors
- Fine forceps
- 2 mosquito hemostats
- Small Senn retractors or skin hook

Centralization of Radial Dysplasia

Step 1 – Patient positioning and extremity setup
Instruments: Hand table, arm board, tourniquet placed but not inflated, padding.
Anticipation: Confirm correct extremity and deformity severity. Ensure tourniquet tubing is routed away from the sterile field.

Step 2 – Prep and sterile draping of extremity
Instruments: Extremity prep supplies, sterile towels and drapes.
Anticipation: Prep must include entire hand and forearm. Keep all digits visible for alignment checks.

Step 3 – Tourniquet inflation if used
Instruments: Tourniquet controlled by anesthesia.
Anticipation: Note inflation time. A bloodless field improves visualization of neurovascular structures.

Step 4 – Skin incision along radial wrist and forearm
Instruments: Scalpel handle with #15 blade, Adsons forceps with teeth.
Anticipation: Incision follows planned correction line. Be ready to pass mosquito hemostats for small bleeders.

Step 5 – Identify and protect neurovascular structures
Instruments: Fine forceps, 2 mosquito hemostats.
Anticipation: Dissection is delicate. Pass instruments slowly and avoid sudden movements.

Step 6 – Release tight soft tissues
Instruments: Metzenbaum scissors, periosteal elevator.
Anticipation: Releases occur incrementally. Anticipate frequent instrument exchanges.

Centralization of Radial Dysplasia

Step 7 – Centralize carpus over ulna
Instruments: Bone holding forceps passed from back table.
Anticipation: Surgeon may pause to assess alignment. Keep fixation instruments ready but unopened.

Step 8 – Fixation of wrist alignment
Instruments: K wires or fixation devices passed from back table.
Anticipation: Confirm size and number before opening. Maintain strict wire control.

Step 9 – Tendon balancing or transfers if indicated
Instruments: Passed from back table when requested.
Anticipation: This step varies. Stay alert to surgeon preference and sequence.

Step 10 – Irrigation and hemostasis
Instruments: Managed from back table.
Anticipation: Assist without placing suction on the Mayo.

Step 11 – Skin closure
Instruments: Brought from back table when requested.
Anticipation: Closure instruments come forward only after fixation is complete.

Step 12 – Apply dressing and splint
Instruments: Dressing supplies, splint materials.
Anticipation: Ensure wrist is held in corrected position during splinting.

Mayo Stand Suggestion:

- Scalpel handle with #15 blade
- Adsons forceps with teeth
- Metzenbaum scissors
- Small Senn retractors
- Periosteal elevator
- Fine forceps
- 2 mosquito hemostats
- K Wires and Drivers

Cheiloplasty or Cleft Lip Repair

Step 1 – Patient positioning and airway confirmation
Instruments: Shoulder roll, headrest, secured endotracheal tube, throat pack if used.
Anticipation: Pediatric airway awareness is critical. Confirm throat pack placement and secure tube away from the operative field.

Step 2 – Facial preparation and careful draping
Instruments: Facial prep supplies, sterile drapes.
Anticipation: Avoid excessive prep solution near mouth and nose. Maintain visibility of lip landmarks.

Step 3 – Verify markings and symmetry
Instruments: Skin marker.
Anticipation: Surgeon may redraw markings after draping. Keep marker immediately available.

Step 4 – Lip incision along markings
Instruments: Scalpel handle with #15 blade, Adsons forceps with teeth.
Anticipation: Incision is precise and cosmetic. Be ready to pass mosquito hemostats immediately for bleeding control.

Cheiloplasty or Cleft Lip Repair

Step 5 – Elevate skin and muscle flaps
Instruments: Fine scissors, 2 mosquito hemostats, fine forceps.
Anticipation: Tissue handling must be delicate. Maintain gentle traction and keep scissors clean.

Step 6 – Reapproximate orbicularis oris muscle
Instruments: Passed from back table when requested.
Anticipation: This is a key functional step. Bring needle driver and sutures only when surgeon commits.

Step 7 – Align vermilion border and philtral landmarks
Instruments: Fine forceps.
Anticipation: Precision is critical. Keep field quiet and uncluttered.

Step 8 – Skin closure
Instruments: Brought from back table when requested.
Anticipation: Closure is layered and cosmetic. Anticipate fine sutures and small needle drivers.

Step 9 – Final symmetry check
Instruments: None additional.
Anticipation: Surgeon may pause to reassess alignment. Maintain sterile stillness.

Step 10 – Apply dressing if indicated
Instruments: Dressing supplies.
Anticipation: Ensure dressing does not distort lip position.

Step 11 – Remove throat pack and airway check
Instruments: Sponge forceps.
Anticipation: Throat pack removal must be verbalized and confirmed before extubation.

Mayo Stand Suggestion:

- Scalpel handle with #15 blade
- Adsons forceps with teeth
- Fine scissors
- Fine forceps
- 2 mosquito hemostats
- Small skin hooks or Senn retractor

Cleft Palate Repair V Y Palatoplasty Technique

Step 1 – Patient positioning and airway protection
Instruments: Shoulder roll, headrest, secured endotracheal tube, throat pack placed.
Anticipation: Pediatric airway awareness is critical. Confirm throat pack placement and ensure tube is secured away from the oral cavity.

Step 2 – Oral cavity preparation and mouth gag placement
Instruments: Dingman or McIvor mouth gag with tongue blade.
Anticipation: Assemble gag before draping. Ensure proper blade size to avoid pressure injury.

Step 3 – Verify palatal landmarks and markings
Instruments: Skin marker or marking pen.
Anticipation: Surgeon may redraw markings intraoperatively. Keep marker accessible without clutter.

Cleft Palate Repair V Y Palatoplasty Technique

Step 4 – Incision along cleft margins and V Y flaps
Instruments: Scalpel handle with #15 blade, Adsons forceps with teeth.
Anticipation: Incisions are precise and bleeding is expected. Be ready to pass mosquito hemostats immediately.

Step 5 – Elevate mucoperiosteal palatal flaps
Instruments: Periosteal elevator, 2 mosquito hemostats, fine forceps.
Anticipation: Gentle elevation preserves blood supply. Maintain organized clamp placement.

Step 6 – Mobilize palatal muscles
Instruments: Fine scissors, periosteal elevator.
Anticipation: This step is delicate and slow. Keep instruments clean and immediately available.

Step 7 – Advance V Y flaps and reposition palate
Instruments: Fine forceps.
Anticipation: Surgeon may pause to assess tension. Maintain a quiet field and avoid rushing handoffs.

Step 8 – Reapproximate nasal mucosa
Instruments: Brought from back table when requested.
Anticipation: This is the transition to suturing. Bring needle driver and fine sutures only when surgeon commits.

Step 9 – Reapproximate oral mucosa
Instruments: Brought from back table when requested.
Anticipation: Layered closure requires multiple suture types. Have correct sutures ready but unopened.

Step 10 – Inspect palate length and symmetry
Instruments: None additional.
Anticipation: Surgeon may reassess flap reach. Keep field uncluttered.

Step 11 – Remove throat pack and final airway check
Instruments: Sponge forceps.
Anticipation: Throat pack removal must be verbalized and confirmed before extubation.

Mayo Stand Suggestion:

- Scalpel handle with #15 blade
- Adsons forceps with teeth
- Periosteal elevator
- Fine scissors
- Fine forceps
- 2 mosquito hemostats
- Small skin hooks or Senn retractor

Endoscopic Brow Lift

Step 1 – Patient positioning and marking verification
Instruments: Headrest, arm boards if needed, skin marker.
Anticipation: Confirm brow markings and symmetry before prep. Head must be positioned to allow endoscopic access without repositioning.

Step 2 – Scalp preparation and sterile draping
Instruments: Scalp prep supplies, sterile drapes, hair isolation materials.
Anticipation: Protect hair from prep solution. Maintain access to incision sites along hairline or scalp.

Endoscopic Brow Lift

Step 3 – Scalp incision for endoscope ports
Instruments: Scalpel handle with #15 blade, Adsons forceps with teeth.
Anticipation: Incisions are small and precise. Be ready to pass mosquito hemostats promptly for bleeding control.

Step 4 – Elevate subperiosteal plane
Instruments: Periosteal elevator, 2 mosquito hemostats.
Anticipation: Elevation proceeds in a controlled plane. Anticipate frequent instrument exchanges.

Step 5 – Insert endoscope and visualize brow structures
Instruments: Endoscope managed .
Anticipation: Confirm camera focus and light before insertion. Keep Mayo clear of cords.

Step 6 – Release brow attachments
Instruments: Endoscopic dissectors passed from back table.
Anticipation: Surgeon may alternate between endoscope and hand instruments. Stay alert to instrument requests.

Step 7 – Elevate brow and confirm position
Instruments: None additional.
Anticipation: Surgeon may pause to assess symmetry. Maintain still field and avoid unnecessary movement.

Step 8 – Fixate brow in new position
Instruments: Fixation devices passed from back table when requested.
Anticipation: Do not open fixation devices until surgeon confirms placement plan.

Step 9 – Remove endoscope and inspect field
Instruments: None additional.
Anticipation: Be ready to assist with irrigation or visualization as needed without adding tubing to the Mayo.

Step 10 – Close scalp incisions
Instruments: Brought from back table when requested.
Anticipation: Closure instruments come to Mayo only after fixation is finalized.

Step 11 – Apply dressing or head wrap
Instruments: Dressing supplies.
Anticipation: Ensure fixation remains stable during dressing application.

Mayo Stand Suggestion:

- Scalpel handle with #15 blade
- Adsons forceps with teeth
- Periosteal elevator
- Fine scissors
- Fine forceps
- 2 mosquito hemostats
- Small skin hooks or Senn retractor

Malar Implants

Step 1 – Patient positioning and marking verification
Instruments: Headrest, arm boards if needed, skin marker.
Anticipation: Confirm implant type, size, and laterality before prep. Ensure facial markings remain visible if surgeon prefers.

Step 2 – Facial or oral preparation and draping
Instruments: Facial or oral prep supplies, sterile drapes.
Anticipation: Prep depends on approach. Intraoral approach requires careful oral isolation.

Step 3 – Incision at chosen approach site
Instruments: Scalpel handle with #15 blade, Adsons forceps with teeth.
Anticipation: Incision is small but precise. Be ready to pass mosquito hemostats promptly for bleeding control.

Step 4 – Elevate periosteal pocket over zygoma
Instruments: Periosteal elevator, 2 mosquito hemostats.
Anticipation: Pocket dissection must be symmetric. Anticipate repeated elevator use and gentle clamp control.

Step 5 – Size implant pocket and assess fit
Instruments: Trial sizer passed from back table if used.
Anticipation: Do not open implant until surgeon confirms pocket size and symmetry.

Step 6 – Insert malar implant
Instruments: Implant passed from back table when requested.
Anticipation: This is a sterile critical moment. Open implant only when surgeon commits to insertion.

Step 7 – Secure implant if fixation used
Instruments: Fixation screws passed from back table.
Anticipation: Confirm fixation method before opening hardware.

Step 8 – Inspect symmetry and contour
Instruments: None additional.
Anticipation: Surgeon may reassess bilaterally. Maintain quiet organized field.

Step 9 – Irrigate and achieve hemostasis
Instruments: Managed from back table.
Anticipation: Assist without placing suction on the Mayo.

Step 10 – Close incision
Instruments: Brought from back table when requested.
Anticipation: Closure instruments come forward only after implant position is finalized.

Step 11 – Apply dressing if indicated
Instruments: Dressing supplies.
Anticipation: Avoid pressure on implants during dressing application.

Mayo Stand Suggestion:

- Scalpel handle with #15 blade
- Adsons forceps with teeth
- Periosteal elevator
- Fine scissors
- 2 mosquito hemostats
- Small Senn retractors or skin hook

Mastopexy Anchor Technique

Step 1 – Patient positioning and marking verification
Instruments: Headrest, arm boards, positioning aids.
Anticipation: Confirm Wise pattern markings and nipple position before prep. Arm symmetry is critical to avoid distortion.

Step 2 – Chest preparation and sterile draping
Instruments: Chest prep supplies, sterile drapes.
Anticipation: Prep widely to allow flap elevation and possible drain placement. Preserve visible markings if surgeon prefers.

Step 3 – Skin incision along anchor markings
Instruments: Scalpel handle with #10 blade, Adsons forceps with teeth.
Anticipation: Incisions are long with predictable bleeding. Be ready to pass mosquito hemostats promptly.

Step 4 – De epithelialization of pedicle
Instruments: Scalpel handle with #15 blade, Adsons forceps with teeth.
Anticipation: This step is meticulous. Keep the blade clean and immediately available.

Step 5 – Elevate skin flaps and shape breast tissue
Instruments: Metzenbaum scissors, 2 mosquito hemostats.
Anticipation: Follow clamp cut rhythm closely. Maintain organized clamp placement.

Step 6 – Reposition nipple areola complex
Instruments: Fine forceps.
Anticipation: Surgeon may pause to confirm symmetry. Keep field quiet and uncluttered.

Step 7 – Excise excess skin and tissue
Instruments: Scalpel handle with #10 blade, scissors.
Anticipation: Specimen removal is imminent. Open specimen container early.

Step 8 – Achieve hemostasis and inspect breast shape
Instruments: Managed from back table.
Anticipation: Bleeding control must be complete before closure.

Step 9 – Place drains if indicated
Instruments: Drains passed from back table.
Anticipation: Confirm drain number and exit sites before placement.

Step 10 – Layered closure
Instruments: Brought from back table when requested.
Anticipation: Bring needle driver and sutures only when surgeon commits to closure.

Step 11 – Apply dressings and support garment
Instruments: Dressing supplies, surgical bra.
Anticipation: Ensure nipple perfusion is not compromised by dressings.

Mayo Stand Suggestion:

- Scalpel handle with #10 blade
- Scalpel handle with #15 blade
- Adsons forceps with teeth
- Allis
- Metzenbaum scissors
- 2 mosquito hemostats
- Small Army Navy or Senn retractor

Mentoplasty

Step 1 – Patient positioning and marking verification
Instruments: Headrest, arm boards if needed, skin marker.
Anticipation: Confirm laterality, implant plan, and markings before prep. Head position affects chin symmetry.

Step 2 – Facial and oral preparation and draping
Instruments: Facial or oral prep supplies, sterile drapes.
Anticipation: Prep depends on approach. Intraoral approach requires careful oral isolation.

Step 3 – Incision at chosen approach site
Instruments: Scalpel handle with #15 blade, Adsons forceps with teeth.
Anticipation: Incision is small and cosmetic. Be ready to pass mosquito hemostats promptly.

Step 4 – Elevate periosteal pocket
Instruments: Periosteal elevator, 2 mosquito hemostats.
Anticipation: Pocket must be symmetric. Anticipate frequent elevator use.

Step 5 – Prepare implant pocket or modify bone
Instruments: Osteotome or rasp passed from back table if needed.
Anticipation: Bone work varies by plan. Do not open bone instruments until requested.

Step 6 – Insert chin implant or reposition bone segment
Instruments: Implant passed from back table when requested.
Anticipation: This is a sterile critical moment. Open implant only when surgeon commits.

Step 7 – Secure implant if fixation used
Instruments: Fixation screws passed from back table.
Anticipation: Confirm fixation plan before opening hardware.

Step 8 – Inspect symmetry and profile
Instruments: None additional.
Anticipation: Surgeon may reassess from multiple angles. Maintain quiet organized field.

Step 9 – Irrigate and achieve hemostasis
Instruments: Managed from back table.
Anticipation: Assist without placing suction on the Mayo.

Step 10 – Close incision
Instruments: Brought from back table when requested.
Anticipation: Closure instruments come forward only after final positioning.

Step 11 – Apply dressing or chin strap
Instruments: Dressing supplies, chin strap.
Anticipation: Ensure implant position is stable before securing dressing.

Mayo Stand Suggestion:

- Scalpel handle with #10 blade
- Scalpel handle with #15 blade
- Adsons forceps with teeth
- Metzenbaum scissors
- 2 mosquito hemostats
- Small Army Navy or Senn retractor

Nipple Reconstruction

Step 1 – Patient positioning and marking verification
Instruments: Headrest, arm boards, skin marker.
Anticipation: Confirm nipple position, laterality, and flap design before prep. Symmetry is critical and markings must remain visible.

Step 2 – Chest preparation and sterile draping
Instruments: Chest prep supplies, sterile drapes.
Anticipation: Prep widely but preserve markings if surgeon prefers to reference them throughout the case.

Step 3 – Incision along flap markings
Instruments: Scalpel handle with #15 blade, Adsons forceps with teeth.
Anticipation: Incisions are small and precise. Be ready to pass mosquito hemostats immediately for bleeding control.

Step 4 – Elevate local skin flaps
Instruments: Fine scissors, 2 mosquito hemostats, fine forceps.
Anticipation: Flaps are delicate. Maintain gentle traction and keep scissors clean and immediately available.

Step 5 – Shape and fold flap to create nipple projection
Instruments: Fine forceps.
Anticipation: Surgeon may pause to assess projection. Maintain a quiet, uncluttered Mayo.

Step 6 – Secure reconstructed nipple
Instruments: Brought from back table when requested.
Anticipation: This signals transition to suturing. Bring needle driver and fine sutures only when surgeon commits.

Step 7 – Inspect symmetry and projection
Instruments: None additional.
Anticipation: Surgeon may reassess alignment. Avoid unnecessary movement in the field.

Step 8 – Apply protective dressing or nipple shield
Instruments: Dressing supplies, nipple protector if used.
Anticipation: Ensure dressing does not compress the newly formed nipple.

Mayo Stand Suggestion:

- Scalpel handle with #15 blade
- Adsons forceps with teeth
- Fine scissors
- Fine forceps
- 2 mosquito hemostats
- Small skin hooks or Senn retractor

Otoplasty

Step 1 – Patient positioning and marking verification
Instruments: Headrest, positioning aids, skin marker.
Anticipation: Confirm operative ear(s), planned correction, and markings before prep. Head position affects ear symmetry.

Step 2 – Ear and scalp preparation and draping
Instruments: Ear and scalp prep supplies, sterile drapes.
Anticipation: Prep must allow access behind the ear. Protect hair and maintain clear exposure of auricular landmarks.

Otoplasty

Step 3 – Posterior auricular skin incision
Instruments: Scalpel handle with #15 blade, Adsons forceps with teeth.
Anticipation: Incision is small but bleeding is expected. Be ready to pass mosquito hemostats promptly.

Step 4 – Elevate skin flap to expose cartilage
Instruments: Fine scissors, 2 mosquito hemostats, fine forceps.
Anticipation: Skin is thin and delicate. Maintain gentle traction and avoid flap tears.

Step 5 – Cartilage scoring or reshaping
Instruments: Cartilage scoring tool or blade passed from back table when requested.
Anticipation: Do not open cartilage tools until surgeon confirms technique.

Step 6 – Place fixation sutures to reshape ear
Instruments: Brought from back table when requested.
Anticipation: This signals transition to suturing. Bring needle driver and sutures only when surgeon commits.

Step 7 – Assess ear position and symmetry
Instruments: None additional.
Anticipation: Surgeon may reassess from multiple angles. Maintain a quiet, still field.

Step 8 – Trim excess skin if indicated
Instruments: Fine scissors.
Anticipation: Skin trimming is conservative. Be ready but do not over anticipate.

Step 9 – Skin closure
Instruments: Brought from back table when requested.
Anticipation: Closure instruments come forward only after final positioning is approved.

Step 10 – Apply dressing and head wrap
Instruments: Dressing supplies, head wrap.
Anticipation: Ensure ears are positioned correctly before wrap application.

Mayo Stand Suggestion:

- Scalpel handle with #15 blade
- Adsons forceps with teeth
- Fine scissors
- Fine forceps
- 2 mosquito hemostats
- Small skin hooks or Senn retractor

Release of Syndactyly

Step 1 – Patient positioning and extremity setup
Instruments: Hand table, arm board, tourniquet placed but not inflated, padding.
Anticipation: Confirm correct hand and digits. Ensure tourniquet tubing is routed away from sterile field.

Step 2 – Prep and sterile draping of extremity
Instruments: Extremity prep supplies, sterile towels and drapes.
Anticipation: Prep must include entire hand and forearm. Keep all digits visible for alignment.

Step 3 – Tourniquet inflation if used
Instruments: Tourniquet controlled by anesthesia.
Anticipation: Note inflation time. Bloodless field improves visualization of neurovascular bundles.

Release of Syndactyly

Step 4 – Zig zag skin incisions between digits
Instruments: Scalpel handle with #15 blade, Adsons forceps with teeth.
Anticipation: Incisions are precise. Be ready to pass mosquito hemostats immediately.

Step 5 – Elevate skin flaps carefully
Instruments: Fine scissors, 2 mosquito hemostats, fine forceps.
Anticipation: Flaps are delicate. Gentle traction and organized clamp placement are critical.

Step 6 – Identify and protect neurovascular bundles
Instruments: Fine forceps.
Anticipation: This is a slow step. Pass instruments deliberately and avoid sudden movements.

Step 7 – Separate digits
Instruments: Fine scissors.
Anticipation: Expect alternating sharp and blunt dissection. Keep scissors clean and ready.

Step 8 – Shape flaps and assess web space
Instruments: Fine forceps.
Anticipation: Surgeon may pause to assess depth and symmetry. Maintain quiet field.

Step 9 – Apply skin graft if required
Instruments: Graft materials passed from back table when requested.
Anticipation: Do not open graft until surgeon confirms need and size.

Step 10 – Secure flaps and grafts
Instruments: Brought from back table when requested.
Anticipation: This signals transition to suturing. Bring needle driver and fine sutures only when surgeon commits.

Step 11 – Apply dressing and splint
Instruments: Dressing and splint supplies.
Anticipation: Ensure digits are positioned correctly and grafts are protected.

Mayo Stand Suggestion:

- Scalpel handle with #15 blade
- Adsons forceps with teeth
- Fine scissors
- Fine forceps
- 2 mosquito hemostats
- Small skin hooks or Senn retractor

Rhinoplasty External Technique

Step 1 – Patient positioning and marking verification
Instruments: Headrest, shoulder roll if used, skin marker.
Anticipation: Confirm operative plan (cosmetic vs functional), markings, and laterality before prep. Head position affects nasal symmetry.

Step 2 – Facial preparation and sterile draping
Instruments: Facial prep supplies, sterile drapes.
Anticipation: Avoid prep pooling in nares and eyes. Maintain full access to nose and upper lip.

Step 3 – Transcolumellar and marginal incisions
Instruments: Scalpel handle with #15 blade, Adsons forceps with teeth.
Anticipation: Incisions are cosmetic and precise. Be ready to pass mosquito hemostats promptly for bleeding control.

Rhinoplasty External Technique

Step 4 – Elevate nasal skin soft tissue envelope
Instruments: Fine scissors, periosteal elevator, 2 mosquito hemostats.
Anticipation: Elevation must be gentle to avoid skin trauma. Maintain organized clamp placement.

Step 5 – Expose nasal cartilages and framework
Instruments: Fine forceps, small retractor (skin hooks or Senn).
Anticipation: Surgeon may alternate between exposure and assessment. Keep retractor readily available.

Step 6 – Cartilage modification and graft harvest if needed
Instruments: Cartilage knife or blade passed from back table.
Anticipation: Do not open graft tools until surgeon confirms need and source.

Step 7 – Osteotomies if indicated
Instruments: Osteotome and mallet passed from back table when requested.
Anticipation: This step is brief but decisive. Have instruments ready but unopened.

Step 8 – Shape nasal tip and dorsum
Instruments: Fine forceps.
Anticipation: Surgeon may pause frequently to assess symmetry. Maintain a quiet field.

Step 9 – Re drape skin envelope and assess contour
Instruments: None additional.
Anticipation: Surgeon may adjust multiple times. Stay attentive without over anticipating.

Step 10 – Close columellar and marginal incisions
Instruments: Brought from back table when requested.
Anticipation: Closure instruments come forward only after final contour is approved.

Step 11 – Apply splint and dressing
Instruments: Nasal splint, dressing supplies.
Anticipation: Ensure splint does not shift nasal alignment during placement.

Mayo Stand Suggestion:

- Scalpel handle with #15 blade
- Adsons forceps with teeth
- Fine scissors
- Periosteal elevator
- Fine forceps
- 2 mosquito hemostats
- Small skin hooks or Senn retractor

Rhytidectomy

Step 1 – Patient positioning and marking verification
Instruments: Headrest, shoulder roll if needed, skin marker.
Anticipation: Confirm incision markings around hairline and ear before prep. Head position affects facial symmetry.

Step 2 – Facial preparation and wide draping
Instruments: Facial prep supplies, sterile drapes.
Anticipation: Prep must include face, neck, and ears. Protect hair and maintain access to postauricular area.

Rhytidectomy

Step 3 – Incisions along pre and postauricular markings
Instruments: Scalpel handle with #15 blade, Adsons forceps with teeth.
Anticipation: Incisions are long and cosmetic. Be ready to pass mosquito hemostats promptly for bleeding control.

Step 4 – Elevate skin and SMAS flap
Instruments: Fine scissors, periosteal or SMAS elevator, 2 mosquito hemostats.
Anticipation: Gentle traction is critical. Follow clamp cut rhythm without crowding the Mayo.

Step 5 – Dissect facial flap to desired extent
Instruments: Fine scissors, small retractor (Senn or skin hooks).
Anticipation: Exposure changes frequently. Keep small retractor immediately accessible.

Step 6 – Reposition and secure SMAS layer
Instruments: Brought from back table when requested.
Anticipation: Transition to suturing phase. Bring needle driver and sutures only when surgeon commits.

Step 7 – Excise excess skin
Instruments: Scalpel handle with #15 blade, scissors.
Anticipation: Skin trimming is incremental. Anticipate repeated passes.

Step 8 – Achieve hemostasis and inspect contour
Instruments: Managed from back table.
Anticipation: Hemostasis must be complete before closure to prevent hematoma.

Step 9 – Layered closure
Instruments: Brought from back table when requested.
Anticipation: Closure is meticulous. Keep the field quiet and organized.

Step 10 – Apply dressings and compression wrap
Instruments: Dressing supplies, facial wrap.
Anticipation: Ensure ears are not folded and pressure is evenly distributed.

Mayo Stand Suggestion:

- Scalpel handle with #15 blade
- Adsons forceps with teeth
- Fine scissors
- Periosteal elevator
- Fine forceps
- 2 mosquito hemostats
- Small skin hooks or Senn retractor

Subtotal Palmar Fasciectomy for Dupuytren Contracture

Step 1 – Patient positioning and extremity setup
Instruments: Hand table, arm board, tourniquet placed but not inflated, padding.
Anticipation: Confirm correct hand and involved digits. Ensure tourniquet tubing is positioned away from the sterile field.

Step 2 – Prep and sterile draping of extremity
Instruments: Extremity prep supplies, sterile towels and drapes.
Anticipation: Prep must include entire hand and forearm. Keep fingers fully visible for alignment checks.

Subtotal Palmar Fasciectomy for Dupuytren Contracture

Step 3 – Tourniquet inflation if used
Instruments: Tourniquet controlled by anesthesia.
Anticipation: Note inflation time. Bloodless field is critical for identifying digital nerves and vessels.

Step 4 – Zig zag palmar skin incisions
Instruments: Scalpel handle with #15 blade, Adsons forceps with teeth.
Anticipation: Incisions are precise and bleeding is expected. Be ready to pass mosquito hemostats promptly.

Step 5 – Elevate skin flaps carefully
Instruments: Fine scissors, 2 mosquito hemostats, fine forceps.
Anticipation: Skin flaps are thin. Gentle traction prevents flap necrosis.

Step 6 – Identify neurovascular bundles
Instruments: Fine forceps.
Anticipation: This step is slow and meticulous. Pass instruments deliberately and avoid crowding the field.

Step 7 – Excise diseased palmar fascia
Instruments: Fine scissors, small retractor (skin hooks or Senn).
Anticipation: Fascia removal is incremental. Keep scissors clean and immediately available.

Step 8 – Extend release into affected digits if needed
Instruments: Fine scissors, fine forceps.
Anticipation: Anticipate deeper dissection near neurovascular structures. Maintain steady exposure.

Step 9 – Assess finger extension and contracture release
Instruments: None additional.
Anticipation: Surgeon may extend and flex fingers repeatedly. Keep the field unobstructed.

Step 10 – Achieve hemostasis and irrigate
Instruments: Managed from back table.
Anticipation: Hemostasis must be complete to reduce hematoma risk.

Step 11 – Skin closure
Instruments: Brought from back table when requested.
Anticipation: Closure instruments come forward only after full release is confirmed.

Step 12 – Apply dressing and splint
Instruments: Dressing supplies, splint materials.
Anticipation: Ensure fingers are positioned in extension during splinting.

Mayo Stand Suggestion:

- Scalpel handle with #15 blade
- Adsons forceps with teeth
- Fine scissors
- Fine forceps
- 2 mosquito hemostats
- Small skin hooks or Senn retractor

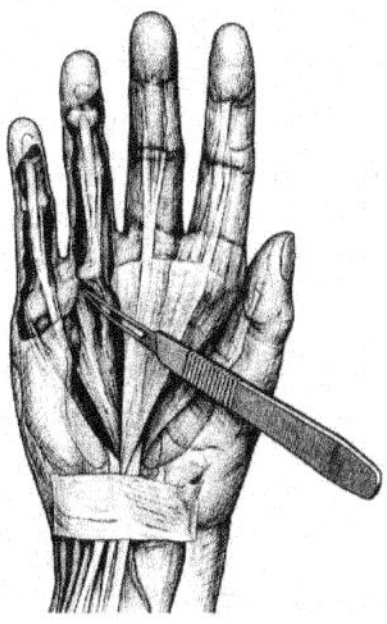

Suction Lipectomy

Step 1 – Patient positioning and marking verification
Instruments: Positioning aids, padding, skin marker (markings usually done preop).
Anticipation: Confirm marked areas and patient positioning allow access to all planned treatment zones without repositioning.

Step 2 – Wide skin preparation and draping
Instruments: Prep supplies, sterile drapes.
Anticipation: Prep must include entire contour area plus adjacent regions for cannula movement.

Step 3 – Small skin access incisions
Instruments: Scalpel handle with #11 or #15 blade, Adsons forceps with teeth.
Anticipation: Incisions are small but multiple. Be ready to pass blade repeatedly.

Step 4 – Infiltration of tumescent solution
Instruments: Managed from back table.
Anticipation: Anticipate fluid shifts and surgeon pauses during infiltration. Keep Mayo uncluttered.

Step 5 – Insert liposuction cannula
Instruments: Cannulas passed from back table when requested.
Anticipation: Cannula selection may change by area. Have sizes ready but unopened.

Step 6 – Perform suction assisted fat removal
Instruments: Cannulas and tubing.
Anticipation: Stay alert to tubing tension and sterile field integrity.

Step 7 – Periodic assessment of contour and symmetry
Instruments: None additional.
Anticipation: Surgeon may stop frequently to assess. Assist with repositioning safely if needed.

Step 8 – Additional passes or cannula changes
Instruments: Alternate cannulas passed from back table.
Anticipation: Anticipate smooth transitions without clutter.

Step 9 – Express residual fluid and inspect sites
Instruments: Gauze, gentle pressure.
Anticipation: Be ready with sponges but avoid aggressive manipulation.

Step 10 – Close access incisions if indicated
Instruments: Brought from back table when requested.
Anticipation: Some incisions remain open. Do not assume closure.

Step 11 – Apply dressings and compression garment
Instruments: Dressing supplies, compression garment.
Anticipation: Ensure cannula sites are not occluded and garment fits evenly.

Mayo Stand Suggestion:

- Scalpel handle with #11 or #15 blade
- Adsons forceps with teeth
- 2 mosquito hemostats
- Gauze sponges
- Liposuction Cannulas

Toe to Hand Transfer

Step 1 – Dual team room setup and positioning
Instruments: Two prep areas, hand tables, padding, tourniquets placed but not inflated.
Anticipation: Confirm which team is donor vs recipient. Keep instrument sets clearly separated to avoid cross contamination.

Step 2 – Prep and drape hand and foot
Instruments: Extremity prep supplies, sterile towels and drapes.
Anticipation: Prep must include full donor toe and recipient hand. Ensure both extremities remain accessible throughout the case.

Step 3 – Tourniquet inflation if used
Instruments: Tourniquet controlled by anesthesia.
Anticipation: Track tourniquet times independently for hand and foot.

Step 4 – Incision at donor toe
Instruments: Scalpel handle with #15 blade, Adsons forceps with teeth.
Anticipation: Dissection is meticulous. Be ready with mosquito hemostats immediately for small vessel control.

Step 5 – Identify and dissect neurovascular structures
Instruments: Fine forceps, 2 mosquito hemostats, fine scissors.
Anticipation: This is microsurgical prep. Pass instruments deliberately and avoid sudden handoffs.

Step 6 – Harvest toe with vessels, nerves, and tendon
Instruments: Fine scissors, periosteal elevator.
Anticipation: Expect pauses while surgeon confirms pedicle length. Maintain quiet organized field.

Step 7 – Prepare recipient hand site
Instruments: Scalpel handle with #15 blade, fine scissors.
Anticipation: Recipient vessels must be identified cleanly. Keep donor toe protected and moist.

Step 8 – Bone fixation of transferred toe
Instruments: Fixation devices passed from back table when requested.
Anticipation: Confirm size and orientation before opening fixation hardware.

Step 9 – Tendon repair
Instruments: Brought from back table when requested.
Anticipation: Transition to suturing. Bring needle driver and sutures only when surgeon commits.

Step 10 – Microvascular anastomosis
Instruments: Microsurgical instruments passed from back table.
Anticipation: Absolute stillness is required. Anticipate surgeon needs without rushing.

Step 11 – Nerve repair
Instruments: Microsurgical sutures and instruments from back table.
Anticipation: Maintain moisture and avoid tension on repaired structures.

Step 12 – Assess perfusion of transferred toe
Instruments: Doppler managed if used.
Anticipation: Watch color, capillary refill, and bleeding. Be prepared to assist immediately if revision is needed.

Toe to Hand Transfer

Step 13 – Donor site closure
Instruments: Brought from back table when requested.
Anticipation: Donor site closure occurs while monitoring recipient perfusion.

Step 14 – Apply dressings and splints
Instruments: Dressing supplies, splints.
Anticipation: Position transferred digit carefully to avoid kinking vessels.

Mayo Stand Suggestion:

- Scalpel handle with #15 blade
- Adsons forceps with teeth
- Fine scissors
- Fine forceps
- 2 mosquito hemostats
- Small skin hooks or Senn retractor

Transverse Rectus Abdominis Musculocutaneous Flap (TRAM)

Step 1 – Patient positioning and marking verification
Instruments: Headrest, arm boards, positioning aids.
Anticipation: Confirm laterality (pedicled vs free TRAM) and flap markings before prep. Ensure arms allow chest and abdomen access.

Step 2 – Chest and abdominal preparation and wide draping
Instruments: Prep supplies, sterile drapes.
Anticipation: Prep must include chest, abdomen, and possible recipient vessels. Keep markings visible if surgeon prefers.

Step 3 – Lower abdominal incision
Instruments: Scalpel handle with #10 blade, Adsons forceps with teeth.
Anticipation: Incision is long with predictable bleeding. Be ready to pass mosquito hemostats promptly.

Step 4 – Elevate abdominal skin and fat flap
Instruments: Metzenbaum scissors, 2 mosquito hemostats, Adsons with teeth.
Anticipation: Follow clamp-cut rhythm closely. Maintain organized clamp placement to avoid clutter.

Step 5 – Identify and dissect rectus muscle and pedicle
Instruments: Metzenbaum scissors, periosteal elevator.
Anticipation: Pedicle preservation is critical. Anticipate careful dissection and slower pacing.

Step 6 – Divide rectus muscle as planned
Instruments: Metzenbaum scissors.
Anticipation: Muscle division marks a key transition. Be ready for specimen handling and pedicle protection.

Step 7 – Transfer flap to chest (tunneled or free)
Instruments: Large instruments passed from back table when requested.
Anticipation: Protect pedicle from torsion or compression during transfer. Maintain a clear Mayo.

Step 8 – Shape flap to reconstruct breast mound
Instruments: Adsons forceps with teeth, Metzenbaum scissors.
Anticipation: Surgeon may repeatedly assess contour. Keep shaping instruments readily available.

Transverse Rectus Abdominis Musculocutaneous Flap (TRAM)

Step 9 – Microvascular anastomosis if free TRAM
Instruments: Microsurgical instruments passed from back table.
Anticipation: Absolute stillness is required. Anticipate needs without rushing.

Step 10 – Inspect flap perfusion and symmetry
Instruments: None additional.
Anticipation: Surgeon may pause for repeated checks. Watch flap color and capillary refill.

Step 11 – Abdominal wall closure and reinforcement
Instruments: Brought from back table when requested.
Anticipation: This marks transition to closure. Confirm mesh use if planned.

Step 12 – Place drains if indicated
Instruments: Drains passed from back table.
Anticipation: Confirm number and exit sites before placement.

Step 13 – Final skin closure and dressing application
Instruments: Brought from back table when requested.
Anticipation: Begin closing counts early. Ensure drains are secured before dressings.

Mayo Stand Suggestion:

- Scalpel handle with #10 blade
- Scalpel handle with #15 blade
- Adsons forceps with teeth
- Metzenbaum scissors
- Periosteal elevator
- 2 mosquito hemostats
- Small Army Navy or Senn retractor

Z Plasty Scar Revision

Step 1 – Patient positioning and marking verification
Instruments: Headrest, positioning aids, skin marker.
Anticipation: Confirm scar orientation and Z limb markings before prep. Markings guide the repair.

Step 2 – Skin preparation and sterile draping
Instruments: Prep supplies, sterile drapes.
Anticipation: Prep must include surrounding tissue to allow flap mobilization without restriction.

Step 3 – Incision along Z plasty markings
Instruments: Scalpel handle with #15 blade, Adsons forceps with teeth.
Anticipation: Incisions are precise and symmetrical. Be ready to pass mosquito hemostats promptly for bleeding control.

Step 4 – Elevate triangular skin flaps
Instruments: Fine scissors, 2 mosquito hemostats, fine forceps.
Anticipation: Flaps must remain viable. Gentle traction and organized clamp placement are critical.

Step 5 – Mobilize flaps to allow transposition
Instruments: Fine scissors, fine forceps.
Anticipation: Surgeon may test flap mobility repeatedly. Keep instruments ready without clutter.

Step 6 – Transpose flaps into new position
Instruments: Fine forceps.
Anticipation: Flap orientation is deliberate. Maintain a quiet field during transposition.

Step 7 – Assess tension and alignment
Instruments: None additional.
Anticipation: Surgeon may pause to reassess tension. Avoid unnecessary movement.

Step 8 – Secure flaps with sutures
Instruments: Brought from back table when requested.
Anticipation: This signals transition to suturing. Bring needle driver and sutures only when surgeon commits.

Step 9 – Final skin closure
Instruments: Brought from back table when requested.
Anticipation: Closure is cosmetic. Keep the field quiet and organized.

Step 10 – Apply dressing if indicated
Instruments: Dressing supplies.
Anticipation: Ensure dressing does not distort flap position.

Mayo Stand Suggestion:

- Scalpel handle with #15 blade
- Adsons forceps with teeth
- Fine scissors
- Fine forceps
- 2 mosquito hemostats
- Small skin hooks or Senn retractor

Section VII:

Genitourinary Procedures

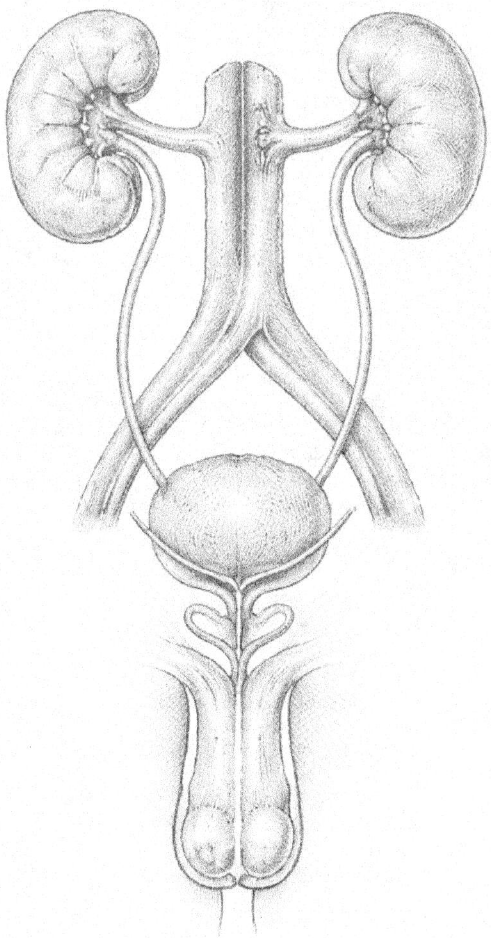

Circumcision

Step 1 – Patient positioning and verification
Instruments: Supine positioning aids, padding.
Anticipation: Confirm patient age, indication, and correct procedure. Pediatric cases require extra attention to positioning and warming.

Step 2 – Genital preparation and sterile draping
Instruments: Prep supplies, fenestrated drape.
Anticipation: Prep must include entire penis and scrotum. Ensure fenestration allows full visualization of the glans.

Step 3 – Foreskin retraction and exposure of glans
Instruments: Adsons forceps with teeth or smooth forceps.
Anticipation: Adhesions may be present. Be ready to assist with gentle traction without tearing tissue.

Step 4 – Mark circumcision line if needed
Instruments: Skin marker.
Anticipation: Surgeon may pause to assess symmetry. Maintain a quiet, uncluttered field.

Step 5 – Clamp foreskin for hemostasis and guidance
Instruments: Straight hemostats or 2 mosquito hemostats.
Anticipation: Follow clamp placement carefully. Clamps define excision margin and bleeding control.

Step 6 – Excise foreskin
Instruments: Scalpel handle with #15 blade, scissors.
Anticipation: Excision is controlled but bleeding can occur quickly. Be ready to pass clamps promptly.

Step 7 – Inspect glans and control bleeding
Instruments: Mosquito hemostats.
Anticipation: Bleeders are small but numerous. Anticipate clamp use without over crowding the Mayo.

Step 8 – Approximate skin edges
Instruments: Brought from back table when requested.
Anticipation: This signals transition to suturing. Bring needle driver and sutures only when surgeon commits.

Step 9 – Final inspection and dressing application
Instruments: Dressing supplies, petroleum gauze if used.
Anticipation: Dressing should not constrict the penis. Ensure glans remains visible if surgeon prefers.

Mayo Stand Suggestion:

- Scalpel handle with #15 blade
- Adsons forceps with teeth or smooth
- Scissors
- 2 mosquito hemostats
- 4 small straight hemostats
- 2 Allis
- Metzenbaum, small

Cystoscopy with Overview of TURBT

Step 1 – Patient positioning and verification
Instruments: Lithotomy stirrups, padding, grounding pad placed by anesthesia.
Anticipation: Confirm lithotomy positioning before prep. Ensure legs are symmetric to avoid nerve injury.

Step 2 – Perineal preparation and sterile draping
Instruments: Perineal prep supplies, cystoscopy drape.
Anticipation: Prep must include penis, scrotum, and perineum. Ensure drape fenestration aligns with urethral meatus.

Step 3 – Assemble cystoscopy equipment
Instruments: Cystoscope sheath and obturator, lens, light cord, camera.
Anticipation: Test light and camera before insertion. Keep cords and organized to prevent contamination.

Step 4 – Urethral lubrication and scope insertion
Instruments: Lubricant, cystoscope with obturator.
Anticipation: Surgeon may pause during insertion. Maintain clear visualization and quiet field.

Step 5 – Remove obturator and insert lens
Instruments: Cystoscope lens.
Anticipation: Be ready to hand lens smoothly to maintain flow without fogging or contamination.

Step 6 – Bladder inspection
Instruments: Irrigation system managed .
Anticipation: Surgeon may request changes in irrigation flow or lens angle. Anticipate camera adjustments.

Step 7 – Identify bladder tumor(s)
Instruments: None additional.
Anticipation: This step guides TURBT planning. Be attentive to surgeon comments regarding tumor location and size.

Step 8 – Overview of TURBT equipment setup
Instruments: Resectoscope components displayed but not used.
Anticipation: Do not open resection loops or cautery accessories unless proceeding to TURBT.

Step 9 – Final inspection and scope removal
Instruments: Cystoscope.
Anticipation: Be prepared to receive scope safely and protect optics immediately.

Step 10 – Apply dressing if indicated
Instruments: Gauze.
Anticipation: Minimal dressing usually required. Maintain patient dignity during undraping.

Mayo Stand Suggestion:

- Lubricant syringe
- Gauze sponges
- 2 mosquito hemostats
- Cystoscope
- Resectoscope

Epispadias Repair (Male Patient)

Step 1 – Patient positioning and verification
Instruments: Supine positioning aids, padding.
Anticipation: Confirm patient age, defect severity, and laterality. Pediatric patients require careful positioning and warming.

Step 2 – Genital preparation and sterile draping
Instruments: Prep supplies, fenestrated pediatric drape.
Anticipation: Prep must include penis, scrotum, and lower abdomen. Ensure unobstructed access to entire phallus.

Step 3 – Catheter placement if used
Instruments: Foley catheter passed from back table.
Anticipation: Catheter size varies by age. Confirm correct size before opening.

Step 4 – Mark urethral reconstruction lines
Instruments: Skin marker.
Anticipation: Surgeon may re mark after draping. Keep marker accessible.

Step 5 – Penile skin incision and flap development
Instruments: Scalpel handle with #15 blade, Adsons forceps with teeth.
Anticipation: Incisions are precise. Be ready to pass mosquito hemostats promptly for bleeding control.

Step 6 – Mobilize urethral plate and surrounding tissues
Instruments: Fine scissors, 2 mosquito hemostats, fine forceps.
Anticipation: Tissue handling must be gentle. Maintain organized clamp placement.

Step 7 – Tubularize or reconstruct urethra
Instruments: Brought from back table when requested.
Anticipation: This signals transition to suturing. Bring needle driver and fine sutures only when surgeon commits.

Step 8 – Correct dorsal chordee if present
Instruments: Fine scissors.
Anticipation: Surgeon may reassess penile straightening multiple times. Keep field clear.

Step 9 – Reapproximate penile skin
Instruments: Brought from back table when requested.
Anticipation: Closure is layered and delicate. Avoid rushing handoffs.

Step 10 – Apply dressing and secure catheter
Instruments: Dressing supplies.
Anticipation: Ensure dressing does not compress urethral repair or catheter.

Mayo Stand Suggestion:

- Scalpel handle with #15 blade
- Adsons forceps with teeth & smooth
- Fine Metzenbaum scissors
- 2 small curved hemostats
- 2 mosquito hemostats
- Small skin hooks
- Allis

Hydrocelectomy

Step 1 – Patient positioning and verification
Instruments: Supine positioning aids, padding.
Anticipation: Confirm patient age, defect severity, and laterality. Pediatric patients require careful positioning and warming.

Step 2 – Genital preparation and sterile draping
Instruments: Prep supplies, fenestrated pediatric drape.
Anticipation: Prep must include penis, scrotum, and lower abdomen. Ensure unobstructed access to entire phallus.

Step 3 – Catheter placement if used
Instruments: Foley catheter passed from back table.
Anticipation: Catheter size varies by age. Confirm correct size before opening.

Step 4 – Mark urethral reconstruction lines
Instruments: Skin marker.
Anticipation: Surgeon may re mark after draping. Keep marker accessible.

Step 5 – Penile skin incision and flap development
Instruments: Scalpel handle with #15 blade, Adsons forceps with teeth.
Anticipation: Incisions are precise. Be ready to pass mosquito hemostats promptly for bleeding control.

Step 6 – Mobilize urethral plate and surrounding tissues
Instruments: Fine scissors, 2 mosquito hemostats, fine forceps.
Anticipation: Tissue handling must be gentle. Maintain organized clamp placement.

Step 7 – Tubularize or reconstruct urethra
Instruments: Brought from back table when requested.
Anticipation: This signals transition to suturing. Bring needle driver and fine sutures only when surgeon commits.

Step 8 – Correct dorsal chordee if present
Instruments: Fine scissors.
Anticipation: Surgeon may reassess penile straightening multiple times. Keep field clear.

Step 9 – Reapproximate penile skin
Instruments: Brought from back table when requested.
Anticipation: Closure is layered and delicate. Avoid rushing handoffs.

Step 10 – Apply dressing and secure catheter
Instruments: Dressing supplies.
Anticipation: Ensure dressing does not compress urethral repair or catheter.

Mayo Stand Suggestion:

- Scalpel handle with #10 or #15 blade
- Adsons forceps with teeth
- Metzenbaum scissors
- 2 curved mosquito hemostats
- 2 right angle
- 2 Allis
- Senn & Army Navy retractor

Hypospadias Repair (Male Patient)

Step 1 – Patient positioning and verification
Instruments: Supine positioning aids, padding, warming devices.
Anticipation: Pediatric cases require careful positioning and temperature management. Confirm defect type and planned repair technique.

Step 2 – Genital preparation and sterile draping
Instruments: Prep supplies, pediatric fenestrated drape.
Anticipation: Prep must include penis, scrotum, and lower abdomen. Ensure full access to shaft and glans.

Step 3 – Urethral catheter placement if used
Instruments: Foley catheter passed from back table.
Anticipation: Catheter size is age dependent. Confirm correct size before opening.

Step 4 – Mark urethral plate and incision lines
Instruments: Skin marker.
Anticipation: Surgeon may re mark after draping. Keep marker readily available.

Step 5 – Penile skin incision and flap elevation
Instruments: Scalpel handle with #15 blade, Adsons forceps with teeth.
Anticipation: Incisions are delicate. Be ready to pass mosquito hemostats immediately for bleeding control.

Step 6 – Mobilize urethral plate and correct chordee
Instruments: Fine scissors, 2 mosquito hemostats, fine forceps.
Anticipation: Gentle handling preserves blood supply. Maintain organized clamp placement.

Step 7 – Tubularize urethra
Instruments: Brought from back table when requested.
Anticipation: Transition to suturing phase. Bring needle driver and fine sutures only when surgeon commits.

Step 8 – Interpose tissue layer if required
Instruments: Passed from back table when requested.
Anticipation: Surgeon may add a protective layer. Do not anticipate without confirmation.

Step 9 – Reapproximate penile skin
Instruments: Brought from back table when requested.
Anticipation: Closure is layered and cosmetic. Avoid rushing handoffs.

Step 10 – Apply dressing and secure catheter
Instruments: Dressing supplies.
Anticipation: Ensure dressing does not compress urethral repair or catheter.

Mayo Stand Suggestion:

- Scalpel handle with #15 blade
- Adsons forceps with teeth & smooth
- Fine Metzenbaum scissors
- 2 small curved hemostats
- 2 mosquito hemostats
- Small skin hooks
- Allis

Insertion of Inflatable Penile Prosthesis

Step 1 – Patient positioning and verification
Instruments: Supine positioning aids, padding.
Anticipation: Confirm implant type and size availability before prep. Position patient to allow perineal and lower abdominal access.

Step 2 – Genital and lower abdominal preparation and draping
Instruments: Prep supplies, fenestrated drape.
Anticipation: Prep must include penis, scrotum, and lower abdomen for reservoir placement.

Step 3 – Foley catheter placement
Instruments: Foley catheter passed from back table.
Anticipation: Catheter protects urethra during corporal dilation. Confirm size before opening.

Step 4 – Incision (penoscrotal or infrapubic)
Instruments: Scalpel handle with #15 blade, Adsons forceps with teeth.
Anticipation: Incision dictates exposure. Be ready with mosquito hemostats for bleeding control.

Step 5 – Expose corpora cavernosa
Instruments: Metzenbaum scissors, 2 mosquito hemostats, small retractor.
Anticipation: Corporal exposure requires steady retraction. Keep clamps organized.

Step 6 – Corporotomy and corporal dilation
Instruments: Dilators passed from back table when requested.
Anticipation: Dilation is sequential. Have sizes ready but unopened.

Step 7 – Measure corporal length
Instruments: Measuring tool passed from back table.
Anticipation: Measurements determine cylinder size. Avoid distraction during this step.

Step 8 – Insert prosthesis cylinders
Instruments: Prosthesis cylinders passed from back table when requested.
Anticipation: This is a sterile critical moment. Open implant only when surgeon commits.

Step 9 – Place pump and reservoir
Instruments: Pump and reservoir passed from back table.
Anticipation: Ensure tubing is not kinked or twisted during placement.

Step 10 – Connect components and test inflation
Instruments: Connection tools passed from back table.
Anticipation: Watch tubing orientation closely. Anticipate saline fill confirmation.

Step 11 – Close corporotomy and incision
Instruments: Brought from back table when requested.
Anticipation: Closure instruments come forward only after prosthesis function is confirmed.

Step 12 – Apply dressing and scrotal support
Instruments: Dressing supplies, scrotal support.
Anticipation: Ensure pump position is correct before final dressing.

Mayo Stand Suggestion:

- Scalpel handle with #15 blade
- Adsons forceps with teeth & smooth
- Metzenbaum scissors
- 2 Allis
- 2 mosquito hemostats
- Senn & Army Navy retractor

Kidney Transplant

Step 1 – Patient positioning and verification
Instruments: Supine positioning aids, padding, arm boards.
Anticipation: Confirm donor kidney side and recipient iliac fossa plan. Ensure wide access to lower abdomen and groin.

Step 2 – Abdominal and groin preparation and draping
Instruments: Prep supplies, large sterile drapes.
Anticipation: Prep must include entire lower abdomen, groin, and thigh for possible vascular access.

Step 3 – Lower quadrant incision
Instruments: Scalpel handle with #10 blade, Adsons forceps with teeth.
Anticipation: Incision is deep with expected bleeding. Be ready to pass mosquito hemostats promptly.

Step 4 – Dissect to expose iliac vessels
Instruments: Metzenbaum scissors, 2 mosquito hemostats, small retractor.
Anticipation: Maintain organized clamp placement. Anticipate gradual exposure of vein first, then artery.

Step 5 – Prepare iliac vessels for anastomosis
Instruments: Vessel loops passed from back table.
Anticipation: Vessel control is critical. Keep loops ready but unopened until requested.

Step 6 – Receive and position donor kidney
Instruments: Kidney handled on sterile basin.
Anticipation: Maintain organ orientation and moisture. Do not allow tension or twisting of vessels.

Step 7 – Venous anastomosis
Instruments: Brought from back table when requested.
Anticipation: Absolute stillness is required. Anticipate suture handoffs without rushing.

Step 8 – Arterial anastomosis
Instruments: Passed from back table when requested.
Anticipation: Be alert for clamp release sequence and immediate reperfusion observation.

Step 9 – Restore blood flow and assess perfusion
Instruments: None additional.
Anticipation: Watch for color change and turgor. Be prepared for rapid response if bleeding occurs.

Step 10 – Ureteral implantation into bladder
Instruments: Passed from back table when requested.
Anticipation: This marks transition to urologic reconstruction. Avoid unnecessary instrument clutter.

Step 11 – Inspect hemostasis and position kidney
Instruments: Managed from back table.
Anticipation: Hemostasis must be meticulous to prevent postoperative bleeding.

Kidney Transplant

Step 12 – Place drains if indicated
Instruments: Drains passed from back table.
Anticipation: Confirm number and exit sites before placement.

Step 13 – Layered closure
Instruments: Brought from back table when requested.
Anticipation: Begin closing counts early. Closure instruments come forward only after surgeon commits.

Mayo Stand Suggestion:

- Scalpel handle with #10 blade
- Adsons forceps with teeth
- Metzenbaum scissors
- 2 mosquito hemostats
- Small retractor

Laparoscopic Prostatectomy with Robot

Step 1 – Patient positioning and safety checks
Instruments: Lithotomy positioning aids, padding, arm tucking supplies.
Anticipation: Steep Trendelenburg is required. Confirm arms, face, and pressure points are well protected before prep.

Step 2 – Abdominal preparation and wide robotic draping
Instruments: Abdominal prep supplies, robotic drapes.
Anticipation: Prep must extend from xiphoid to mid thighs. Ensure access for assistant port and camera.

Step 3 – Establish pneumoperitoneum
Instruments: Veress needle or optical trocar passed from back table.
Anticipation: Confirm insufflator is tested and ready. Be alert for pressure alarms.

Step 4 – Trocar placement
Instruments: Laparoscopic trocars passed from back table.
Anticipation: Trocar placement is precise for robotic arm spacing. Hand trocars deliberately and keep caps controlled.

Step 5 – Dock robotic system
Instruments: Robot docked by team.
Anticipation: Ensure cords and tubing are clear before docking. Mayo should be cleared during docking.

Step 6 – Console dissection of prostate
Instruments: Robotic instruments controlled at console.
Anticipation: Anticipate instrument exchanges and coordinate with circulator for smooth swaps.

Step 7 – Control dorsal venous complex
Instruments: Passed from back table if assistant instruments are needed.
Anticipation: Bleeding control is critical. Be ready with clips or sutures as requested.

Step 8 – Nerve sparing dissection if indicated
Instruments: Managed from back table.
Anticipation: Surgeon may slow pace significantly. Maintain quiet, focused field.

Laparoscopic Prostatectomy with Robot

Step 9 – Transect urethra and remove prostate
Instruments: Specimen retrieval bag passed from back table when requested.
Anticipation: Open bag only when surgeon confirms specimen ready for extraction.

Step 10 – Vesicourethral anastomosis
Instruments: Passed from back table when requested.
Anticipation: This is a suturing intensive step. Anticipate suture changes without rushing.

Step 11 – Undock robot and inspect field
Instruments: None additional.
Anticipation: Ensure all robotic instruments are accounted for before undocking.

Step 12 – Close port sites
Instruments: Brought from back table when requested.
Anticipation: Closure instruments come forward only after undocking is complete.

Mayo Stand Suggestion:

- Scalpel handle with #11 blade
- Adsons forceps with teeth
- 2 mosquito hemostats
- Gauze sponges

Laparoscopic Simple Nephrectomy

Step 1 – Patient positioning and safety verification
Instruments: Lateral decubitus positioning aids, padding, bean bag, axillary roll.
Anticipation: Confirm operative side is up. Protect pressure points and ensure patient is fully secured before table rotation.

Step 2 – Abdominal preparation and wide draping
Instruments: Prep supplies, laparoscopic drapes.
Anticipation: Prep from mid chest to mid thigh. Maintain access for possible specimen extraction incision.

Step 3 – Establish pneumoperitoneum
Instruments: Veress needle or optical entry device passed from back table.
Anticipation: Confirm insufflator function and pressure settings before insertion.

Step 4 – Trocar placement
Instruments: Laparoscopic trocars passed from back table.
Anticipation: Trocar placement is strategic. Hand trocars deliberately and control caps.

Step 5 – Mobilize colon to expose kidney
Instruments: Managed via laparoscopic instruments.
Anticipation: Be ready to assist with retraction through assistant port if requested.

Step 6 – Identify ureter and renal hilum
Instruments: Managed .
Anticipation: Surgeon may request clips or stapler preparation. Do not open until confirmed.

Step 7 – Control renal vessels
Instruments: Clips or vascular stapler passed from back table when requested.
Anticipation: Vessel control is critical. Maintain strict implant discipline.

Laparoscopic Simple Nephrectomy

Step 8 – Divide ureter
Instruments: Passed from back table when requested.
Anticipation: Confirm clip placement sequence before division.

Step 9 – Free kidney from surrounding attachments
Instruments: Managed .
Anticipation: Dissection proceeds circumferentially. Maintain clear communication.

Step 10 – Place kidney in specimen retrieval bag
Instruments: Specimen bag passed from back table when requested.
Anticipation: Open bag only when kidney is fully mobilized.

Step 11 – Enlarge extraction site and remove specimen
Instruments: Scalpel handle with #10 or #15 blade passed from back table.
Anticipation: Incision enlargement may be brief. Be ready with blade promptly.

Step 12 – Inspect hemostasis and irrigate
Instruments: Managed .
Anticipation: Assist without introducing suction to Mayo.

Step 13 – Close port sites
Instruments: Brought from back table when requested.
Anticipation: Closure instruments come forward only after final inspection.

Mayo Stand Suggestion:

- Scalpel handle with #11 blade
- Adsons forceps with teeth
- 2 mosquito hemostats
- Gauze sponges

Marshall Marchetti Krantz Procedure

Step 1 – Patient positioning and verification
Instruments: Supine positioning aids, padding, Foley catheter placed by anesthesia or surgeon.
Anticipation: Confirm procedure and indication. Ensure bladder is decompressed before incision.

Step 2 – Lower abdominal preparation and sterile draping
Instruments: Prep supplies, abdominal drapes.
Anticipation: Prep must include lower abdomen and perineum. Maintain access to urethra and bladder neck region.

Step 3 – Pfannenstiel or lower midline incision
Instruments: Scalpel handle with #10 blade, Adsons forceps with teeth.
Anticipation: Incision is controlled but deep. Be ready to pass mosquito hemostats promptly.

Step 4 – Dissect to retropubic space
Instruments: Metzenbaum scissors, 2 mosquito hemostats, small retractor.
Anticipation: Bladder and urethra are nearby. Gentle dissection and clear visualization are critical.

Step 5 – Identify bladder neck and periurethral tissue
Instruments: Fine forceps.
Anticipation: Surgeon may palpate Foley balloon to localize anatomy. Maintain quiet field.

Marshall Marchetti Krantz Procedure

Step 6 – Place sutures to suspend urethra to pubic symphysis
Instruments: Brought from back table when requested.
Anticipation: This is a key functional step. Bring needle driver and sutures only when surgeon commits.

Step 7 – Confirm urethral support and bladder integrity
Instruments: None additional.
Anticipation: Surgeon may request bladder filling or manipulation. Be ready to assist indirectly.

Step 8 – Inspect hemostasis
Instruments: Mosquito hemostats if needed.
Anticipation: Hemostasis is critical to prevent retropubic hematoma.

Step 9 – Layered closure
Instruments: Brought from back table when requested.
Anticipation: Begin closing counts early. Closure instruments come forward only after surgeon commits.

Mayo Stand Suggestion:

- Scalpel handle with #10 blade
- Adsons forceps with teeth
- Metzenbaum scissors
- 2 mosquito hemostats
- Small retractor

Open Simple Nephrectomy

Step 1 – Patient positioning and verification
Instruments: Lateral decubitus positioning aids, bean bag, axillary roll, padding.
Anticipation: Confirm operative side is up. Secure patient fully before table flexion.

Step 2 – Abdominal or flank preparation and draping
Instruments: Prep supplies, large sterile drapes.
Anticipation: Prep widely to allow extension of incision if exposure becomes difficult.

Step 3 – Flank or subcostal incision
Instruments: Scalpel handle with #10 blade, Adsons forceps with teeth.
Anticipation: Incision is deep with muscle layers. Be ready to pass mosquito hemostats promptly.

Step 4 – Divide muscle layers and enter retroperitoneum
Instruments: Metzenbaum scissors, 2 mosquito hemostats, Adsons forceps.
Anticipation: Follow clamp-cut rhythm. Maintain organized clamp placement to control bleeding

Step 5 – Retract tissues to expose kidney
Instruments: Small handheld retractor if repeatedly used.
Anticipation: Exposure deepens quickly. Keep Mayo uncluttered and pass large retractor from back table only when requested.

Step 6 – Identify ureter and renal hilum
Instruments: Metzenbaum scissors.
Anticipation: Surgeon may isolate ureter first. Anticipate vessel control instruments but do not open until confirmed.

Open Simple Nephrectomy

Step 7 – Ligate and divide renal vessels
Instruments: Passed from back table when requested.
Anticipation: Vessel ligation sequence matters. Be alert to clamp and tie order.

Step 8 – Free kidney from surrounding attachments
Instruments: Metzenbaum scissors.
Anticipation: Expect slow circumferential dissection. Keep scissors clean and ready.

Step 9 – Remove kidney specimen
Instruments: Specimen container opened early.
Anticipation: Coordinate specimen handling promptly to maintain sterile field.

Step 10 – Inspect hemostasis and irrigate
Instruments: Managed from back table.
Anticipation: Bleeding control is critical. Assist without adding suction to Mayo.

Step 11 – Place drain if indicated
Instruments: Drain passed from back table.
Anticipation: Confirm exit site before placement.

Step 12 – Layered closure
Instruments: Brought from back table when requested.
Anticipation: Begin closing counts early. Closure instruments come forward only after surgeon commits.

Mayo Stand Suggestion:

- Scalpel handle with #10 blade
- Adsons forceps with teeth
- Metzenbaum scissors
- Vessel Loops
- 2 mosquito hemostats
- Army Navy retractor
- Richardson retractor

Orchiopexy

Step 1 – Patient positioning and verification
Instruments: Supine positioning aids, padding, warming devices.
Anticipation: Pediatric patients require careful positioning and temperature control. Confirm laterality before prep.

Step 2 – Inguinal and scrotal preparation and draping
Instruments: Prep supplies, pediatric fenestrated drape.
Anticipation: Prep must include lower abdomen, groin, and scrotum to allow testicular mobilization.

Step 3 – Inguinal incision
Instruments: Scalpel handle with #15 blade, Adsons forceps with teeth.
Anticipation: Incision is small but vascular. Be ready to pass mosquito hemostats promptly.

Step 4 – Dissect through inguinal canal
Instruments: Metzenbaum scissors, 2 mosquito hemostats, Adsons forceps.
Anticipation: Tissue planes are delicate. Maintain organized clamp placement.

Orchiopexy

Step 5 – Identify and mobilize undescended testicle
Instruments: Fine forceps, Metzenbaum scissors.
Anticipation: Gentle handling preserves blood supply. Avoid excessive traction.

Step 6 – Ligate patent processus vaginalis if present
Instruments: Passed from back table when requested.
Anticipation: This step mirrors hernia repair. Anticipate suture readiness without opening early.

Step 7 – Create scrotal pouch
Instruments: Scalpel handle with #15 blade, Metzenbaum scissors.
Anticipation: Coordinate timing between inguinal and scrotal fields smoothly.

Step 8 – Deliver and secure testicle into scrotum
Instruments: Passed from back table when requested.
Anticipation: Ensure cord is not twisted. Surgeon may check tension repeatedly.

Step 9 – Inspect hemostasis
Instruments: Mosquito hemostats.
Anticipation: Bleeding control prevents postoperative hematoma.

Step 10 – Close incisions
Instruments: Brought from back table when requested.
Anticipation: Begin closing counts early. Closure instruments come forward only after surgeon commits.

Mayo Stand Suggestion:

- Scalpel handle with #10 blade
- Adsons forceps with teeth
- Metzenbaum scissors
- 2 mosquito hemostats
- Handheld retractor

Penectomy

Step 1 – Patient positioning and verification
Instruments: Supine positioning aids, padding, grounding pad placed by anesthesia.
Anticipation: Confirm partial vs total penectomy and planned urinary diversion before prep. Position must allow perineal access if urethrostomy is planned.

Step 2 – Genital and perineal preparation and draping
Instruments: Prep supplies, wide fenestrated drape.
Anticipation: Prep must include penis, scrotum, and perineum. Maintain exposure for possible perineal urethrostomy.

Step 3 – Foley catheter placement
Instruments: Foley catheter passed from back table.
Anticipation: Catheter helps identify urethra. Confirm size before opening.

Step 4 – Mark level of resection
Instruments: Skin marker.
Anticipation: Surgeon may reassess margins before incision. Keep marker available.

Penectomy

Step 5 – Circumferential skin incision
Instruments: Scalpel handle with #10 or #15 blade, Adsons forceps with teeth.
Anticipation: Bleeding is expected early. Be ready with mosquito hemostats immediately.

Step 6 – Dissect through corporal bodies
Instruments: Metzenbaum scissors, 2 mosquito hemostats, Adsons forceps.
Anticipation: Follow clamp-cut rhythm closely. Organized clamp placement prevents confusion.

Step 7 – Identify and transect urethra
Instruments: Metzenbaum scissors.
Anticipation: Surgeon may pause to confirm margins. Maintain quiet field.

Step 8 – Control corporal and dorsal vessels
Instruments: Mosquito hemostats.
Anticipation: Vascular control is critical. Anticipate repeated clamp placement.

Step 9 – Remove specimen
Instruments: Specimen container opened early.
Anticipation: Coordinate specimen handling promptly and maintain sterility.

Step 10 – Create urethral meatus or perineal urethrostomy
Instruments: Passed from back table when requested.
Anticipation: This marks transition to reconstruction. Closure instruments come forward only when surgeon commits.

Step 11 – Inspect hemostasis
Instruments: Mosquito hemostats if needed.
Anticipation: Hemostasis must be meticulous to prevent postoperative bleeding.

Step 12 – Layered closure and dressing
Instruments: Brought from back table when requested.
Anticipation: Begin closing counts early. Ensure catheter is secured before dressing application.

Mayo Stand Suggestion:

- Scalpel handle with #10 blade
- Adsons forceps with teeth
- Metzenbaum scissors
- 2 mosquito hemostats
- Handheld retractor

Percutaneous Implantation of Radioactive Seeds in the Prostate Gland

Step 1 – Patient positioning and verification
Instruments: Lithotomy stirrups, padding, grounding pad placed by anesthesia.
Anticipation: Confirm seed count with radiation safety protocols before prep.

Step 2 – Perineal preparation and sterile draping
Instruments: Perineal prep supplies, brachytherapy drape.
Anticipation: Prep must include perineum, scrotum, and lower abdomen. Maintain clear access for ultrasound probe and needle grid.

Step 3 – Insert transrectal ultrasound probe
Instruments: Ultrasound probe and cover managed .
Anticipation: Confirm probe cover integrity and secure cords to avoid contamination.

Percutaneous Implantation of Radioactive Seeds in the Prostate Gland

Step 4 – Attach template grid to perineum
Instruments: Template grid system.
Anticipation: Ensure grid alignment is correct before needle insertion begins.

Step 5 – Load implantation needles
Instruments: Needles passed from back table when requested.
Anticipation: Seeds remain shielded until immediately before use. Maintain radiation safety awareness at all times.

Step 6 – Percutaneous needle insertion through template
Instruments: Implant needles.
Anticipation: Needle placement is sequential. Track needle count carefully.

Step 7 – Deploy radioactive seeds into prostate
Instruments: Seed deployment devices.
Anticipation: Confirm seed count and placement verbally if required. Maintain quiet, focused environment.

Step 8 – Remove needles and confirm placement
Instruments: None additional.
Anticipation: Watch for bleeding at needle sites. Be ready with sponges for gentle pressure.

Step 9 – Final ultrasound assessment
Instruments: Ultrasound probe.
Anticipation: Surgeon may pause to reassess dosimetry. Do not rush workflow.

Step 10 – Remove equipment and apply dressing
Instruments: Dressing supplies.
Anticipation: Ensure no radioactive material remains on field before break down.

Mayo Stand Suggestion:

- Gauze Sponges
- 2 Mosquito Hemostats

Pyelolithotomy

Step 1 – Patient positioning and verification
Instruments: Lateral decubitus positioning aids, bean bag, axillary roll, padding.
Anticipation: Confirm operative side is up. Secure patient fully before table flexion.

Step 2 – Flank or subcostal preparation and draping
Instruments: Prep supplies, large sterile drapes.
Anticipation: Prep widely to allow extension of incision if needed for exposure.

Step 3 – Flank or subcostal incision
Instruments: Scalpel handle with #10 blade, Adsons forceps with teeth.
Anticipation: Incision is deep with muscle layers. Be ready with mosquito hemostats immediately.

Step 4 – Divide muscle layers and enter retroperitoneum
Instruments: Metzenbaum scissors, 2 mosquito hemostats, Adsons forceps.
Anticipation: Follow clamp-cut rhythm closely. Maintain organized clamp placement.

Pyelolithotomy

Step 5 – Retract tissues to expose kidney and renal pelvis
Instruments: Small handheld retractor if repeatedly used.
Anticipation: Exposure deepens quickly. Large retractor are passed from back table only when requested.

Step 6 – Identify renal pelvis and stone location
Instruments: Metzenbaum scissors.
Anticipation: Surgeon may palpate kidney to localize stone. Maintain quiet field.

Step 7 – Incise renal pelvis
Instruments: Scalpel handle with #15 blade, fine scissors.
Anticipation: Anticipate controlled bleeding. Be ready to pass mosquito hemostats promptly.

Step 8 – Remove stone(s)
Instruments: Stone forceps passed from back table when requested.
Anticipation: Open specimen container early. Multiple stones may be removed sequentially.

Step 9 – Inspect renal pelvis for residual stones
Instruments: None additional.
Anticipation: Surgeon may irrigate or palpate again. Avoid cluttering the field.

Step 10 – Close renal pelvis
Instruments: Brought from back table when requested.
Anticipation: This marks transition to fine suturing. Bring needle driver and sutures only when surgeon commits.

Step 11 – Inspect hemostasis and place drain if indicated
Instruments: Drain passed from back table when requested.
Anticipation: Confirm drain exit site before placement.

Step 12 – Layered closure
Instruments: Brought from back table when requested.
Anticipation: Begin closing counts early. Closure instruments come forward only after surgeon commits.

Mayo Stand Suggestion:

- Scalpel handle with #10 blade
- Scalpel handle with #15 blade
- Adsons forceps with teeth
- Metzenbaum scissors
- 2 mosquito hemostats
- Small handheld retractor

Radical Cystectomy with Ileal Conduit – Male Patient

Step 1 – Patient positioning and verification
Instruments: Supine positioning aids, padding, arm boards.
Anticipation: Confirm diversion type and stoma site marking pre-prep. Position must allow access to pelvis and right lower quadrant.

Step 2 – Abdominal preparation and wide draping
Instruments: Prep supplies, large abdominal drapes.
Anticipation: Prep from nipples to mid-thighs. Preserve visibility of stoma site.

Radical Cystectomy with Ileal Conduit – Male Patient

Step 3 – Midline abdominal incision
Instruments: Scalpel handle with #10 blade, Adsons forceps with teeth.
Anticipation: Incision is long with early bleeding. Have mosquito hemostats ready immediately.

Step 4 – Enter abdomen and expose pelvis
Instruments: Metzenbaum scissors, 2 mosquito hemostats, small handheld retractor.
Anticipation: Exposure deepens quickly. Pass large retractor from back table only when requested.

Step 5 – Mobilize bladder and identify ureters
Instruments: Metzenbaum scissors, fine forceps.
Anticipation: Ureters are isolated early. Be ready for vessel loops or clips from back table.

Step 6 – Control and divide ureters
Instruments: Passed from back table when requested.
Anticipation: Specimen handling begins. Open labeled specimen containers early.

Step 7 – Dissect and remove bladder and prostate
Instruments: Metzenbaum scissors, mosquito hemostats.
Anticipation: Expect alternating dissection and vascular control. Maintain clamp–cut rhythm.

Step 8 – Pelvic lymph node dissection if performed
Instruments: Passed from back table when requested.
Anticipation: Node packets must be clearly labeled. Track specimens carefully.

Step 9 – Isolate ileal segment for conduit
Instruments: Scalpel handle with #10 blade passed from back table.
Anticipation: Bowel work begins. Ensure bowel is protected with moist laps.

Step 10 – Create ileal conduit
Instruments: Passed from back table when requested.
Anticipation: This is a reconstruction phase. Keep Mayo uncluttered.

Step 11 – Uretero-ileal anastomosis
Instruments: Passed from back table when requested.
Anticipation: Fine suturing. Anticipate stents without opening early.

Step 12 – Mature stoma through abdominal wall
Instruments: Passed from back table when requested.
Anticipation: Confirm stoma orientation before final fixation.

Step 13 – Inspect hemostasis and place drains
Instruments: Drains passed from back table.
Anticipation: Confirm number and exit sites before placement.

Step 14 – Layered abdominal closure
Instruments: Brought from back table when requested.
Anticipation: Begin closing counts early. Closure instruments move forward only after surgeon commits.

Radical Cystectomy with Ileal Conduit – Male Patient

Mayo Stand Suggestion:

- Scalpel handle with #10 blade
- Adsons forceps with teeth
- Metzenbaum scissors
- 2 mosquito hemostats
- Small handheld retractor

Simple Orchiectomy

Step 1 – Patient positioning and verification
Instruments: Supine positioning aids, padding.
Anticipation: Confirm operative side and indication. Position must allow groin and scrotal access.

Step 2 – Inguinal or scrotal preparation and draping
Instruments: Prep supplies, fenestrated drape.
Anticipation: Prep must include groin and scrotum. Maintain exposure in case incision extends.

Step 3 – Inguinal or scrotal incision
Instruments: Scalpel handle with #10 or #15 blade, Adsons forceps with teeth.
Anticipation: Bleeding can occur early. Be ready with mosquito hemostats immediately.

Step 4 – Dissect to expose spermatic cord and testicle
Instruments: Metzenbaum scissors, 2 mosquito hemostats, Adsons forceps.
Anticipation: Follow clamp-cut rhythm. Keep clamp placement organized to avoid tangling the cord.

Step 5 – Mobilize and deliver testicle
Instruments: Gentle traction with forceps or manual handling.
Anticipation: Avoid excessive traction on cord structures.

Step 6 – Clamp and divide spermatic cord
Instruments: Passed from back table when requested.
Anticipation: Cord division sequence matters. Anticipate clamp placement and specimen handling.

Step 7 – Remove testicle specimen
Instruments: Specimen container opened early.
Anticipation: Coordinate specimen handling promptly to maintain sterility.

Step 8 – Inspect hemostasis
Instruments: Mosquito hemostats if needed.
Anticipation: Cord stump bleeding must be controlled to prevent hematoma.

Step 9 – Close incision
Instruments: Brought from back table when requested.
Anticipation: Closure instruments come forward only after surgeon commits.

Step 10 – Apply dressing and scrotal support
Instruments: Dressing supplies, scrotal support.
Anticipation: Ensure compression is adequate without compromising circulation.

Mayo Stand Suggestion:

- Scalpel handle with #10 or #15 blade
- Adsons forceps with teeth
- Metzenbaum scissors
- 2 mosquito hemostats
- Small handheld retractor

Suprapubic Prostatectomy

Step 1 – Patient positioning and verification
Instruments: Supine positioning aids, padding, arm boards.
Anticipation: Confirm indication (BPH) and bladder status. Position must allow lower abdominal and perineal access.

Step 2 – Lower abdominal preparation and sterile draping
Instruments: Prep supplies, abdominal drapes.
Anticipation: Prep from umbilicus to mid-thighs. Maintain clear access to suprapubic region.

Step 3 – Lower midline or Pfannenstiel incision
Instruments: Scalpel handle with #10 blade, Adsons forceps with teeth.
Anticipation: Incision is deep with expected bleeding. Be ready with mosquito hemostats immediately.

Step 4 – Dissect to expose bladder
Instruments: Metzenbaum scissors, 2 mosquito hemostats, Adsons forceps.
Anticipation: Maintain clamp-cut rhythm. Exposure deepens quickly; large retractor are passed from the back table only when requested.

Step 5 – Open bladder (cystotomy)
Instruments: Scalpel handle with #15 blade, Metzenbaum scissors.
Anticipation: Anticipate urine spillage. Keep sponges ready without introducing suction onto the Mayo.

Step 6 – Identify prostate adenoma through bladder neck
Instruments: Metzenbaum scissors.
Anticipation: Surgeon may palpate digitally. Maintain a quiet, unobstructed field.

Step 7 – Enucleate prostate adenoma
Instruments: Metzenbaum scissors, mosquito hemostats.
Anticipation: Bleeding can increase during enucleation. Be ready for rapid clamp placement.

Step 8 – Remove prostate specimen
Instruments: Specimen container opened early.
Anticipation: Coordinate specimen handling promptly and label correctly.

Step 9 – Inspect and control bleeding in prostatic fossa
Instruments: Mosquito hemostats.
Anticipation: Hemostasis is critical to prevent postoperative hemorrhage.

Step 10 – Insert Foley catheter and bladder irrigation tubing
Instruments: Passed from back table when requested.
Anticipation: Confirm catheter size and balloon volume before opening.

Step 11 – Close bladder
Instruments: Brought from back table when requested.
Anticipation: This marks transition to suturing. Bring needle driver and sutures only when surgeon commits.

Step 12 – Place drain if indicated
Instruments: Drain passed from back table.
Anticipation: Confirm exit site before placement.

Suprapubic Prostatectomy

Step 13 – Layered abdominal closure
Instruments: Brought from back table when requested.
Anticipation: Begin closing counts early. Closure instruments move forward only after surgeon commits.

Mayo Stand Suggestion:

- Scalpel handle with #10 or #15 blade
- Adsons forceps with teeth
- Metzenbaum scissors
- 2 mosquito hemostats
- Small handheld retractor

Transurethral Resection of the Prostate (TURP)

Step 1 – Patient positioning and verification
Instruments: Lithotomy stirrups, padding, grounding pad placed by anesthesia.
Anticipation: Confirm monopolar vs bipolar system (affects irrigation fluid). Verify leg symmetry and pressure points.

Step 2 – Perineal preparation and sterile draping
Instruments: Perineal prep supplies, TUR drape.
Anticipation: Prep includes penis, scrotum, perineum. Ensure fenestration aligns with urethral meatus.

Step 3 – Assemble and test resectoscope system
Instruments: Resectoscope sheath, obturator, lens, camera, light cord ().
Anticipation: Test optics and light before insertion. Ensure correct loop and irrigation tubing are available but unopened.

Step 4 – Insert resectoscope into urethra
Instruments: Lubricant syringe.
Anticipation: Surgeon may pause during insertion. Maintain quiet field and protect optics.

Step 5 – Remove obturator and insert lens with loop
Instruments: Resectoscope lens and loop ().
Anticipation: Confirm loop orientation and electrical connection before activation.

Step 6 – Begin systematic prostate resection
Instruments: Resectoscope loop and irrigation system ().
Anticipation: Expect repeated requests for loop changes. Keep replacements ready but unopened.

Step 7 – Evacuate resected chips periodically
Instruments: Ellik evacuator managed .
Anticipation: Coordinate chip evacuation smoothly to maintain visualization.

Step 8 – Inspect prostatic fossa and achieve hemostasis
Instruments: Managed via resectoscope system.
Anticipation: Bleeding control is critical. Be attentive to changes in irrigation clarity.

Step 9 – Final bladder inspection
Instruments: Resectoscope.
Anticipation: Surgeon confirms no residual chips or bleeding sites.

Transurethral Resection of the Prostate (TURP)

Step 10 – Remove scope and insert Foley catheter
Instruments: Foley catheter passed from back table.
Anticipation: Confirm catheter size and balloon volume. Continuous bladder irrigation may follow.

Step 11 – Apply dressing and secure catheter
Instruments: Gauze, catheter securement.
Anticipation: Ensure catheter tubing is not kinked before patient repositioning.

Mayo Stand Suggestion:

- No Mayo Stand, Typically just working from backtable

Ureteroscopy (Male Patient)

Step 1 – Patient positioning and verification
Instruments: Lithotomy stirrups, padding, grounding pad placed by anesthesia.
Anticipation: Confirm side and indication (diagnostic vs stone removal). Ensure legs are symmetric to prevent nerve injury.

Step 2 – Perineal preparation and sterile draping
Instruments: Perineal prep supplies, cystoscopy/ureteroscopy drape.
Anticipation: Prep must include penis, scrotum, and perineum. Ensure clear access to urethral meatus.

Step 3 – Assemble and test endoscopic equipment
Instruments: Cystoscope, ureteroscope, camera, light source
Anticipation: Test optics and white balance before insertion. Keep cords organized and off the Mayo.

Step 4 – Cystoscopic access to ureteral orifice
Instruments: Cystoscope with obturator
Anticipation: Surgeon may need lens or scope angle changes. Be ready to assist without crowding the field.

Step 5 – Insert guidewire into ureter
Instruments: Guidewire passed from back table when requested.
Anticipation: Do not open wires early. Maintain sterility and track wire length carefully.

Step 6 – Advance ureteroscope over guidewire
Instruments: Ureteroscope
Anticipation: Scope advancement is delicate. Protect optics and avoid tension on the wire.

Step 7 – Identify pathology (stone or stricture)
Instruments: None additional.
Anticipation: Surgeon may pause for visualization. Maintain quiet, stable field.

Step 8 – Treat pathology if indicated
Instruments: Stone basket or laser fiber passed from back table when requested.
Anticipation: Confirm correct accessory before opening. Track all devices placed into the urinary tract.

Ureteroscopy (Male Patient)

Step 9 – Retrieve stone fragments if present
Instruments: Basket device
Anticipation: Specimen cup should be opened early but kept .

Step 10 – Place ureteral stent if indicated
Instruments: Stent passed from back table when requested.
Anticipation: Confirm stent size and laterality before opening.

Step 11 – Remove scope and complete procedure
Instruments: Endoscope.
Anticipation: Be ready to receive scope safely and protect optics immediately.

Step 12 – Foley catheter placement if ordered
Instruments: Foley catheter passed from back table.
Anticipation: Confirm catheter size and balloon volume before opening.

Mayo Stand Suggestion:

- No Mayo Stand, Typically just working from backtable

Wilms Tumor Excision

Step 1 – Patient positioning and verification
Instruments: Supine positioning aids, padding, warming devices.
Anticipation: Pediatric patient—confirm side and tumor size. Maintain normothermia and protect pressure points.

Step 2 – Abdominal preparation and wide sterile draping
Instruments: Prep supplies, large pediatric drapes.
Anticipation: Prep from chest to groin. Wide exposure is needed in case of tumor extension.

Step 3 – Abdominal incision (transverse or midline)
Instruments: Scalpel handle with #10 blade, Adsons forceps with teeth.
Anticipation: Incision may be extended. Be ready with mosquito hemostats early.

Step 4 – Enter abdomen and explore
Instruments: Metzenbaum scissors, 2 mosquito hemostats, Adsons forceps.
Anticipation: Tumor rupture must be avoided. Gentle tissue handling is critical.

Step 5 – Mobilize colon to expose kidney
Instruments: Metzenbaum scissors.
Anticipation: Exposure is gradual. Large retractor are passed from back table only when requested.

Step 6 – Identify and control renal vessels early
Instruments: Passed from back table when requested.
Anticipation: Early vascular control reduces tumor bleeding. Anticipate clamp sequence without opening early.

Step 7 – Mobilize kidney with intact tumor capsule
Instruments: Metzenbaum scissors, mosquito hemostats.
Anticipation: Avoid tumor spillage. Keep dissection slow and controlled.

Wilms Tumor Excision

Step 8 – Ligate and divide ureter
Instruments: Passed from back table when requested.
Anticipation: Specimen handling begins—open specimen container early.

Step 9 – Remove kidney and tumor en bloc
Instruments: Specimen container.
Anticipation: Handle specimen gently. Coordinate immediate transfer to pathology.

Step 10 – Inspect operative field for tumor spillage or bleeding
Instruments: Mosquito hemostats if needed.
Anticipation: Assist with visualization so the surgeon can inspect the operative field.

Step 11 – Place drain if indicated
Instruments: Drain passed from back table.
Anticipation: Confirm exit site before placement.

Step 12 – Layered abdominal closure
Instruments: Brought from back table when requested.
Anticipation: Begin closing counts early. Closure instruments move forward only after surgeon commits.

Mayo Stand Suggestion:

- Scalpel handle with #10 blade
- Adsons forceps with teeth
- Metzenbaum scissors
- Vascular Clamps
- 2 mosquito hemostats
- Small handheld retractor
- Large retractor
- Mayo Scissors

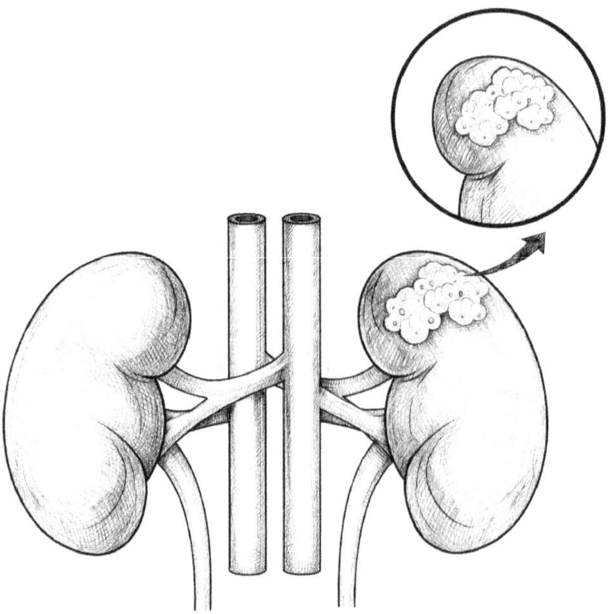

Section VIII:

Orthopedic Procedures

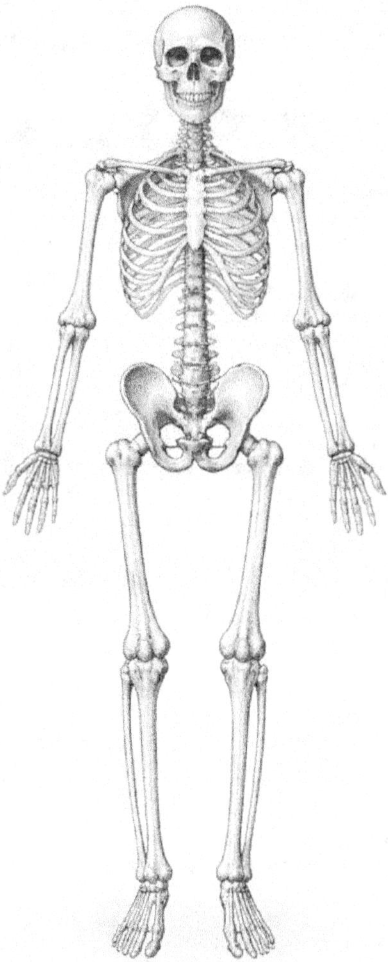

Above the Knee Amputation (AKA)

Step 1 – Patient positioning and verification
Instruments: Supine positioning aids, padding, tourniquet placed but not inflated.
Anticipation: Confirm level of amputation and side. Ensure stump positioning allows straight flap closure.

Step 2 – Extremity preparation and wide draping
Instruments: Prep supplies, sterile towels, extremity drape.
Anticipation: Prep well proximal to planned incision to allow flap adjustment if needed.

Step 3 – Skin marking and flap design
Instruments: Skin marker.
Anticipation: Surgeon may adjust flap length based on tissue quality. Keep marker accessible.

Step 4 – Circumferential skin and subcutaneous incision
Instruments: Scalpel handle with #10 blade, Adsons forceps with teeth.
Anticipation: Incision is long and vascular. Be ready with mosquito hemostats immediately.

Step 5 – Divide muscle layers to femur
Instruments: Metzenbaum scissors, 2 mosquito hemostats, Adsons forceps.
Anticipation: Follow clamp cut rhythm. Maintain organized clamp placement to control bleeding.

Step 6 – Identify and ligate major vessels
Instruments: Passed from back table when requested.
Anticipation: Femoral vessels are controlled individually. Anticipate vessel sequence without opening early.

Step 7 – Transect femur
Instruments: Oscillating saw passed from back table.
Anticipation: Protect soft tissues during bone cut. Clear Mayo and field before saw use.

Step 8 – Smooth bone edges and shape muscle flaps
Instruments: Rasp passed from back table.
Anticipation: Surgeon may test stump contour.

Step 9 – Achieve hemostasis and inspect stump
Instruments: Mosquito hemostats.
Anticipation: Bleeding control is critical before closure.

Step 10 – Place drain if indicated
Instruments: Drain passed from back table.
Anticipation: Confirm exit site before placement.

Step 11 – Layered closure of muscle and skin
Instruments: Brought from back table when requested.
Anticipation: Begin closing counts early. Closure instruments come forward only after surgeon commits.

Step 12 – Apply sterile dressing and compression
Instruments: Dressing supplies, compression wrap.
Anticipation: Ensure even pressure to prevent hematoma without compromising circulation.

Above the Knee Amputation (AKA)

Mayo Stand Suggestion:

- Scalpel handle with #10 blade
- Adsons forceps with teeth
- Metzenbaum scissors
- 2 mosquito hemostats
- Oscillating Saw
- Small handheld retractor
- Large retractor
- Bone Rasp

Acromioplasty, Arthroscopic

Step 1 – Patient positioning and verification
Instruments: Beach chair or lateral decubitus positioning equipment, padding, arm holder or traction device.
Anticipation: Confirm positioning choice and operative shoulder. Secure head and protect pressure points before prep.

Step 2 – Shoulder preparation and sterile draping
Instruments: Prep supplies, arthroscopy drapes.
Anticipation: Prep must include shoulder, upper arm, and scapula. Ensure access for posterior and lateral portals.

Step 3 – Establish posterior viewing portal
Instruments: Scalpel handle with #11 blade, trocar passed from back table.
Anticipation: Portal placement is precise. Hand blade promptly and keep trocar caps controlled.

Step 4 – Insert arthroscope and perform diagnostic survey
Instruments: Arthroscope and camera ().
Anticipation: Confirm camera clarity and white balance before insertion.

Step 5 – Establish lateral working portal
Instruments: Scalpel handle with #11 blade, cannula passed from back table.
Anticipation: Anticipate second portal quickly to maintain visualization.

Step 6 – Bursectomy and exposure of acromion
Instruments: Shaver passed from back table.
Anticipation: Expect frequent instrument exchanges. Coordinate smoothly with circulator.

Step 7 – Resect undersurface of acromion
Instruments: Burr passed from back table when requested.
Anticipation: Burr use is sequential. Keep additional burrs unopened.

Step 8 – Inspect decompression and smooth edges
Instruments: Burr or shaver.
Anticipation: Surgeon may alternate viewing angles. Be attentive to scope orientation.

Step 9 – Final inspection and lavage
Instruments: Managed via arthroscopy system.
Anticipation: Ensure visualization remains clear to confirm adequate decompression.

Step 10 – Remove instruments and close portals
Instruments: Brought from back table when requested.
Anticipation: Closure instruments come forward only after scope removal.

Acromioplasty, Arthroscopic

Step 11 – Apply sterile dressing and immobilizer
Instruments: Dressing supplies, sling.
Anticipation: Ensure arm is positioned correctly in sling before leaving field.

Mayo Stand Suggestion:

- Scalpel handle with #11 blade
- Adsons forceps with teeth
- 2 mosquito hemostats
- Gauze sponges
- Arthroscope
- Shaver
- Burr
- Cannulas and trocars

Acromioplasty, Open

Step 1 – Patient positioning and verification
Instruments: Beach chair or lateral decubitus positioning aids, padding, arm holder.
Anticipation: Confirm operative shoulder and positioning preference. Ensure head and cervical alignment are secure before prep.

Step 2 – Shoulder preparation and sterile draping
Instruments: Prep supplies, shoulder drapes.
Anticipation: Prep must include clavicle, acromion, and proximal humerus. Maintain access for possible extension of incision.

Step 3 – Skin incision over anterolateral shoulder
Instruments: Scalpel handle with #10 blade, Adsons forceps with teeth.
Anticipation: Incision is small but vascular. Be ready with mosquito hemostats immediately.

Step 4 – Dissect through deltoid to acromion
Instruments: Metzenbaum scissors, 2 mosquito hemostats, Adsons forceps.
Anticipation: Follow clamp–cut rhythm. Protect deltoid fibers to preserve function.

Step 5 – Retract deltoid to expose acromion
Instruments: Small handheld retractor if repeatedly used.
Anticipation: Exposure deepens quickly. Pass larger retractor from the back table only when requested.

Step 6 – Resect anteroinferior acromion
Instruments: Osteotome and mallet or oscillating saw passed from back table when requested.
Anticipation: Clear the field before bone work. Protect soft tissue and rotator cuff.

Step 7 – Smooth bone edges
Instruments: Bone rasp passed from back table.
Anticipation: Surgeon may reassess repeatedly.

Step 8 – Inspect subacromial space
Instruments: None additional.
Anticipation: Surgeon confirms adequate decompression. Maintain quiet field.

Step 9 – Achieve hemostasis
Instruments: Mosquito hemostats if needed.
Anticipation: Bleeding control is critical prior to closure.

Acromioplasty, Open

Step 10 – Reapproximate deltoid
Instruments: Brought from back table when requested.
Anticipation: Transition to suturing. Bring needle driver and sutures only when surgeon commits.

Step 11 – Skin closure
Instruments: Brought from back table when requested.
Anticipation: Begin closing counts early.

Step 12 – Apply dressing and sling
Instruments: Dressing supplies, shoulder immobilizer.
Anticipation: Ensure arm is positioned correctly before final dressing.

Mayo Stand Suggestion:

- Scalpel handle with #11 blade
- Adsons forceps with teeth
- 2 mosquito hemostats
- Saw
- Osteotomes
- Bone Rasp
- Mallet

Acromioplasty, Open

Step 1 – Patient positioning and verification
Instruments: Beach chair or lateral decubitus positioning aids, padding, arm holder.
Anticipation: Confirm operative shoulder and positioning preference. Ensure head and cervical alignment are secure before prep.

Step 2 – Shoulder preparation and sterile draping
Instruments: Prep supplies, shoulder drapes.
Anticipation: Prep must include clavicle, acromion, and proximal humerus. Maintain access for possible extension of incision.

Step 3 – Skin incision over anterolateral shoulder
Instruments: Scalpel handle with #10 blade, Adsons forceps with teeth.
Anticipation: Incision is small but vascular. Be ready with mosquito hemostats immediately.

Step 4 – Dissect through deltoid to acromion
Instruments: Metzenbaum scissors, 2 mosquito hemostats, Adsons forceps.
Anticipation: Follow clamp-cut rhythm. Protect deltoid fibers to preserve function.

Step 5 – Retract deltoid to expose acromion
Instruments: Small handheld retractor if repeatedly used.
Anticipation: Exposure deepens quickly. Pass larger retractor from the back table only when requested.

Step 6 – Resect anteroinferior acromion
Instruments: Osteotome and mallet or oscillating saw passed from back table when requested.
Anticipation: Clear the field before bone work. Protect soft tissue and rotator cuff.

Step 7 – Smooth bone edges
Instruments: Bone rasp passed from back table.
Anticipation: Surgeon may reassess repeatedly. Keep bone tools until requested.

Acromioplasty, Open

Step 8 – Inspect subacromial space
Instruments: None additional.
Anticipation: Surgeon confirms adequate decompression. Maintain quiet field.

Step 9 – Achieve hemostasis
Instruments: Mosquito hemostats if needed.
Anticipation: Bleeding control is critical prior to closure.

Step 10 – Reapproximate deltoid
Instruments: Brought from back table when requested.
Anticipation: Transition to suturing. Bring needle driver and sutures only when surgeon commits.

Step 11 – Skin closure
Instruments: Brought from back table when requested.
Anticipation: Begin closing counts early.

Step 12 – Apply dressing and sling
Instruments: Dressing supplies, shoulder immobilizer.
Anticipation: Ensure arm is positioned correctly before final dressing.

Mayo Stand Suggestion:

- Scalpel handle with #10 blade
- Adsons forceps with teeth
- Metzenbaum scissors
- 2 mosquito hemostats
- Osteotomes
- Bone Rasp
- Mallet
- Saw

Achilles Tendon Repair

Step 1 – Patient positioning and verification
Instruments: Prone positioning aids, chest rolls, padding, foot support.
Anticipation: Confirm operative side and rupture location. Ensure toes hang free to allow ankle manipulation.

Step 2 – Lower extremity preparation and draping
Instruments: Prep supplies, extremity drape.
Anticipation: Prep from mid-calf to foot. Keep heel and posterior ankle fully exposed.

Step 3 – Posteromedial longitudinal incision
Instruments: Scalpel handle with #10 or #15 blade, Adsons forceps with teeth.
Anticipation: Skin is thin posteriorly. Be ready with mosquito hemostats for early bleeding.

Step 4 – Dissect through subcutaneous tissue and paratenon
Instruments: Metzenbaum scissors, 2 mosquito hemostats, Adsons forceps.
Anticipation: Preserve paratenon for closure. Follow clamp–cut rhythm carefully.

Step 5 – Identify proximal and distal tendon ends
Instruments: Metzenbaum scissors.
Anticipation: Tendon ends may be frayed. Maintain gentle handling to preserve tissue quality.

Step 6 – Debride tendon ends if needed
Instruments: Metzenbaum scissors.
Anticipation: Debridement is conservative. Avoid over-anticipating additional instruments.

Achilles Tendon Repair

Step 7 – Tendon repair (Krackow or similar stitch)
Instruments: Brought from back table when requested.
Anticipation: This is a critical step. Bring needle driver and sutures only when surgeon commits to repair.

Step 8 – Approximate tendon ends with ankle plantarflexed
Instruments: None additional.
Anticipation: Surgeon may adjust ankle position repeatedly. Maintain clear field.

Step 9 – Close paratenon
Instruments: Brought from back table when requested.
Anticipation: Paratenon closure improves healing. Anticipate fine sutures.

Step 10 – Inspect repair and hemostasis
Instruments: Mosquito hemostats if needed.
Anticipation: Ensure no gapping or bleeding before closure.

Step 11 – Subcutaneous and skin closure
Instruments: Brought from back table when requested.
Anticipation: Begin closing counts early. Closure instruments move forward only after surgeon commits.

Step 12 – Apply dressing and splint or cast
Instruments: Dressing supplies, splint or cast materials.
Anticipation: Foot must remain plantarflexed during immobilization.

Mayo Stand Suggestion:

- Scalpel handle with #10 or #15 blade
- Adsons forceps with teeth
- Metzenbaum scissors
- 2 mosquito hemostats
- Small handheld retractor
- Suture and Needle Driver

ACL Repair

Step 1 – Patient positioning and verification
Instruments: Supine positioning aids, lateral post, foot support, padding.
Anticipation: Confirm operative knee and graft choice. Ensure tourniquet placement and leg positioning allow full knee flexion.

Step 2 – Lower extremity preparation and sterile draping
Instruments: Prep supplies, arthroscopy drapes.
Anticipation: Prep from mid-thigh to foot. Keep landmarks visible for portal placement.

Step 3 – Establish anterolateral viewing portal
Instruments: Scalpel handle with #11 blade, trocar passed from back table.
Anticipation: Portal placement is precise. Hand blade promptly and control trocar caps.

Step 4 – Insert arthroscope and perform diagnostic survey
Instruments: Arthroscope and camera ().
Anticipation: Confirm camera clarity and white balance before insertion.

Step 5 – Establish anteromedial working portal
Instruments: Scalpel handle with #11 blade, cannula passed from back table.
Anticipation: Anticipate second portal quickly to maintain visualization.

ACL Repair

Step 6 – Debride torn ACL stump
Instruments: Shaver passed from back table.
Anticipation: Expect frequent instrument exchanges. Coordinate smoothly with circulator.

Step 7 – Prepare graft if autograft used
Instruments: Graft preparation tools managed .
Anticipation: Do not open graft instruments until surgeon confirms graft choice.

Step 8 – Drill femoral and tibial tunnels
Instruments: Drill guides and reamers passed from back table.
Anticipation: Clear field before drilling. Protect soft tissue and maintain orientation.

Step 9 – Pass graft through tunnels
Instruments: Passing devices passed from back table.
Anticipation: Confirm graft orientation before fixation.

Step 10 – Fixate graft (screws or suspensory device)
Instruments: Fixation devices passed from back table when requested.
Anticipation: Implant discipline is critical. Open devices only when surgeon commits.

Step 11 – Cycle knee and assess stability
Instruments: None additional.
Anticipation: Surgeon may flex and extend knee repeatedly. Maintain unobstructed field.

Step 12 – Close portals
Instruments: Brought from back table when requested.
Anticipation: Closure instruments come forward only after scope removal.

Step 13 – Apply dressing and brace
Instruments: Dressing supplies, knee brace.
Anticipation: Ensure brace is applied with knee in correct position.

Mayo Stand Suggestion:

- Scalpel handle with #11 blade
- Adsons forceps with teeth
- 2 mosquito hemostats
- Gauze Sponges
- Fixation Devices
- Drill

Arthroscopy of the Knee Joint with Repair of Torn Meniscus

Step 1 – Patient positioning and verification
Instruments: Supine positioning aids, lateral post, foot holder, padding.
Anticipation: Confirm operative knee and repair vs partial meniscectomy. Ensure leg positioning allows full flexion and valgus stress.

Step 2 – Lower extremity preparation and sterile draping
Instruments: Prep supplies, arthroscopy drapes.
Anticipation: Prep from mid-thigh to foot. Keep landmarks visible for portal placement.

Step 3 – Establish anterolateral viewing portal
Instruments: Scalpel handle with #11 blade, trocar passed from back table.
Anticipation: Portal placement is precise. Hand blade promptly and manage trocar caps carefully.

Arthroscopy of the Knee Joint with Repair of Torn Meniscus

Step 4 – Insert arthroscope and perform diagnostic survey
Instruments: Arthroscope and camera
Anticipation: Confirm image clarity before proceeding. Anticipate camera orientation changes.

Step 5 – Establish anteromedial working portal
Instruments: Scalpel handle with #11 blade, cannula passed from back table.
Anticipation: Portal placement may be adjusted based on tear location.

Step 6 – Identify and probe meniscal tear
Instruments: Probe passed from back table.
Anticipation: Surgeon determines repairability here. Do not open repair devices until confirmed.

Step 7 – Prepare meniscal edges
Instruments: Shaver or rasp passed from back table.
Anticipation: Expect alternating use of probe and shaver. Keep exchanges smooth.

Step 8 – Meniscus repair (inside-out, outside-in, or all-inside)
Instruments: Repair devices passed from back table when requested.
Anticipation: Implant discipline is critical. Open only the system selected.

Step 9 – Secure sutures and assess stability
Instruments: Managed via arthroscopy system.
Anticipation: Surgeon may stress the knee repeatedly. Maintain clear field.

Step 10 – Final inspection and lavage
Instruments: Arthroscopy system.
Anticipation: Ensure clear visualization to confirm repair integrity.

Step 11 – Remove instruments and close portals
Instruments: Brought from back table when requested.
Anticipation: Closure instruments come forward only after scope removal.

Step 12 – Apply dressing and brace if ordered
Instruments: Dressing supplies, knee brace.
Anticipation: Brace positioning is surgeon-specific—confirm settings.

Mayo Stand Suggestion:

- Scalpel handle with #11 blade
- Adsons forceps with teeth
- 2 mosquito hemostats
- Gauze Sponges
- Arthroscope
- Shaver

Bankart Procedure – Arthroscopic with Suture Anchors

Step 1 – Patient positioning and verification
Instruments: Beach chair or lateral decubitus positioning equipment, padding, arm holder or traction device.
Anticipation: Confirm operative shoulder and instability direction. Ensure head and neck alignment before prep.

Step 2 – Shoulder preparation and sterile draping
Instruments: Prep supplies, arthroscopy drapes.
Anticipation: Prep must include shoulder, axilla, and upper arm. Maintain access for anterior and posterior portals.

Bankart Procedure – Arthroscopic with Suture Anchors

Step 3 – Establish posterior viewing portal
Instruments: Scalpel handle with #11 blade, trocar passed from back table.
Anticipation: Portal placement is precise. Hand blade promptly and control trocar caps.

Step 4 – Insert arthroscope and perform diagnostic survey
Instruments: Arthroscope and camera
Anticipation: Confirm camera clarity and orientation before proceeding.

Step 5 – Establish anterior working portal(s)
Instruments: Scalpel handle with #11 blade, cannula passed from back table.
Anticipation: Portal number and location depend on tear extent. Be ready for additional cannulas.

Step 6 – Mobilize labrum and prepare glenoid rim
Instruments: Shaver or rasp passed from back table.
Anticipation: Surgeon will decide anchor number after mobilization. Do not open anchors yet.

Step 7 – Place suture anchors into glenoid
Instruments: Suture anchors passed from back table when requested.
Anticipation: Implant discipline is critical. Open anchors one at a time only after position confirmed.

Step 8 – Pass sutures through labrum and capsule
Instruments: Suture passer passed from back table.
Anticipation: Expect alternating suture and camera movements. Keep sutures organized.

Step 9 – Tie arthroscopic knots
Instruments: Knot pusher passed from back table.
Anticipation: Surgeon may retension sutures. Avoid crowding field.

Step 10 – Assess stability and labral position
Instruments: None additional.
Anticipation: Surgeon may rotate arm to test repair. Maintain clear operative field.

Step 11 – Final inspection and lavage
Instruments: Arthroscopy system.
Anticipation: Ensure visualization remains clear to confirm repair integrity.

Step 12 – Remove instruments and close portals
Instruments: Brought from back table when requested.
Anticipation: Closure instruments come forward only after scope removal.

Step 13 – Apply sterile dressing and immobilizer
Instruments: Dressing supplies, shoulder immobilizer.
Anticipation: Immobilizer position is critical for repair protection.

Mayo Stand Suggestion:

- Scalpel handle with #11 blade
- Adsons forceps with teeth
- 2 mosquito hemostats
- Cannulas
- Arthroscope
- Shaver
- Knot Pusher

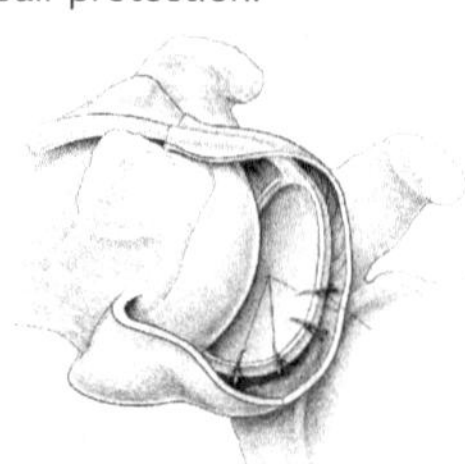

Bankart Procedure – Open

Step 1 – Patient positioning and verification
Instruments: Beach chair or supine positioning aids, padding, arm holder.
Anticipation: Confirm operative shoulder and incision location. Ensure head and neck alignment before prep.

Step 2 – Shoulder preparation and sterile draping
Instruments: Prep supplies, shoulder drapes.
Anticipation: Prep must include clavicle, shoulder, and upper arm. Maintain access to anterior shoulder.

Step 3 – Anterior deltopectoral skin incision
Instruments: Scalpel handle with #10 blade, Adsons forceps with teeth.
Anticipation: Incision is vascular. Be ready with mosquito hemostats immediately.

Step 4 – Dissect through deltopectoral interval
Instruments: Metzenbaum scissors, 2 mosquito hemostats, Adsons forceps.
Anticipation: Identify and protect cephalic vein. Follow clamp-cut rhythm.

Step 5 – Expose subscapularis tendon
Instruments: Metzenbaum scissors, small handheld retractor.
Anticipation: Surgeon may split or detach subscapularis. Keep retractor available but minimal.

Step 6 – Incise capsule and expose glenoid rim
Instruments: Scalpel handle with #15 blade.
Anticipation: Capsulotomy is precise. Be ready to manage small bleeders.

Step 7 – Identify Bankart lesion and prepare glenoid
Instruments: Metzenbaum scissors.
Anticipation: Surgeon assesses labral mobility. Do not open anchors until confirmed.

Step 8 – Place suture anchors or transosseous sutures
Instruments: Passed from back table when requested.
Anticipation: Implant discipline is critical. Open anchors one at a time only after position confirmed.

Step 9 – Repair labrum and capsule
Instruments: Brought from back table when requested.
Anticipation: Transition to suturing phase. Bring needle driver and sutures only when surgeon commits.

Step 10 – Reapproximate subscapularis
Instruments: Passed from back table when requested.
Anticipation: Subscapularis repair tension is important. Avoid rushing handoffs.

Step 11 – Inspect stability and hemostasis
Instruments: Mosquito hemostats if needed.
Anticipation: Surgeon may range shoulder to test stability.

Step 12 – Layered closure
Instruments: Brought from back table when requested.
Anticipation: Begin closing counts early. Closure instruments come forward only after surgeon commits.

Bankart Procedure – Open

Step 13 – Apply dressing and immobilizer
Instruments: Dressing supplies, shoulder immobilizer.
Anticipation: Immobilizer positioning is critical to protect repair.

Mayo Stand Suggestion:

- Scalpel handle with #10 blade
- Adsons forceps with teeth
- Metzenbaum scissors
- 2 mosquito hemostats
- Oscillating Saw
- Bone Rasp
- Large retractor

Below the Knee Amputation (BKA)

Step 1 – Patient positioning and verification
Instruments: Supine positioning aids, padding, tourniquet placed but not inflated.
Anticipation: Confirm level of amputation and side. Ensure knee can be flexed during flap formation.

Step 2 – Extremity preparation and wide draping
Instruments: Prep supplies, sterile towels, extremity drape.
Anticipation: Prep well proximal to incision to allow flap modification if tissue quality is poor.

Step 3 – Skin marking and flap design (posterior flap)
Instruments: Skin marker.
Anticipation: Surgeon may adjust flap length based on vascular status. Keep marker accessible.

Step 4 – Skin and subcutaneous incision
Instruments: Scalpel handle with #10 blade, Adsons forceps with teeth.
Anticipation: Incision is long and vascular. Be ready with mosquito hemostats immediately.

Step 5 – Divide anterior muscle compartments
Instruments: Metzenbaum scissors, 2 mosquito hemostats, Adsons forceps.
Anticipation: Follow clamp–cut rhythm. Maintain organized clamp placement to control bleeding.

Step 6 – Identify and ligate anterior tibial vessels and nerves
Instruments: Passed from back table when requested.
Anticipation: Vessel control is critical. Anticipate sequence without opening instruments early.

Step 7 – Transect tibia and fibula
Instruments: Oscillating saw passed from back table.
Anticipation: Clear the field before bone cutting. Protect soft tissues and posterior flap.

Step 8 – Smooth bone edges and bevel anterior tibia
Instruments: Bone rasp passed from back table.
Anticipation: Proper bevel prevents skin breakdown. Keep bone tools until requested.

Step 9 – Divide posterior compartment and shape flap
Instruments: Metzenbaum scissors, mosquito hemostats.
Anticipation: Preserve posterior flap bulk for padding. Avoid excessive traction.

Step 10 – Inspect hemostasis and muscle balance
Instruments: Mosquito hemostats if needed.
Anticipation: Bleeding control is critical prior to closure.

Below the Knee Amputation (BKA)

Step 11 – Place drain if indicated
Instruments: Drain passed from back table.
Anticipation: Confirm exit site before placement.

Step 12 – Layered closure of fascia, muscle, and skin
Instruments: Brought from back table when requested.
Anticipation: Begin closing counts early. Closure instruments come forward only after surgeon commits.

Step 13 – Apply sterile dressing and compression
Instruments: Dressing supplies, compression wrap.
Anticipation: Ensure even compression without compromising circulation.

Mayo Stand Suggestion:

- Scalpel handle with #10 blade
- Adsons forceps with teeth
- Metzenbaum scissors
- 2 mosquito hemostats
- Oscillating Saw
- Bone Rasp
- Large retractor

Bunionectomy

Step 1 – Patient positioning and verification
Instruments: Supine positioning aids, padding, foot support.
Anticipation: Confirm operative foot and specific bunion technique planned (simple exostectomy vs osteotomy).

Step 2 – Foot preparation and sterile draping
Instruments: Prep supplies, extremity drape.
Anticipation: Prep from ankle to toes. Keep entire forefoot exposed for alignment assessment.

Step 3 – Medial longitudinal incision over first MTP joint
Instruments: Scalpel handle with #15 blade, Adsons forceps with teeth.
Anticipation: Incision is small but vascular. Be ready with mosquito hemostats promptly.

Step 4 – Dissect through subcutaneous tissue and capsule
Instruments: Metzenbaum scissors, 2 mosquito hemostats, Adsons forceps.
Anticipation: Follow clamp-cut rhythm carefully. Preserve capsule for later repair.

Step 5 – Expose medial eminence of first metatarsal
Instruments: Small handheld retractor if repeatedly used.
Anticipation: Exposure must be clean for bone work. Avoid cluttering the field.

Step 6 – Resect medial eminence (exostectomy)
Instruments: Osteotome and mallet or sagittal saw passed from back table when requested.
Anticipation: Clear Mayo and field before bone work. Protect surrounding soft tissue.

Step 7 – Perform osteotomy if indicated
Instruments: Saw and fixation devices passed from back table when requested.
Anticipation: Implant discipline is critical. Open fixation only when surgeon commits.

Bunionectomy

Step 8 – Realign metatarsal and assess correction
Instruments: None additional.
Anticipation: Surgeon may manually correct toe position several times.

Step 9 – Smooth bone edges
Instruments: Bone rasp passed from back table.
Anticipation: Proper smoothing reduces postoperative irritation.

Step 10 – Repair capsule and soft tissues
Instruments: Brought from back table when requested.
Anticipation: Transition to suturing phase—bring needle driver and sutures only when surgeon commits.

Step 11 – Skin closure
Instruments: Brought from back table when requested.
Anticipation: Begin closing counts early.

Step 12 – Apply dressing and postoperative shoe
Instruments: Dressing supplies, postoperative shoe or wrap.
Anticipation: Ensure toe alignment is maintained during dressing application.

Mayo Stand Suggestion:

- Scalpel handle with #15 blade
- Adsons forceps with teeth
- Metzenbaum scissors
- 2 mosquito hemostats
- Small Handheld retractor
- Bone Rasp
- Osteotome
- Saw

External Fixation of a Colles' Fracture

Step 1 – Patient positioning and verification
Instruments: Supine positioning aids, hand table, padding.
Anticipation: Confirm operative side and fracture pattern. Ensure C-arm access before prep.

Step 2 – Upper extremity preparation and sterile draping
Instruments: Prep supplies, extremity drape.
Anticipation: Prep from mid-forearm to hand. Keep fingers visible to assess alignment.

Step 3 – Fracture reduction under fluoroscopy
Instruments: Manual traction.
Anticipation: Surgeon may reduce fracture before pin placement. Maintain clear field for imaging.

Step 4 – Mark pin insertion sites
Instruments: Skin marker.
Anticipation: Pin placement is precise. Keep marker accessible for adjustments.

Step 5 – Small skin incisions for pins
Instruments: Scalpel handle with #15 blade, Adsons forceps with teeth.
Anticipation: Incisions are small but bleed. Be ready with mosquito hemostats immediately.

Step 6 – Insert proximal and distal fixation pins
Instruments: Drill and pins passed from back table when requested.
Anticipation: Protect tendons and neurovascular structures. Clear Mayo before power use.

External Fixation of a Colles' Fracture

Step 7 – Assemble external fixator frame
Instruments: Fixator bars and clamps passed from back table.
Anticipation: Components are assembled sequentially. Keep unused parts organized .

Step 8 – Adjust distraction and alignment
Instruments: Fixator adjustment tools.
Anticipation: Surgeon may check alignment repeatedly under fluoroscopy.

Step 9 – Tighten fixator and confirm stability
Instruments: Fixator wrench.
Anticipation: Ensure all connections are secure before final imaging.

Step 10 – Inspect pin sites for bleeding
Instruments: Mosquito hemostats if needed.
Anticipation: Minor bleeding is common. Control before dressing.

Step 11 – Apply sterile dressings around pins
Instruments: Dressing supplies.
Anticipation: Pin sites must be padded without compromising stability.

Step 12 – Final fluoroscopic confirmation
Instruments: C-arm.
Anticipation: Confirm alignment before drapes are removed.

Mayo Stand Suggestion:

- Scalpel handle with #15 blade
- Adsons forceps with teeth
- Metzenbaum scissors
- 2 mosquito hemostats
- Drill and Pins
- External fixation device
- Skin Marker

ORIF Radius

Step 1 – Patient positioning and verification
Instruments: Supine positioning aids, hand table, padding, tourniquet placed but not inflated.
Anticipation: Confirm operative side, fracture location, and plate system.

Step 2 – Upper extremity preparation and sterile draping
Instruments: Prep supplies, extremity drape.
Anticipation: Prep from mid-forearm to hand. Fingers must remain visible for alignment checks.

Step 3 – Volar (or dorsal) incision
Instruments: Scalpel handle with #15 blade, Adsons forceps with teeth.
Anticipation: Incision is controlled but vascular. Be ready with mosquito hemostats immediately.

Step 4 – Dissect through subcutaneous tissue and fascia
Instruments: Metzenbaum scissors, 2 mosquito hemostats, Adsons forceps.
Anticipation: Follow clamp–cut rhythm. Protect superficial nerves and vessels.

Step 5 – Expose radius and fracture site
Instruments: Small handheld retractor if repeatedly used.
Anticipation: Exposure must be clean for plate placement. Large retractor come from back table only if requested.

ORIF Radius

Step 6 – Reduce fracture
Instruments: Reduction forceps passed from back table when requested.
Anticipation: Surgeon may reduce fracture multiple times under fluoroscopy. Maintain uncluttered field.

Step 7 – Apply plate to radius
Instruments: Plate passed from back table.
Anticipation: Confirm plate orientation before opening screws.

Step 8 – Drill and insert fixation screws
Instruments: Drill, depth gauge, screws passed from back table.
Anticipation: Implant discipline is critical. Open screws sequentially as requested.

Step 9 – Confirm reduction and fixation with fluoroscopy
Instruments: C-arm.
Anticipation: Clear Mayo and field for imaging. Surgeon may request multiple views.

Step 10 – Inspect hemostasis
Instruments: Mosquito hemostats if needed.
Anticipation: Bleeding must be controlled before closure.

Step 11 – Layered closure
Instruments: Brought from back table when requested.
Anticipation: Begin closing counts early. Closure instruments move forward only after surgeon commits.

Step 12 – Apply sterile dressing and splint
Instruments: Dressing supplies, splint materials.
Anticipation: Ensure wrist alignment is maintained during immobilization.

Mayo Stand Suggestion:

- Scalpel handle with #15 blade
- Adsons forceps with teeth
- Metzenbaum scissors
- 2 mosquito hemostats
- Drill and Pins
- Plates and screws
- Small handheld retractor

ORIF Hip Fracture

Step 1 – Patient positioning and verification
Instruments: Fracture table or radiolucent table, padding, traction boots.
Anticipation: Confirm fracture type and operative side. Ensure C-arm access and traction alignment before prep.

Step 2 – Lower extremity preparation and sterile draping
Instruments: Prep supplies, hip drapes.
Anticipation: Prep from iliac crest to knee. Maintain access to groin for traction adjustments.

Step 3 – Fracture reduction under fluoroscopy
Instruments: Manual traction via fracture table.
Anticipation: Reduction may take time. Maintain quiet field and protect sterile drapes during imaging.

ORIF Hip Fracture

Step 4 – Lateral thigh incision
Instruments: Scalpel handle with #10 blade, Adsons forceps with teeth.
Anticipation: Incision is deep and vascular. Be ready with mosquito hemostats immediately.

Step 5 – Dissect through fascia and muscle
Instruments: Metzenbaum scissors, 2 mosquito hemostats, Adsons forceps.
Anticipation: Follow clamp-cut rhythm. Protect underlying neurovascular structures.

Step 6 – Expose proximal femur and fracture site
Instruments: Small handheld retractor if repeatedly used.
Anticipation: Exposure must be clean for hardware placement. Large retractor come from back table only when requested.

Step 7 – Confirm reduction with fluoroscopy
Instruments: C-arm.
Anticipation: Surgeon may request multiple views before implant placement.

Step 8 – Insert guidewire or lag screw
Instruments: Guidewire passed from back table when requested.
Anticipation: Guidewire placement is critical. Confirm trajectory before opening additional implants.

Step 9 – Apply fixation device (plate, screw, or nail)
Instruments: Fixation device passed from back table.
Anticipation: Implant discipline is essential. Open only what is immediately needed.

Step 10 – Secure fixation and reassess alignment
Instruments: Drill and screws passed from back table.
Anticipation: Expect alternating drilling and imaging. Keep Mayo uncluttered.

Step 11 – Inspect hemostasis
Instruments: Mosquito hemostats if needed.
Anticipation: Bleeding control is critical prior to closure.

Step 12 – Layered closure
Instruments: Brought from back table when requested.
Anticipation: Begin closing counts early. Closure instruments move forward only after surgeon commits.

Step 13 – Apply sterile dressing
Instruments: Dressing supplies.
Anticipation: Maintain leg alignment during dressing application.

Mayo Stand Suggestion:

- Scalpel handle with #15 blade
- Adsons forceps with teeth
- Bonnie Forceps
- Metzenbaum scissors
- 2 mosquito hemostats
- 2 Straight Oschner
- Senn, Volkman rake, Hohmann, Gelpi
- Rongeur, Curettes

Repair of Femoral Shaft Fracture AO Titanium Femoral Nail System

Step 1 – Patient positioning and verification
Instruments: Fracture table or radiolucent table, traction boots, padding.
Anticipation: Confirm operative side and nail system.

Step 2 – Lower extremity preparation and sterile draping
Instruments: Prep supplies, hip/thigh drapes.
Anticipation: Prep from iliac crest to knee. Maintain access to groin for traction adjustments.

Step 3 – Fracture reduction under fluoroscopy
Instruments: Manual traction via fracture table.
Anticipation: Reduction may take time. Protect sterile field during repeated imaging.

Step 4 – Proximal incision for nail entry point
Instruments: Scalpel handle with #10 blade, Adsons forceps with teeth.
Anticipation: Incision is small but deep. Be ready with mosquito hemostats immediately.

Step 5 – Dissect to greater trochanter entry site
Instruments: Metzenbaum scissors, 2 mosquito hemostats, Adsons forceps.
Anticipation: Maintain clean exposure for guidewire placement.

Step 6 – Insert guidewire into femoral canal
Instruments: Guidewire passed from back table when requested.
Anticipation: Guidewire trajectory is critical. Confirm placement before advancing.

Step 7 – Ream femoral canal
Instruments: Reamers passed from back table sequentially.
Anticipation: Reaming proceeds incrementally. Open only the next size requested.

Step 8 – Insert intramedullary nail
Instruments: AO titanium nail passed from back table.
Anticipation: Confirm correct length and diameter before opening.

Step 9 – Proximal locking screw placement
Instruments: Drill and locking screws passed from back table.
Anticipation: Coordinate drill use with C-arm imaging. Keep Mayo clear.

Step 10 – Distal locking screw placement
Instruments: Drill and screws passed from back table.
Anticipation: Distal locking often requires multiple images. Maintain organized implant control.

Step 11 – Confirm alignment and fixation
Instruments: C-arm.
Anticipation: Surgeon may request final images before closure.

Step 12 – Inspect hemostasis
Instruments: Mosquito hemostats if needed.
Anticipation: Control bleeding prior to closure.

Step 13 – Layered closure
Instruments: Brought from back table when requested.
Anticipation: Begin closing counts early. Closure instruments come forward only after surgeon commits.

Repair of Femoral Shaft Fracture AO Titanium Femoral Nail System

Step 14 – Apply sterile dressing
Instruments: Dressing supplies.
Anticipation: Maintain leg alignment during dressing application.

Mayo Stand Suggestion:

- Scalpel handle with #10 blade
- Adsons forceps with teeth
- Metzenbaum scissors
- 2 mosquito hemostats
- Reamers and drills
- AO nails and locking screws
- Large retractor

Shoulder Arthroscopy

Step 1 – Patient positioning and verification
Instruments: Beach chair or lateral decubitus positioning equipment, padding, arm holder or traction device.
Anticipation: Confirm operative shoulder and positioning preference. Secure head and neck and protect pressure points before prep.

Step 2 – Shoulder preparation and sterile draping
Instruments: Prep supplies, arthroscopy drapes.
Anticipation: Prep must include shoulder, axilla, scapula, and upper arm. Ensure portal sites remain accessible.

Step 3 – Establish posterior viewing portal
Instruments: Scalpel handle with #11 blade, trocar passed from back table.
Anticipation: Portal placement is precise. Hand blade promptly and control trocar caps.

Step 4 – Insert arthroscope and perform diagnostic survey
Instruments: Arthroscope and camera
Anticipation: Confirm white balance and image clarity before insertion.

Step 5 – Establish anterior and/or lateral working portal(s)
Instruments: Scalpel handle with #11 blade, cannula passed from back table.
Anticipation: Portal number depends on pathology. Be ready for additional cannulas without opening early.

Step 6 – Systematic evaluation of intra-articular structures
Instruments: Probe passed from back table.
Anticipation: Surgeon may request probe repeatedly. Keep exchanges smooth and controlled.

Step 7 – Perform indicated procedure (debridement, repair, etc.)
Instruments: Shaver, burr, or repair devices passed from back table when requested.
Anticipation: Procedure-specific instruments vary—open only what is confirmed.

Step 8 – Reassess joint and achieve hemostasis arthroscopically
Instruments: Arthroscopy system.
Anticipation: Monitor fluid clarity and pressure to maintain visualization.

Step 9 – Final inspection and lavage
Instruments: Arthroscopy system.
Anticipation: Ensure clear visualization to confirm completion of procedure.

Shoulder Arthroscopy

Step 10 – Remove instruments and close portals
Instruments: Brought from back table when requested.
Anticipation: Closure instruments come forward only after scope removal.

Step 11 – Apply sterile dressing and immobilizer
Instruments: Dressing supplies, sling or immobilizer.
Anticipation: Immobilizer positioning must match surgeon preference.

Mayo Stand Suggestion:

- Scalpel handle with #15 blade
- Adsons forceps with teeth
- Metzenbaum scissors
- Arthroscope, Shaver, Burr
- Cannulas and Trocars
- 2 Curved hemostats

Total Hip Arthroplasty – Posterolateral Approach

Step 1 – Patient positioning and verification
Instruments: Lateral decubitus positioning aids, bean bag, padding, axillary roll.
Anticipation: Confirm operative side and implant system. Ensure pelvis is stable and landmarks are visible before prep.

Step 2 – Hip and lower extremity preparation and draping
Instruments: Prep supplies, hip drapes.
Anticipation: Prep from iliac crest to knee. Maintain access for leg manipulation and trialing.

Step 3 – Posterolateral skin incision
Instruments: Scalpel handle with #10 blade, Adsons forceps with teeth.
Anticipation: Incision is long and vascular. Be ready with mosquito hemostats immediately.

Step 4 – Dissect through fascia and split gluteus maximus
Instruments: Metzenbaum scissors, 2 mosquito hemostats, Adsons forceps.
Anticipation: Follow clamp–cut rhythm. Protect underlying sciatic nerve.

Step 5 – Identify and detach short external rotators
Instruments: Metzenbaum scissors, mosquito hemostats.
Anticipation: Rotators are tagged for later repair. Be attentive to suture requests from back table.

Step 6 – Capsulotomy and hip dislocation
Instruments: Metzenbaum scissors.
Anticipation: Surgeon will manipulate leg extensively. Maintain clear field.

Step 7 – Femoral neck osteotomy
Instruments: Oscillating saw passed from back table when requested.
Anticipation: Clear Mayo and field before bone cutting. Protect soft tissues.

Step 8 – Acetabular exposure and preparation
Instruments: Reamers passed from back table sequentially.
Anticipation: Reaming progresses incrementally. Open only next size requested.

Step 9 – Insert acetabular component
Instruments: Cup and impactor passed from back table.
Anticipation: Confirm size and orientation before opening liner.

Total Hip Arthroplasty – Posterolateral Approach

Step 10 – Prepare femoral canal
Instruments: Broaches passed from back table.
Anticipation: Broaching proceeds stepwise. Keep sizes organized.

Step 11 – Trial reduction and leg length assessment
Instruments: Trial components passed from back table.
Anticipation: Surgeon may trial multiple combinations. Track components carefully.

Step 12 – Implant final femoral and acetabular components
Instruments: Final implants passed from back table when requested.
Anticipation: Implant discipline is critical. Open one component at a time.

Step 13 – Repair capsule and short external rotators
Instruments: Brought from back table when requested.
Anticipation: Transition to suturing phase. Bring needle driver and sutures only when surgeon commits.

Step 14 – Inspect stability and hemostasis
Instruments: Mosquito hemostats if needed.
Anticipation: Surgeon will range hip to confirm stability.

Step 15 – Layered closure
Instruments: Brought from back table when requested.
Anticipation: Begin closing counts early.

Step 16 – Apply sterile dressing and abduction pillow
Instruments: Dressing supplies, abduction pillow.
Anticipation: Ensure leg positioning protects posterior precautions.

Mayo Stand Suggestion:

- Scalpel handle with #10 blade
- Ferris-Smith , Bonney Forceps
- 2 curved hemostats
- 2 straight Oschner
- Metzenbaum scissors
- Large Gelpi
- Large Rake
- Hohmann
- Curved, Straight Mayo
- Meyerding
- Rongeur Large, Small
- Curettes
- Mallet
- Osteotomes

Total Knee Arthroplasty (TKA)

Step 1 – Patient positioning and verification
Instruments: Supine positioning aids, padding, tourniquet placed but not inflated, foot support.
Anticipation: Confirm operative knee, implant system, and laterality. Ensure leg holder allows full flexion and extension.

Step 2 – Lower extremity preparation and sterile draping
Instruments: Prep supplies, knee drapes.
Anticipation: Prep from mid-thigh to foot. Keep landmarks visible for alignment checks.

Step 3 – Midline anterior skin incision
Instruments: Scalpel handle with #10 blade, Adsons forceps with teeth.
Anticipation: Incision is long and vascular. Be ready with mosquito hemostats immediately.

Total Knee Arthroplasty (TKA)

Step 4 – Medial parapatellar arthrotomy
Instruments: Metzenbaum scissors, 2 mosquito hemostats, Adsons forceps.
Anticipation: Follow clamp–cut rhythm. Arthrotomy exposure determines visualization for the entire case.

Step 5 – Evert or sublux patella and expose joint
Instruments: Small handheld retractor if repeatedly used.
Anticipation: Patella handling is critical. Avoid excessive traction that risks tendon injury.

Step 6 – Resect distal femur
Instruments: Cutting guides and saw passed from back table when requested.
Anticipation: Clear Mayo completely before bone cuts. Protect soft tissues during sawing.

Step 7 – Prepare proximal tibia
Instruments: Tibial cutting guides and saw passed from back table.
Anticipation: Alignment is checked repeatedly. Expect guide adjustments before final cut.

Step 8 – Remove osteophytes and balance ligaments
Instruments: Osteotomes and rongeurs passed from back table.
Anticipation: Bone trimming occurs intermittently. Do not stage rongeurs on Mayo.

Step 9 – Trial femoral and tibial components
Instruments: Trial components passed from back table.
Anticipation: Multiple trials may be used. Track sizes carefully and keep unused trials .

Step 10 – Assess range of motion and stability
Instruments: None additional.
Anticipation: Surgeon cycles knee repeatedly. Maintain clear field and awareness of limb position.

Step 11 – Prepare patella if resurfaced
Instruments: Patellar reamer and guide passed from back table.
Anticipation: Confirm resurfacing plan before opening patellar components.

Step 12 – Cement and implant final components
Instruments: Cement system and implants passed from back table when requested.
Anticipation: Timing is critical. Open cement only when bone surfaces are ready.

Step 13 – Final reduction and stability check
Instruments: None additional.
Anticipation: Surgeon confirms alignment and tracking before closure.

Step 14 – Inspect hemostasis
Instruments: Mosquito hemostats if needed.
Anticipation: Bleeding control before closure reduces hematoma risk.

Step 15 – Layered closure
Instruments: Brought from back table when requested.
Anticipation: Begin closing counts early. Closure instruments move forward only after surgeon commits.

Total Knee Arthroplasty (TKA)

Step 16 – Apply sterile dressing and compression
Instruments: Dressing supplies, compression wrap.
Anticipation: Maintain knee extension during dressing application per surgeon preference.

Mayo Stand Suggestion:

- Scalpel handle with #10 blade
- Bonney Forceps
- 2 curved hemostats
- 2 straight Oschner
- Metzenbaum scissors
- Large Gelpi
- Volkman Rake
- Hohmann Curved
- Curved, Straight Mayo
- Hohmann Blunt
- Z retractors
- Rongeur Large, Small
- Curettes
- Mallet
- Osteotomes

Total Shoulder Arthroplasty

Step 1 – Patient positioning and verification
Instruments: Beach chair positioning equipment, padding, headrest, arm holder.
Anticipation: Confirm operative shoulder and implant system. Ensure head and neck alignment and secure positioning before prep.

Step 2 – Shoulder preparation and sterile draping
Instruments: Prep supplies, shoulder arthroplasty drapes.
Anticipation: Prep must include shoulder, axilla, and upper arm. Maintain access for arm manipulation and imaging.

Step 3 – Deltopectoral skin incision
Instruments: Scalpel handle with #10 blade, Adsons forceps with teeth.
Anticipation: Incision is moderately vascular. Be ready with mosquito hemostats immediately.

Step 4 – Dissect through deltopectoral interval
Instruments: Metzenbaum scissors, 2 mosquito hemostats, Adsons forceps.
Anticipation: Identify and protect the cephalic vein. Follow clamp-cut rhythm.

Step 5 – Expose subscapularis tendon
Instruments: Metzenbaum scissors, small handheld retractor if repeatedly used.
Anticipation: Surgeon may tenotomize or peel subscapularis. Anticipate later repair.

Step 6 – Capsulotomy and humeral head dislocation
Instruments: Metzenbaum scissors.
Anticipation: Arm manipulation increases at this point. Maintain clear field and protect drapes.

Step 7 – Resect humeral head
Instruments: Oscillating saw passed from back table when requested.
Anticipation: Clear Mayo before bone cutting. Protect surrounding soft tissue.

Step 8 – Prepare humeral canal
Instruments: Reamers and broaches passed from back table sequentially.
Anticipation: Sizing progresses incrementally. Open only the next size requested.

Step 9 – Expose and prepare glenoid
Instruments: Glenoid retractor, reamers, and guides passed from back table.
Anticipation: Glenoid exposure is technically demanding. Expect pauses for visualization.

Total Shoulder Arthroplasty

Step 10 – Trial humeral and glenoid components
Instruments: Trial components passed from back table.
Anticipation: Multiple trials may be used. Track components carefully.

Step 11 – Implant final components
Instruments: Final implants passed from back table when requested.
Anticipation: Implant discipline is critical. Open one component at a time.

Step 12 – Reduce shoulder and assess stability and range
Instruments: None additional.
Anticipation: Surgeon will range shoulder repeatedly. Maintain unobstructed field.

Step 13 – Repair subscapularis and capsule
Instruments: Brought from back table when requested.
Anticipation: Transition to suturing phase. Bring needle driver and sutures only when surgeon commits.

Step 14 – Inspect hemostasis
Instruments: Mosquito hemostats if needed.
Anticipation: Bleeding control is critical prior to closure.

Step 15 – Layered closure
Instruments: Brought from back table when requested.
Anticipation: Begin closing counts early.

Step 16 – Apply sterile dressing and immobilizer
Instruments: Dressing supplies, shoulder immobilizer.
Anticipation: Immobilizer positioning protects repair.

Mayo Stand Suggestion:

- Scalpel handle with #10 blade
- Bonney Forceps
- 2 curved hemostats
- 2 straight Oschner
- Metzenbaum scissors
- Gelpi
- Army Navy retractors
- Hohmann
- Curved, Straight Mayo

Triple Arthrodesis

Step 1 – Patient positioning and verification
Instruments: Supine positioning aids, bump under ipsilateral hip, padding, foot support.
Anticipation: Confirm operative foot and deformity correction plan. Position must allow medial and lateral foot access.

Step 2 – Foot and ankle preparation and sterile draping
Instruments: Prep supplies, extremity drape.
Anticipation: Prep from mid-calf to toes. Leave heel fully accessible for alignment checks.

Step 3 – Lateral incision over sinus tarsi
Instruments: Scalpel handle with #15 blade, Adsons forceps with teeth.
Anticipation: Incision is small but vascular. Be ready with mosquito hemostats immediately.

Step 4 – Dissect to expose subtalar and calcaneocuboid joints
Instruments: Metzenbaum scissors, 2 mosquito hemostats, Adsons forceps.
Anticipation: Follow clamp–cut rhythm. Protect peroneal tendons and sural nerve.

Step 5 – Medial incision to expose talonavicular joint
Instruments: Scalpel handle with #15 blade, Metzenbaum scissors.
Anticipation: Two-incision workflow requires clean organization and instrument discipline.

Step 6 – Expose all three joints
Instruments: Small handheld retractor.
Anticipation: Exposure determines fusion success. Large retractor are passed from back table only when requested.

Step 7 – Remove cartilage from fusion surfaces
Instruments: Osteotomes, curettes, rongeurs passed from back table.
Anticipation: Bone preparation is sequential. Do not stage bone instruments on Mayo.

Step 8 – Correct deformity and position foot
Instruments: Manual manipulation.
Anticipation: Surgeon may reposition foot multiple times.

Step 9 – Fixate joints with screws or staples
Instruments: Guidewires, drill, fixation hardware passed from back table.
Anticipation: Implant discipline is critical. Open only fixation requested.

Step 10 – Confirm alignment and fixation
Instruments: C-arm.
Anticipation: Multiple images are common. Clear Mayo and field for fluoroscopy.

Step 11 – Inspect hemostasis
Instruments: Mosquito hemostats if needed.
Anticipation: Bleeding control before closure reduces postoperative complications.

Step 12 – Layered closure of incisions
Instruments: Brought from back table when requested.
Anticipation: Begin closing counts early. Closure instruments move forward only after surgeon commits.

Step 13 – Apply sterile dressing and cast or splint
Instruments: Dressing supplies, cast or splint materials.
Anticipation: Maintain corrected foot position during immobilization.

Mayo Stand Suggestion:

- Scalpel handle with #15 blade
- Bonney Forceps
- 2 curved hemostats
- 2 straight Oschner
- Metzenbaum scissors
- Mayo straight
- Senn retractor
- Army Navy
- Hohmann

Section IX:

Cardiothoracic Procedures

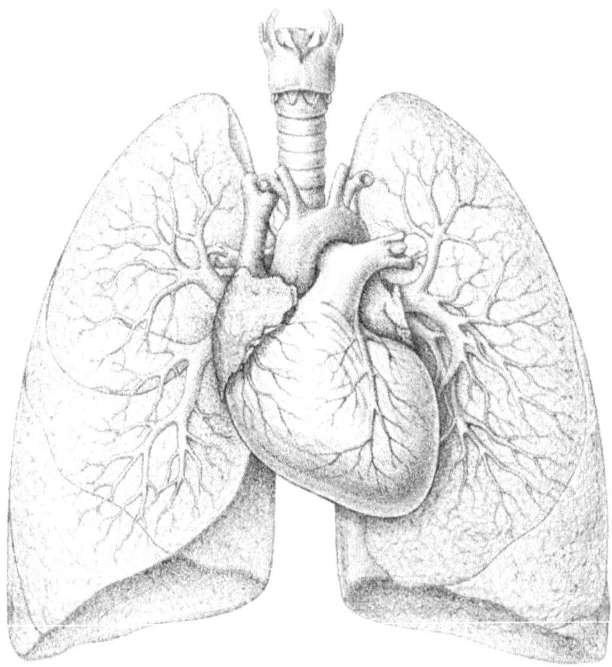

Aortic Valve Replacement (AVR)

Step 1 – Patient positioning and verification
Instruments: Supine positioning aids, shoulder roll, padding.
Anticipation: Confirm valve type and size range available. Verify perfusion setup and cross-clamp readiness.

Step 2 – Chest preparation and sterile draping
Instruments: Prep supplies, cardiac drapes.
Anticipation: Wide prep from neck to groin for possible femoral access.

Step 3 – Median sternotomy
Instruments: Scalpel handle with #10 blade, Adsons forceps with teeth.
Anticipation: Incision is long and vascular. Be ready with mosquito hemostats immediately.

Step 4 – Open sternum and expose mediastinum
Instruments: Metzenbaum scissors, 2 mosquito hemostats.
Anticipation: Sternal retractors comes from back table only when requested. Maintain organized clamp placement.

Step 5 – Pericardiotomy and pericardial stay sutures
Instruments: Metzenbaum scissors.
Anticipation: Surgeon will place traction sutures—anticipate needle driver from back table only when asked.

Step 6 – Systemic heparinization and cannulation
Instruments: Cannulas passed from back table when requested.
Anticipation: Coordinate with perfusion. Maintain quiet, uncluttered field.

Step 7 – Initiate cardiopulmonary bypass and apply aortic cross clamp
Instruments: Aortic cross clamp passed from back table.
Anticipation: Timing is critical. Ensure clamps are ready but unopened until call.

Step 8 – Aortotomy
Instruments: Scalpel handle with #15 blade, Metzenbaum scissors.
Anticipation: Precise incision—be ready for small bleeders.

Step 9 – Excise native aortic valve
Instruments: Valve scissors, rongeurs, punches passed from back table.
Anticipation: Tissue fragments must be controlled. Keep field clear and organized.

Step 10 – Size annulus and select prosthetic valve
Instruments: Valve sizers passed from back table.
Anticipation: Do not open valve until size is confirmed aloud.

Step 11 – Place annular sutures and seat valve
Instruments: Sutures and needle driver brought from back table when requested.
Anticipation: This marks transition to suturing phase—counts and suture organization are critical.

Step 12 – Close aortotomy
Instruments: Passed from back table when requested.
Anticipation: Ensure suture material matches surgeon preference.

Aortic Valve Replacement (AVR)

Step 13 – De air heart and remove cross clamp
Instruments: None additional.
Anticipation: Communicate readiness; protect sterile field during de-airing maneuvers.

Step 14 – Wean from bypass and assess valve function
Instruments: None additional.
Anticipation: Be prepared for pacing wires or adjustments as requested.

Step 15 – Achieve hemostasis and place chest tubes
Instruments: Chest tubes passed from back table.
Anticipation: Tube size and number vary—confirm before opening.

Step 16 – Sternal closure
Instruments: Sternal wires and drivers passed from back table.
Anticipation: Heavy instruments introduced only at this phase.

Step 17 – Layered soft tissue and skin closure
Instruments: Brought from back table when requested.
Anticipation: Begin closing counts early and confirm final counts before dressings.

Step 18 – Apply sterile dressing
Instruments: Dressing supplies.
Anticipation: Maintain chest tube security and line organization.

Mayo Stand Suggestion:

- 2 Scalpel handle with #10 blade
- Debakey, Russian Forceps
- Potts-Smith, Adsons Brown
- 2 mosquitos
- 2 mosquito with suture boots
- 4 curved hemostat
- 4 Crile, 4 Right Angle, 4 Kelly
- 4 tubing clamps
- 2 Crafoord, 2 Satinsky
- 2 Cooley
- 2 straight vascular clamp
- Metzenbaum, Mayo
- Jameson, Coronary
- Sternum retractors
- 2 Richardson
- 2 vein retractor

Bronchoscopy

Step 1 – Patient positioning and verification
Instruments: Supine positioning aids, headrest.
Anticipation: Confirm indication (diagnostic vs biopsy), route (oral vs nasal), and anesthesia type. Ensure bite block availability if oral approach.

Step 2 – Airway preparation and monitoring setup
Instruments: None sterile at this phase.
Anticipation: Coordinate with anesthesia. Oxygenation and ventilation take priority—maintain a clear sterile field.

Step 3 – Assemble and test bronchoscope system
Instruments: Bronchoscope, camera, light source ().
Anticipation: Verify image clarity and light before insertion. Ensure backup scope availability if required.

Step 4 – Insert bronchoscope into airway
Instruments: Bronchoscope ().
Anticipation: Protect scope from torque and tension. Maintain quiet field during insertion.

Bronchoscopy

Step 5 – Systematic examination of trachea and bronchi
Instruments: None additional.
Anticipation: Surgeon may pause frequently to inspect anatomy. Avoid unnecessary movement around the field.

Step 6 – Perform bronchoalveolar lavage if indicated
Instruments: Lavage supplies managed .
Anticipation: Be ready to receive specimen containers promptly and label correctly.

Step 7 – Obtain biopsy or brushings if indicated
Instruments: Biopsy forceps or cytology brush passed from back table when requested.
Anticipation: Do not open biopsy instruments early. Track specimen count carefully.

Step 8 – Control minor bleeding if present
Instruments: Managed via bronchoscope.
Anticipation: Bleeding is usually minimal but requires clear visualization—avoid introducing clutter.

Step 9 – Complete airway survey and withdraw scope
Instruments: Bronchoscope.
Anticipation: Protect optics immediately upon removal.

Step 10 – Secure airway and conclude procedure
Instruments: None sterile.
Anticipation: Assist with specimen handling and ensure equipment is powered down safely.

Mayo Stand Suggestion:

- Biopsy forceps
- light cord
- lubricant
- Lukens Specimen Trap

Closure of Patent Ductus Arteriosus (PDA)

Step 1 – Patient positioning and verification
Instruments: Right lateral decubitus positioning aids, padding, axillary roll.
Anticipation: Confirm patient age (neonate vs child), side of approach (left thoracotomy), and availability of vascular clips or ties.

Step 2 – Left chest preparation and sterile draping
Instruments: Prep supplies, thoracic drapes.
Anticipation: Prep from axilla to mid-abdomen. Maintain wide exposure for possible extension.

Step 3 – Left posterolateral thoracotomy incision
Instruments: Scalpel handle with #10 blade, Adsons forceps with teeth.
Anticipation: Incision is vascular. Be ready with mosquito hemostats immediately.

Step 4 – Dissect through muscle layers and enter pleural space
Instruments: Metzenbaum scissors, 2 mosquito hemostats, Adsons forceps.
Anticipation: Follow clamp–cut rhythm. Protect underlying lung.

Closure of Patent Ductus Arteriosus (PDA)

Step 5 – Place rib spreader and expose mediastinum
Instruments: Rib spreader passed from back table when requested.
Anticipation: Exposure is delicate in small patients. Maintain organized instrument flow.

Step 6 – Identify aorta, pulmonary artery, and ductus arteriosus
Instruments: Metzenbaum scissors.
Anticipation: Anatomy may be small and fragile. Maintain a quiet field.

Step 7 – Carefully dissect around ductus
Instruments: Right-angle clamp passed from back table.
Anticipation: This is a critical step—anticipate clamp positioning without opening early.

Step 8 – Ligate or clip ductus arteriosus
Instruments: Vascular clips or ties passed from back table when requested.
Anticipation: Confirm ligation method before opening clips or sutures.

Step 9 – Divide ductus if indicated
Instruments: Passed from back table if requested.
Anticipation: Bleeding risk increases—be ready with clamps immediately.

Step 10 – Inspect for hemostasis
Instruments: Mosquito hemostats if needed.
Anticipation: Even small bleeds are significant in pediatric patients.

Step 11 – Re-expand lung and place chest tube if ordered
Instruments: Chest tube passed from back table.
Anticipation: Confirm tube size before opening.

Step 12 – Close thoracotomy incision
Instruments: Brought from back table when requested.
Anticipation: Begin closing counts early. Closure instruments move forward only after surgeon commits.

Step 13 – Apply sterile dressing
Instruments: Dressing supplies.
Anticipation: Secure chest tube and maintain line organization.

Mayo Stand Suggestion:

- 2 Scalpel handle with #10 blade
- Debakey, Russian Forceps
- Potts-Smith, Adsons Brown
- 2 mosquitos
- 2 mosquito with suture boots
- 4 curved hemostat
- 4 Crile, 4 Right Angle, 4 Kelly
- 4 tubing clamps
- 2 Crawford, 2 Satinsky
- 2 Cooley
- 2 straight vascular clamp
- Metzenbaum, Mayo
- Jameson, Coronary
- Rib spreader

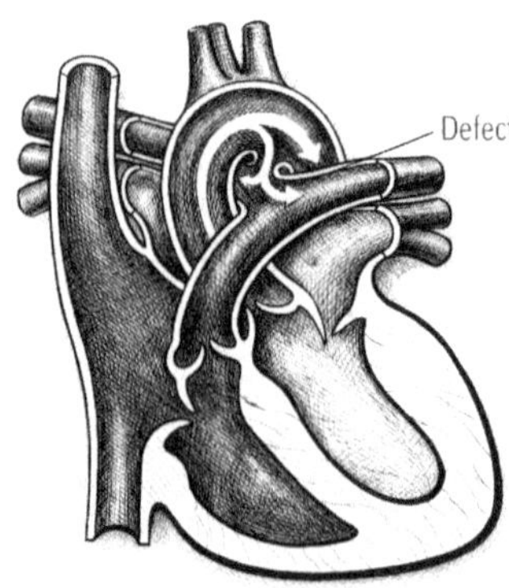

Coronary Artery Bypass with Grafting (CABG)

Step 1 – Patient positioning and verification
Instruments: Supine positioning aids, shoulder roll, padding.
Anticipation: Confirm number of grafts planned and conduit type (LIMA, saphenous vein, radial). Verify perfusion readiness.

Step 2 – Chest and conduit site preparation and draping
Instruments: Prep supplies, cardiac drapes.
Anticipation: Prep from chin to knees if vein harvest planned. Maintain access to chest and leg.

Step 3 – Median sternotomy
Instruments: Scalpel handle with #10 blade, Adsons forceps with teeth.
Anticipation: Incision is long and vascular. Be ready with mosquito hemostats immediately.

Step 4 – Open sternum and expose mediastinum
Instruments: Metzenbaum scissors, 2 mosquito hemostats.
Anticipation: Sternal retractors comes from back table only when requested. Maintain organized clamp placement.

Step 5 – Pericardiotomy and pericardial stay sutures
Instruments: Metzenbaum scissors.
Anticipation: Stay sutures placed early—anticipate needle driver from back table only when requested.

Step 6 – Harvest graft conduit(s)
Instruments: Passed from back table when requested.
Anticipation: Vein or artery harvest may occur simultaneously. Track graft handling and orientation carefully.

Step 7 – Systemic heparinization and cannulation
Instruments: Cannulas passed from back table when requested.
Anticipation: Coordinate with perfusion. Maintain quiet, uncluttered field.

Step 8 – Initiate cardiopulmonary bypass and apply cross clamp
Instruments: Aortic cross clamp passed from back table.
Anticipation: Timing is critical—clamps must be ready but unopened until called for.

Step 9 – Perform distal coronary anastomoses
Instruments: Sutures and needle driver brought from back table when requested.
Anticipation: Anastomosis sequence matters. Organize sutures by graft site.

Step 10 – Perform proximal graft anastomoses
Instruments: Aortic punch and clamps passed from back table when requested.
Anticipation: Confirm graft length and orientation before opening punch.

Step 11 – De air heart and remove cross clamp
Instruments: None additional.
Anticipation: Protect sterile field during de-airing and cardiac manipulation.

Step 12 – Wean from bypass and assess graft flow
Instruments: None additional.
Anticipation: Be prepared for pacing wires or adjustments as requested.

Coronary Artery Bypass with Grafting (CABG)

Step 13 – Achieve hemostasis and place chest tubes
Instruments: Chest tubes passed from back table.
Anticipation: Confirm tube size and number before opening.

Step 14 – Sternal closure
Instruments: Sternal wires and drivers passed from back table.
Anticipation: Heavy instruments introduced only at this phase.

Step 15 – Soft tissue and skin closure
Instruments: Brought from back table when requested.
Anticipation: Begin closing counts early and confirm final counts.

Step 16 – Apply sterile dressing
Instruments: Dressing supplies.
Anticipation: Secure chest tubes and lines before leaving field.

Mayo Stand Suggestion:

- 2 Scalpel handle with #10 blade
- Debakey, Russian Forceps
- Potts-Smith, Adsons Brown
- 2 mosquitos
- 2 mosquito with suture boots
- 4 curved hemostat
- 4 Crile, 4 Right Angle, 4 Kelly
- 4 tubing clamps
- 2 Crafoord, 2 Satinsky
- 2 Cooley
- 2 straight vascular clamp
- Metzenbaum, Mayo
- Jameson, Coronary
- Sternum retractors
- 2 Richardson
- 2 vein retractor

Decortication of the Lung

Step 1 – Patient positioning and verification
Instruments: Lateral decubitus positioning aids, axillary roll, padding.
Anticipation: Confirm operative side and whether approach is open thoracotomy or VATS. Ensure chest tube sizes are available.

Step 2 – Chest preparation and sterile draping
Instruments: Prep supplies, thoracic drapes.
Anticipation: Prep widely from axilla to iliac crest to allow incision extension.

Step 3 – Posterolateral thoracotomy or VATS port incision
Instruments: Scalpel handle with #10 blade, Adsons forceps with teeth.
Anticipation: Incision is muscular and vascular. Be ready with mosquito hemostats immediately.

Step 4 – Dissect through chest wall and enter pleural space
Instruments: Metzenbaum scissors, 2 mosquito hemostats, Adsons forceps.
Anticipation: Follow clamp–cut rhythm. Protect underlying lung on entry.

Step 5 – Place rib spreader or thoracoscopic access
Instruments: Rib spreader passed from back table when requested.
Anticipation: Rib spreading may cause bleeding. Keep clamps organized.

Step 6 – Identify pleural peel and lung surface
Instruments: Metzenbaum scissors.
Anticipation: Surgeon assesses thickness and extent of peel before removal.

Decortication of the Lung

Step 7 – Elevate and remove fibrous pleural peel
Instruments: Penfield dissector, rongeurs passed from back table.
Anticipation: Peel removal is slow and methodical. Do not stage bone or peel instruments on Mayo.

Step 8 – Assist with lung re-expansion checks
Instruments: None additional.
Anticipation: Anesthesia may perform recruitment maneuvers—maintain clear field.

Step 9 – Control bleeding from pleural surfaces
Instruments: Mosquito hemostats if needed.
Anticipation: Bleeding is common. Anticipate clamp placement quickly.

Step 10 – Irrigate and inspect lung expansion
Instruments: Managed .
Anticipation: Surgeon confirms full expansion before closure.

Step 11 – Place chest tubes
Instruments: Chest tubes passed from back table when requested.
Anticipation: Confirm tube size and number before opening.

Step 12 – Close thoracotomy or port sites
Instruments: Brought from back table when requested.
Anticipation: Begin closing counts early. Closure instruments move forward only after surgeon commits.

Step 13 – Apply sterile dressing
Instruments: Dressing supplies.
Anticipation: Secure chest tubes and maintain line organization.

Mayo Stand Suggestion:

- Scalpel handle with #10 blade
- Adsons Forceps with teeth
- 2 curved hemostats
- Metzenbaum scissors
- Rib Spreader
- Rongeurs
- Penfield Dissector

Double Lung Transplant

Step 1 – Patient positioning and verification
Instruments: Supine positioning aids, shoulder roll, padding.
Anticipation: Confirm donor lung arrival status, ABO compatibility, and laterality sequence. Coordinate closely with perfusion and anesthesia.

Step 2 – Chest preparation and wide sterile draping
Instruments: Prep supplies, transplant drapes.
Anticipation: Prep from neck to groin for possible femoral cannulation. Maintain access to both hemithoraces.

Step 3 – Bilateral thoracotomy or clamshell incision
Instruments: Scalpel handle with #10 blade, Adsons forceps with teeth.
Anticipation: Incision is extensive and vascular. Be ready with mosquito hemostats immediately.

Step 4 – Enter chest and place rib spreaders
Instruments: Metzenbaum scissors, 2 mosquito hemostats.
Anticipation: Rib spreaders are passed from back table only when requested. Maintain organized clamp placement.

Step 5 – Systemic heparinization and initiate cardiopulmonary bypass or ECMO if needed
Instruments: Cannulas passed from back table when requested.
Anticipation: Timing and communication with perfusion are critical. Keep Mayo uncluttered.

Step 6 – Pneumonectomy of first native lung
Instruments: Vascular clamps and staplers passed from back table.
Anticipation: Bronchus, pulmonary artery, and veins are divided sequentially. Anticipate order without opening early.

Step 7 – Prepare recipient bronchus, artery, and veins
Instruments: Metzenbaum scissors.
Anticipation: Anastomotic sites must be clean. Avoid clutter near field.

Step 8 – Implant first donor lung
Instruments: Sutures and needle driver brought from back table when requested.
Anticipation: Anastomoses occur in order: bronchus, artery, then veins. Organize sutures by structure.

Step 9 – Reperfuse and ventilate transplanted lung
Instruments: None additional.
Anticipation: Coordinate with anesthesia during reperfusion. Be alert for bleeding at anastomoses.

Step 10 – Repeat pneumonectomy and implantation on contralateral side
Instruments: Passed from back table as requested.
Anticipation: Workflow repeats but fatigue increases—maintain strict instrument discipline.

Step 11 – Inspect hemostasis and airway integrity
Instruments: Mosquito hemostats if needed.
Anticipation: Bleeding control is critical before chest closure.

Step 12 – Place bilateral chest tubes
Instruments: Chest tubes passed from back table.
Anticipation: Confirm size and number before opening.

Step 13 – Wean from bypass or ECMO if used
Instruments: None additional.
Anticipation: Maintain clear field during hemodynamic adjustments.

Step 14 – Close chest incision
Instruments: Brought from back table when requested.
Anticipation: Begin closing counts early. Heavy instruments introduced only at closure phase.

Step 15 – Apply sterile dressing and secure lines
Instruments: Dressing supplies.
Anticipation: Secure chest tubes, pacing wires, and lines carefully.

Double Lung Transplant

Mayo Stand Suggestion:

- Scalpel handle with #10 blade
- Adsons Forceps with teeth
- 2 curved hemostats
- Metzenbaum scissors
- Rib Spreader
- Vascular clamps
- Cannulas

Intra-aortic Balloon Pump (IABP) Insertion

Step 1 – Patient positioning and verification
Instruments: Supine positioning aids, padding.
Anticipation: Confirm indication (cardiogenic shock, peri-CABG support), insertion site (usually femoral), and balloon size based on patient height.

Step 2 – Groin preparation and sterile draping
Instruments: Prep supplies, vascular drape.
Anticipation: Prep widely from umbilicus to mid-thigh. Maintain access for possible contralateral access.

Step 3 – Identify femoral artery (percutaneous or cutdown)
Instruments: Ultrasound probe cover (if used) or palpation landmarks.
Anticipation: Clarify percutaneous vs open cutdown approach before opening instruments.

Step 4 – Percutaneous arterial access or surgical cutdown
Instruments:
• **Percutaneous:** introducer needle and sheath ()
• **Cutdown:** scalpel handle with #10 blade, Adsons forceps with teeth, 2 mosquito hemostats, Metzenbaum scissors
Anticipation: Only open cutdown instruments if surgeon commits to open approach.

Step 5 – Advance guidewire into aorta
Instruments: Guidewire passed from back table when requested.
Anticipation: Maintain strict wire control—do not open early or allow contamination.

Step 6 – Insert introducer sheath
Instruments: Sheath passed from back table.
Anticipation: Confirm sheath size matches balloon catheter.

Step 7 – Advance balloon catheter to correct position
Instruments: Balloon catheter ().
Anticipation: Positioning is confirmed by fluoroscopy or waveform—maintain quiet field.

Step 8 – Confirm balloon position and remove sheath dilator
Instruments: None additional.
Anticipation: Balloon tip should sit distal to left subclavian artery—verify before securing.

Step 9 – Secure catheter at insertion site
Instruments: Sutures and needle driver passed from back table only if required.
Anticipation: Not all IABPs require sutures—confirm surgeon preference.

Step 10 – Connect balloon catheter to console
Instruments: Console tubing ().
Anticipation: Coordinate timing with anesthesia/perfusion to avoid premature inflation.

Intra-aortic Balloon Pump (IABP) Insertion

Step 11 – Initiate balloon pumping and verify timing
Instruments: None sterile.
Anticipation: Assist with line organization and ensure catheter is not kinked.

Step 12 – Apply sterile dressing and secure lines
Instruments: Dressing supplies.
Anticipation: Secure tubing to prevent migration during patient transfer

Mayo Stand Suggestion:

- Scalpel handle with #10 blade
- Adsons Forceps with teeth
- 2 mosquito hemostats
- Metzenbaum scissors

Mediastinoscopy

Step 1 – Patient positioning and verification
Instruments: Supine positioning aids, shoulder roll to extend neck, head ring.
Anticipation: Confirm indication (staging vs diagnosis) and laterality of lymph node targets. Ensure neck extension is adequate before prep.

Step 2 – Neck and upper chest preparation and draping
Instruments: Prep supplies, thoracic/neck drapes.
Anticipation: Prep from mandible to upper chest. Maintain access to suprasternal notch.

Step 3 – Suprasternal skin incision
Instruments: Scalpel handle with #15 blade, Adsons forceps with teeth.
Anticipation: Incision is small but vascular. Be ready with mosquito hemostats immediately.

Step 4 – Dissect through platysma and pretracheal fascia
Instruments: Metzenbaum scissors, 2 mosquito hemostats, Adsons forceps.
Anticipation: Follow clamp–cut rhythm. Protect anterior jugular veins.

Step 5 – Blunt dissection to enter mediastinum
Instruments: Finger dissection or blunt instrument passed from back table.
Anticipation: Maintain a clear, uncluttered field. Surgeon relies on tactile feedback.

Step 6 – Insert mediastinoscope
Instruments: Mediastinoscope
Anticipation: Protect scope optics and cables. Ensure light source is functioning.

Step 7 – Identify anatomic landmarks
Instruments: None additional.
Anticipation: Surgeon may pause to orient—avoid unnecessary movement.

Step 8 – Biopsy mediastinal lymph nodes
Instruments: Biopsy forceps passed from back table when requested.
Anticipation: Open biopsy instruments only when target node is identified. Track specimen count carefully.

Mediastinoscopy

Step 9 – Control minor bleeding
Instruments: Mosquito hemostats if needed.
Anticipation: Bleeding is usually minimal but must be addressed promptly.

Step 10 – Withdraw mediastinoscope and inspect tract
Instruments: None additional.
Anticipation: Ensure no retained specimens or instruments.

Step 11 – Close neck incision
Instruments: Brought from back table when requested.
Anticipation: Begin closing counts early. Closure instruments come forward only after surgeon commits.

Step 12 – Apply sterile dressing
Instruments: Dressing supplies.
Anticipation: Keep dressing secure due to neck movement.

Mayo Stand Suggestion:

- Scalpel handle with #15 blade
- Adsons Forceps with teeth
- Debakey
- 2 mosquito hemostats
- 2 Right Angle
- 1 Oschner
- 2 Senn
- 2 Army Navy
- 1 Gelpi
- 2 Richardson
- Metzenbaum scissors
- Straight Mayo

MID CABG

Step 1 – Patient positioning and verification
Instruments: Supine positioning aids with left chest elevation, padding.
Anticipation: Confirm target vessel (often LAD) and conduit (LIMA). Ensure defibrillator pads and TEE readiness per anesthesia.

Step 2 – Left chest preparation and sterile draping
Instruments: Prep supplies, cardiac/thoracic drapes.
Anticipation: Prep from neck to upper abdomen. Maintain access to left chest and possible groin site if conversion needed.

Step 3 – Left anterior thoracotomy incision
Instruments: Scalpel handle with #10 blade, Adsons forceps with teeth.
Anticipation: Incision is smaller but deep. Be ready with mosquito hemostats immediately.

Step 4 – Dissect through intercostal muscles and enter pleural space
Instruments: Metzenbaum scissors, 2 mosquito hemostats, Adsons forceps.
Anticipation: Follow clamp-cut rhythm. Protect lung on entry.

Step 5 – Place rib retractors and expose heart
Instruments: Rib retractors passed from back table when requested.
Anticipation: Exposure is narrow. Keep the Mayo minimal to avoid crowding.

Step 6 – Harvest LIMA
Instruments: Passed from back table when requested.
Anticipation: Harvest is delicate, maintain organized instrument flow and avoid opening extras.

MID CABG

Step 7 – Identify LAD and prepare target site
Instruments: Passed from back table when requested.
Anticipation: Surgeon may request stabilizer and coronary shunt, do not open until called.

Step 8 – Apply coronary stabilizer and perform anastomosis
Instruments: Stabilizer and sutures passed from back table when requested.
Anticipation: Anastomosis timing is critical. Organize sutures and keep field quiet.

Step 9 – Assess graft flow and hemostasis
Instruments: None additional.
Anticipation: Be ready for adjustments. Maintain clear field for visualization.

Step 10 – Place chest tube if ordered
Instruments: Chest tube passed from back table.
Anticipation: Confirm tube size before opening.

Step 11 – Close thoracotomy incision
Instruments: Brought from back table when requested.
Anticipation: Begin closing counts early. Closure instruments move forward only after surgeon commits.

Step 12 – Apply sterile dressing
Instruments: Dressing supplies.
Anticipation: Secure chest tube and lines before drape removal.

Mayo Stand Suggestion:

- 2 Scalpel handle with #10 blade
- Debakey, Russian Forceps
- Potts-Smith, Adsons Brown
- 2 mosquitos
- 2 mosquito with suture boots
- 4 curved hemostat
- 4 Crile, 4 Right Angle, 4 Kelly
- 4 tubing clamps
- 2 Crafoord, 2 Satinsky
- 2 Cooley
- 2 straight vascular clamp
- Metzenbaum, Mayo
- Jameson, Coronary
- Sternum retractors
- 2 Richardson
- 2 vein retractor

Nuss Pectus Excavatum Repair by VATS

Step 1 – Patient positioning and verification
Instruments: Supine positioning aids with arms abducted, padding.
Anticipation: Confirm bar size availability, number of bars planned, and laterality of thoracoscopic access. Verify patient age and chest wall rigidity.

Step 2 – Chest preparation and wide sterile draping
Instruments: Prep supplies, thoracic drapes.
Anticipation: Prep from neck to umbilicus and laterally to mid-axillary lines. Maintain bilateral chest access.

Step 3 – Mark bar entry and exit sites
Instruments: Skin marker.
Anticipation: Symmetry is critical. Keep marker available for adjustments before incision.

Step 4 – Lateral chest wall incisions
Instruments: Scalpel handle with #15 blade, Adsons forceps with teeth.
Anticipation: Incisions are small but deep. Be ready with mosquito hemostats immediately.

Nuss Pectus Excavatum Repair by VATS

Step 5 – Establish thoracoscopic access
Instruments: Trocar and thoracoscope ().
Anticipation: Confirm camera and light before insertion. Protect optics at all times.

Step 6 – Create substernal tunnel
Instruments: Nuss introducer passed from back table when requested.
Anticipation: This is a critical step. Maintain absolute focus and do not introduce unnecessary instruments.

Step 7 – Pass Nuss bar through substernal tunnel
Instruments: Nuss bar passed from back table.
Anticipation: Confirm correct bar orientation before passing. Do not open extra bars prematurely.

Step 8 – Rotate bar to elevate sternum
Instruments: Bar flipper passed from back table.
Anticipation: Rotation changes chest wall dynamics—maintain clear field and communicate readiness.

Step 9 – Secure bar with stabilizers
Instruments: Stabilizers and fixation hardware passed from back table.
Anticipation: Confirm side and fixation method before opening hardware.

Step 10 – Reinspect thoracic cavity
Instruments: Thoracoscope.
Anticipation: Surgeon checks for bleeding and lung expansion. Avoid unnecessary movement.

Step 11 – Place chest tube if ordered
Instruments: Chest tube passed from back table.
Anticipation: Not always required—confirm before opening.

Step 12 – Close incisions
Instruments: Brought from back table when requested.
Anticipation: Begin closing counts early. Closure instruments come forward only after surgeon commits.

Step 13 – Apply sterile dressings and secure bar
Instruments: Dressing supplies.
Anticipation: Ensure bar ends are padded and protected to prevent skin breakdown.

NUSS PECTUS

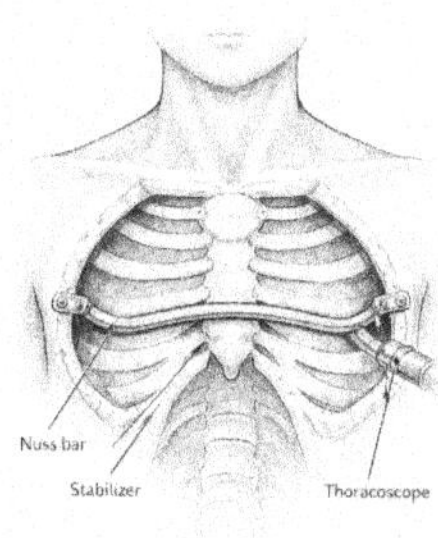

Off-Pump Coronary Artery Bypass (OPCAB)

Step 1 – Patient positioning and verification
Instruments: Supine positioning aids, shoulder roll, padding.
Anticipation: Confirm target vessels, number of grafts, and stabilizer system availability. Be prepared for rapid conversion to on-pump if needed.

Step 2 – Chest and conduit site preparation and draping
Instruments: Prep supplies, cardiac drapes.
Anticipation: Prep from chin to knees if vein harvest is planned. Maintain leg access without contaminating chest field.

Step 3 – Median sternotomy
Instruments: Scalpel handle with #10 blade, Adsons forceps with teeth.
Anticipation: Incision is long and vascular. Be ready with mosquito hemostats immediately.

Step 4 – Open sternum and expose mediastinum
Instruments: Metzenbaum scissors, 2 mosquito hemostats.
Anticipation: Sternal retractors comes from back table only when requested. Maintain clean clamp organization.

Step 5 – Pericardiotomy and stay sutures
Instruments: Metzenbaum scissors.
Anticipation: Surgeon may place multiple traction sutures—anticipate needle driver from back table only when asked.

Step 6 – Harvest graft conduit(s)
Instruments: Passed from back table when requested.
Anticipation: LIMA harvest and coronary exposure may overlap—stay aware of workflow split.

Step 7 – Position heart for target vessel exposure
Instruments: Heart positioner and stabilizer passed from back table.
Anticipation: Hemodynamics may change with heart manipulation—maintain quiet, controlled field.

Step 8 – Apply coronary stabilizer and shunt if used
Instruments: Stabilizer, shunt passed from back table.
Anticipation: Do not open shunts until vessel is exposed and surgeon commits.

Step 9 – Perform distal coronary anastomosis
Instruments: Sutures and needle driver brought from back table when requested.
Anticipation: Organize sutures by graft site. Avoid unnecessary instruments on Mayo.

Step 10 – Repeat positioning and anastomoses as needed
Instruments: Passed from back table.
Anticipation: Each graft may require repositioning—stay alert and adaptive.

Step 11 – Assess graft patency and hemostasis
Instruments: None additional.
Anticipation: Be prepared for additional sutures or adjustments.

Step 12 – Place chest tubes if ordered
Instruments: Chest tubes passed from back table.
Anticipation: Confirm tube size and number before opening.

Off-Pump Coronary Artery Bypass (OPCAB)

Step 13 – Sternal closure
Instruments: Sternal wires and drivers passed from back table.
Anticipation: Heavy instruments introduced only at this phase.

Step 14 – Soft tissue and skin closure
Instruments: Brought from back table when requested.
Anticipation: Begin closing counts early and confirm final counts.

Step 15 – Apply sterile dressing
Instruments: Dressing supplies.
Anticipation: Secure tubes and lines before drape removal

Mayo Stand Suggestion:

- 2 Scalpel handle with #10 blade
- Debakey, Russian Forceps
- Potts-Smith, Adsons Brown
- 2 mosquitos
- 2 mosquito with suture boots
- 4 curved hemostat
- 4 Crile, 4 Right Angle, 4 Kelly
- 4 tubing clamps
- 2 Crafoord, 2 Satinsky
- 2 Cooley
- 2 straight vascular clamp
- Metzenbaum, Mayo
- Jameson, Coronary
- Sternum retractors
- 2 Richardson
- 2 vein retractor

Pulmonary Thromboendarterectomy

Step 1 – Patient positioning and verification
Instruments: Supine positioning aids, shoulder roll, padding.
Anticipation: Confirm diagnosis, laterality sequence, and availability of hypothermia and bypass equipment. This is a long, high-risk case—organization is critical.

Step 2 – Chest preparation and wide sterile draping
Instruments: Prep supplies, cardiac drapes.
Anticipation: Prep from chin to groin for possible femoral access. Maintain access for perfusion lines.

Step 3 – Median sternotomy
Instruments: Scalpel handle with #10 blade, Adsons forceps with teeth.
Anticipation: Incision is long and vascular. Be ready with mosquito hemostats immediately.

Step 4 – Open sternum and expose mediastinum
Instruments: Metzenbaum scissors, 2 mosquito hemostats.
Anticipation: Sternal retractors comes from back table only when requested. Maintain clear clamp organization.

Step 5 – Pericardiotomy and stay sutures
Instruments: Metzenbaum scissors.
Anticipation: Anticipate stay sutures early—needle driver stays until requested.

Step 6 – Systemic heparinization and cannulation
Instruments: Cannulas passed from back table when requested.
Anticipation: Coordinate closely with perfusion. Maintain quiet, uncluttered field.

Step 7 – Initiate cardiopulmonary bypass and cool patient
Instruments: None additional.
Anticipation: Cooling phase is prolonged. Maintain readiness without opening instruments prematurely.

Pulmonary Thromboendarterectomy

Step 8 – Apply aortic cross clamp and achieve circulatory arrest
Instruments: Cross clamp passed from back table.
Anticipation: Absolute timing matters—do not distract the field.

Step 9 – Pulmonary arteriotomy
Instruments: Scalpel handle with #15 blade, Metzenbaum scissors.
Anticipation: Precise incision—be ready for small bleeders.

Step 10 – Identify and remove organized thrombus
Instruments: Endarterectomy dissectors and forceps passed from back table.
Anticipation: This step is delicate and methodical. Do not stage these instruments early.

Step 11 – Repeat endarterectomy on contralateral side
Instruments: Passed from back table when requested.
Anticipation: Workflow repeats under time pressure—stay focused and organized.

Step 12 – Close pulmonary arteriotomies
Instruments: Sutures and needle driver brought from back table when requested.
Anticipation: Transition to suturing phase—counts and suture control are critical.

Step 13 – Rewarm patient and wean from bypass
Instruments: None additional.
Anticipation: Be alert for requests for pacing wires or adjustments.

Step 14 – Inspect hemostasis and place chest tubes
Instruments: Chest tubes passed from back table.
Anticipation: Confirm tube size and number before opening.

Step 15 – Sternal closure
Instruments: Sternal wires and drivers passed from back table.
Anticipation: Heavy instruments introduced only at this phase.

Step 16 – Soft tissue and skin closure
Instruments: Brought from back table when requested.
Anticipation: Begin closing counts early and confirm final counts.

Step 17 – Apply sterile dressing
Instruments: Dressing supplies.
Anticipation: Secure tubes and lines before drape removal.

Mayo Stand Suggestion:

- Scalpel handle with #10 blade
- Debakey, Russian Forceps
- Gerald, Adsons Brown Forceps
- 2 Cooley Clamps
- Satinsky Occlusion Clamps
- Bulldog and Fogarty Clamps
- Pulmonary Endarterectomy Dissector
- Nerve Hooks
- Freer Elevator
- Frazier Suction
- Vessel Loops
- Finochietto Sternal retractors

Pneumonectomy

Step 1 – Patient positioning and verification
Instruments: Lateral decubitus positioning aids, axillary roll, padding.
Anticipation: Confirm operative side, bronchial stump management plan, and chest tube requirements. Ensure double-lumen tube placement is confirmed by anesthesia.

Step 2 – Chest preparation and sterile draping
Instruments: Prep supplies, thoracic drapes.
Anticipation: Prep widely from axilla to iliac crest to allow incision extension.

Step 3 – Posterolateral thoracotomy incision
Instruments: Scalpel handle with #10 blade, Adsons forceps with teeth.
Anticipation: Incision is muscular and vascular. Be ready with mosquito hemostats immediately.

Step 4 – Dissect through muscle layers and enter pleural space
Instruments: Metzenbaum scissors, 2 mosquito hemostats, Adsons forceps.
Anticipation: Follow clamp-cut rhythm. Protect underlying lung during entry.

Step 5 – Place rib spreader and expose lung
Instruments: Rib spreader passed from back table when requested.
Anticipation: Exposure is extensive. Maintain organized instrument flow.

Step 6 – Mobilize lung and divide pulmonary ligament
Instruments: Metzenbaum scissors.
Anticipation: Surgeon may reposition lung frequently; keep field clear.

Step 7 – Isolate and divide pulmonary vessels
Instruments: Vascular clamps and staplers passed from back table when requested.
Anticipation: Division sequence (artery, vein) varies—confirm before opening staplers.

Step 8 – Divide main bronchus
Instruments: Bronchial stapler passed from back table.
Anticipation: Confirm correct bronchus and stump length before firing.

Step 9 – Remove lung specimen
Instruments: Specimen bag passed from back table if used.
Anticipation: Clear path for specimen removal. Open container before division.

Step 10 – Inspect bronchial stump and hemostasis
Instruments: Mosquito hemostats if needed.
Anticipation: Bronchial stump integrity is critical; be ready for reinforcement.

Step 11 – Place chest tube if ordered
Instruments: Chest tube passed from back table.
Anticipation: Not always placed after pneumonectomy; confirm before opening.

Step 12 – Close thoracotomy incision
Instruments: Brought from back table when requested.
Anticipation: Begin closing counts early. Closure instruments.

Step 13 – Apply sterile dressing
Instruments: Dressing supplies.
Anticipation: Secure chest tube and maintain line organization.

Pneumonectomy

Mayo Stand Suggestion:

- Scalpel handle with #10 blade
- Debakey, Russian Forceps
- Gerald, Adsons Brown Forceps
- Right Angle, Curved Kelly Clamps
- Satinsky Occlusion Clamps
- Bulldog and Tonsil Clamps
- Bronchial and GIA Stapler

Repair of Atrial Septal Defect (ASD)

Step 1 – Patient positioning and verification
Instruments: Supine positioning aids, shoulder roll, padding.
Anticipation: Confirm ASD type (secundum, primum, sinus venosus), patient size, and patch material availability if needed.

Step 2 – Chest preparation and sterile draping
Instruments: Prep supplies, cardiac drapes.
Anticipation: Prep from chin to groin for potential femoral cannulation.

Step 3 – Median sternotomy
Instruments: Scalpel handle with #10 blade, Adsons forceps with teeth.
Anticipation: Incision is long and vascular. Be ready with mosquito hemostats immediately.

Step 4 – Open sternum and expose mediastinum
Instruments: Metzenbaum scissors, 2 mosquito hemostats.
Anticipation: Sternal retractors is passed from back table only when requested.

Step 5 – Pericardiotomy and stay sutures
Instruments: Metzenbaum scissors.
Anticipation: Anticipate stay sutures early; needle driver stays until requested.

Step 6 – Systemic heparinization and cannulation
Instruments: Cannulas passed from back table when requested.
Anticipation: Coordinate with perfusion. Maintain uncluttered field.

Step 7 – Initiate cardiopulmonary bypass and apply cross-clamp
Instruments: Aortic cross-clamp passed from back table.
Anticipation: Timing is critical. Maintain quiet field.

Step 8 – Right atriotomy
Instruments: Scalpel handle with #15 blade, Metzenbaum scissors.
Anticipation: Precise incision; be ready for small bleeders.

Step 9 – Identify and expose atrial septal defect
Instruments: Atrial retractor passed from back table.
Anticipation: Exposure determines repair quality. Keep Mayo clear.

Step 10 – Close ASD with sutures or patch
Instruments: Sutures, needle driver, and patch passed from back table when requested.
Anticipation: Confirm patch type and size before opening.

Step 11 – Close atriotomy
Instruments: Passed from back table when requested.
Anticipation: Suture organization and counts are critical.

Repair of Atrial Septal Defect (ASD)

Step 12 – De-air heart and remove cross-clamp
Instruments: None additional.
Anticipation: Protect sterile field during de-airing.

Step 13 – Wean from bypass and assess repair
Instruments: None additional.
Anticipation: Be prepared for pacing wires or revision if needed.

Step 14 – Achieve hemostasis and place chest tubes
Instruments: Chest tubes passed from back table.
Anticipation: Confirm size and number before opening.

Step 15 – Sternal closure
Instruments: Sternal wires and drivers passed from back table.
Anticipation: Heavy instruments introduced only at this phase.

Step 16 – Soft tissue and skin closure
Instruments: Brought from back table when requested.
Anticipation: Begin closing counts early and confirm final counts.

Step 17 – Apply sterile dressing
Instruments: Dressing supplies.
Anticipation: Secure chest tubes and pacing wires.

Mayo Stand Suggestion:

- Scalpel handle with #10 blade
- Debakey, Russian Forceps
- Gerald, Adsons Brown Forceps
- Right Angle, Curved Kelly Clamps
- Satinsky Occlusion Clamps
- Bulldog and Tonsil Clamps
- Atrial retractor
- Nerve Hooks
- Potts-Smith Scissors
- Metzenbaum Scissors
- Tenotomy Scissors

Repair of Coarctation of the Aorta

Step 1 – Patient positioning and verification
Instruments: Right lateral decubitus positioning aids, axillary roll, padding.
Anticipation: Confirm repair method (end to end anastomosis, patch aortoplasty, subclavian flap) and patient age. Ensure vascular clamp sizes appropriate for patient.

Step 2 – Left chest preparation and sterile draping
Instruments: Prep supplies, thoracic drapes.
Anticipation: Prep widely from axilla to iliac crest. Maintain access for possible extension and for monitoring lines.

Step 3 – Left posterolateral thoracotomy incision
Instruments: Scalpel handle with #10 blade, Adsons forceps with teeth.
Anticipation: Incision is vascular. Be ready with mosquito hemostats immediately.

Step 4 – Dissect through muscle layers and enter pleural space
Instruments: Metzenbaum scissors, 2 mosquito hemostats, Adsons forceps.
Anticipation: Follow clamp-cut rhythm. Protect underlying lung on entry.

Step 5 – Place rib spreader and expose descending thoracic aorta
Instruments: Rib spreader passed from back table when requested.
Anticipation: Exposure is narrow in pediatrics; keep field minimal and organized.

Repair of Coarctation of the Aorta

Step 6 – Mobilize aorta and identify coarctation segment
Instruments: Metzenbaum scissors.
Anticipation: Maintain a quiet field; dissection is close to critical structures.

Step 7 – Apply proximal and distal vascular clamps
Instruments: Vascular clamps passed from back table when requested.
Anticipation: Clamp choice depends on anatomy. Do not open extra clamps early.

Step 8 – Resect narrowed segment or open aorta for patch
Instruments: Scalpel handle with #15 blade, Metzenbaum scissors.
Anticipation: Precise vascular work—be ready for controlled instrument handoffs.

Step 9 – Perform repair (end to end anastomosis or patch)
Instruments: Sutures and needle driver brought from back table when requested; patch graft if used.
Anticipation: Confirm patch material before opening. Organize sutures carefully.

Step 10 – Release clamps and inspect for bleeding
Instruments: Mosquito hemostats if needed.
Anticipation: Bleeding control is critical. Be ready to pass additional sutures quickly.

Step 11 – Re-expand lung and place chest tube if ordered
Instruments: Chest tube passed from back table.
Anticipation: Confirm tube size before opening.

Step 12 – Close thoracotomy incision
Instruments: Brought from back table when requested.
Anticipation: Begin closing counts early. Closure instruments move forward only after surgeon commits.

Step 13 – Apply sterile dressing
Instruments: Dressing supplies.
Anticipation: Secure chest tube and line organization.

Mayo Stand Suggestion:

- Scalpel handle with #10 blade
- Debakey, Russian Forceps
- Gerald, Adsons Brown Forceps
- Right Angle Clamps
- Satinsky Occlusion Clamps
- Bulldog and Tonsil Clamps
- Atrial retractor
- Nerve Hooks
- Potts-Smith Scissors
- Metzenbaum Scissors
- Tenotomy Scissors
- Penfield #1 and #3

Repair of Tetralogy of Fallot (TOF)

Step 1 – Patient positioning and verification
Instruments: Supine positioning aids, shoulder roll, padding.
Anticipation: Confirm planned repair components (VSD patch, RVOT relief, possible transannular patch, possible PA patch). Ensure correct pediatric cannula sizes and patch materials are available.

Step 2 – Chest preparation and wide sterile draping
Instruments: Prep supplies, cardiac drapes.
Anticipation: Prep from chin to groin for potential femoral access. Keep line management tidy for a high-line pediatric case.

Repair of Tetralogy of Fallot (TOF)

Step 3 – Median sternotomy
Instruments: Scalpel handle with #10 blade, Adsons forceps with teeth.
Anticipation: Long midline incision. Be ready with mosquito hemostats early for subcutaneous bleeders.

Step 4 – Open sternum and expose mediastinum
Instruments: Metzenbaum scissors, 2 mosquito hemostats.
Anticipation: Sternal retractors is passed from back table only when requested. Maintain a clean, uncluttered Mayo.

Step 5 – Pericardiotomy and pericardial stay sutures
Instruments: Metzenbaum scissors.
Anticipation: Stay sutures are often multiple. Keep suture organization tight and prepare to pass needle driver from back table only when asked.

Step 6 – Systemic heparinization and cannulation
Instruments: Aortic and venous cannulas passed from back table when requested.
Anticipation: Pediatric cannulation is sensitive to size and sequence. Confirm cannula sizes are correct before they are opened/handed off.

Step 7 – Initiate cardiopulmonary bypass and myocardial protection
Instruments: Aortic cross clamp passed from back table when requested.
Anticipation: Timing is critical. Keep the field quiet during cross clamp and cardioplegia delivery.

Step 8 – Right atriotomy and exposure of VSD
Instruments: Scalpel handle with #15 blade, Metzenbaum scissors.
Anticipation: Exposure drives repair quality. Atrial retractor come from back table.

Step 9 – VSD closure with patch (or primary closure if small)
Instruments: Patch material, sutures, needle driver passed from back table when requested.
Anticipation: Do not open patch until surgeon confirms size/shape needed. Have sutures staged on back table by type (pledgeted vs nonpledgeted) and pass only as requested.

Step 10 – Relief of RV outflow tract obstruction
Instruments: Passed from back table when requested.
Anticipation: Surgeon may address muscle bundles/infundibular stenosis and then reassess. Be ready for a change in plan (transannular patch vs valve-sparing approach).

Step 11 – Pulmonary valve/PA repair if required
Instruments: Patch material and sutures passed from back table when requested.
Anticipation: Patch work often shifts quickly between RVOT and PA. Keep patch options controlled and unopened until committed.

Step 12 – Close atriotomy and any ventriculotomy/arteriotomy
Instruments: Sutures and needle driver passed from back table when requested.
Anticipation: Confirm suture type and needle size for each closure layer. Maintain strict needle counts.

Step 13 – De-air heart and remove cross clamp
Instruments: None additional.
Anticipation: De-airing is high-focus. Minimize movement and be ready to pass requested items quickly without prompting.

Repair of Tetralogy of Fallot (TOF)

Step 14 – Wean from bypass and assess repair
Instruments: None additional.
Anticipation: Be prepared for pacing wires if requested and for rapid hemostasis needs as pressures normalize.

Step 15 – Hemostasis and chest tubes
Instruments: Chest tubes passed from back table when requested.
Anticipation: Confirm tube size/quantity before opening. Secure tubes and keep line organization clean.

Step 16 – Sternal closure
Instruments: Sternal wires and wire driver passed from back table when requested.
Anticipation: Heavy instruments come forward only now. Ensure counts are progressing and communicated clearly.

Step 17 – Soft tissue and skin closure
Instruments: Brought from back table when requested.
Anticipation: Closure sequence may be fast after a long case. Stay disciplined: only bring closure instruments forward when surgeon commits.

Step 18 – Dressing and secure lines
Instruments: Dressing supplies.
Anticipation: Final check: chest tubes secured, pacing wires secured if present, no line tension before drapes come down.

Mayo Stand Suggestion:

- #7 Knife Handle with #15 blade
- Potts-Smith Scissors
- Metzenbaum Scissors
- Debakey Forceps
- Gerald Forceps (without teeth)
- Right-Angle Clamp (Mixter)
- Atraumatic Bulldog Clamp
- Castroviejo Needle driver
- Debakey Needle driver
- Frazier Suction Tip
- Nerve Hook
- Pledget Forceps

Upper Lobectomy

Step 1 – Patient positioning and verification
Instruments: Lateral decubitus positioning aids, axillary roll, padding.
Anticipation: Confirm operative side and approach (open vs VATS). Verify double-lumen tube placement with anesthesia.

Step 2 – Chest preparation and sterile draping
Instruments: Prep supplies, thoracic drapes.
Anticipation: Prep widely from axilla to iliac crest. Ensure room for incision extension.

Step 3 – Thoracotomy incision or VATS port incisions
Instruments: Scalpel handle with #10 blade, Adsons forceps with teeth.
Anticipation: Incisions are muscular and vascular. Be ready with mosquito hemostats immediately.

Step 4 – Dissect through chest wall and enter pleural space
Instruments: Metzenbaum scissors, 2 mosquito hemostats, Adsons forceps.
Anticipation: Follow clamp–cut rhythm. Protect lung on entry.

Upper Lobectomy

Step 5 – Place rib spreader or establish thoracoscopic access
Instruments: Rib spreader or trocars passed from back table when requested.
Anticipation: Exposure changes quickly; keep Mayo minimal.

Step 6 – Explore thoracic cavity and identify upper lobe structures
Instruments: None additional.
Anticipation: Surgeon assesses anatomy and tumor location; avoid crowding field.

Step 7 – Mobilize and divide pulmonary vein to upper lobe
Instruments: Vascular clamp and stapler passed from back table when requested.
Anticipation: Confirm vessel before opening stapler load.

Step 8 – Divide pulmonary artery branches to upper lobe
Instruments: Vascular stapler or clips passed from back table.
Anticipation: Multiple branches may require multiple loads; open sequentially.

Step 9 – Divide upper lobe bronchus
Instruments: Bronchial stapler passed from back table.
Anticipation: Confirm correct bronchus and stump length before firing.

Step 10 – Divide fissure and complete lobectomy
Instruments: Stapler loads passed from back table.
Anticipation: Fissure work can be variable. Keep additional loads available but unopened.

Step 11 – Remove specimen
Instruments: Specimen retrieval bag or container passed from back table.
Anticipation: Open specimen container before lobe is freed.

Step 12 – Inspect bronchial stump and air leak test
Instruments: None additional.
Anticipation: Surgeon may request reinforcements. Be ready for suture requests from back table.

Step 13 – Irrigate and achieve hemostasis
Instruments: Managed .
Anticipation: Bleeding control is critical before chest tubes.

Step 14 – Place chest tube(s)
Instruments: Chest tubes passed from back table.
Anticipation: Confirm tube size and number before opening.

Step 15 – Close thoracotomy or port sites
Instruments: Brought from back table when requested.
Anticipation: Begin closing counts early. Closure instruments move forward only after surgeon commits.

Step 16 – Apply sterile dressing
Instruments: Dressing supplies.
Anticipation: Secure chest tubes and keep line organization clean.

Upper Lobectomy

Mayo Stand Suggestion:

- Knife Handle with #10 blade
- Metzenbaum Scissors
- Long Metzenbaum Scissors
- Potts-Smith Scissors
- Debakey Forceps
- Gerald Forceps (with teeth)
- Right-Angle Clamp (Mixter)
- Debakey Vascular Clamp
- Duval Lung Forceps
- Mayo-Hegar Needle Driver
- Frazier Suction Tip
- Foerster Sponge Forceps

Ventricular Aneurysm Repair

Step 1 – Patient positioning and verification
Instruments: Supine positioning aids, shoulder roll, padding.
Anticipation: Confirm aneurysm location (usually LV apex or anterior wall), patch material availability, and whether repair is linear or patch-based.

Step 2 – Chest preparation and wide sterile draping
Instruments: Prep supplies, cardiac drapes.
Anticipation: Prep from chin to groin for potential femoral cannulation. Keep line management organized for bypass workflow.

Step 3 – Median sternotomy
Instruments: Scalpel handle with #10 blade, Adsons forceps with teeth.
Anticipation: Long, vascular incision. Be ready with mosquito hemostats immediately for skin and subcutaneous bleeders.

Step 4 – Open sternum and expose mediastinum
Instruments: Metzenbaum scissors, 2 mosquito hemostats.
Anticipation: Sternal retractors is passed from the back table only when requested. Maintain a clean, uncluttered Mayo.

Step 5 – Pericardiotomy and pericardial stay sutures
Instruments: Metzenbaum scissors.
Anticipation: Anticipate multiple stay sutures. Needle driver ready.

Step 6 – Systemic heparinization and cannulation
Instruments: Aortic and venous cannulas passed from back table when requested.
Anticipation: Coordinate closely with perfusion. Confirm cannula size and sequence before passing.

Step 7 – Initiate cardiopulmonary bypass and apply cross clamp
Instruments: Aortic cross clamp.
Anticipation: Timing is critical. Maintain a quiet, distraction-free field during clamping.

Step 8 – Identify ventricular aneurysm and perform ventriculotomy
Instruments: Scalpel handle with #15 blade, Metzenbaum scissors.
Anticipation: Precise incision into weakened myocardium. Be prepared for controlled suctioning by anesthesia/perfusion.

Step 9 – Remove aneurysmal tissue and thrombus
Instruments: Passed when requested.
Anticipation: Thrombus may be present. Ensure specimen container is ready before tissue removal

Step 10 – Ventricular reconstruction (linear closure or patch repair)
Instruments: Patch material, sutures, needle driver passed from back table when requested.
Anticipation: Do not open patch until surgeon confirms size and technique. Organize sutures carefully by needle type and length.

Step 11 – Close ventriculotomy and reinforce repair
Instruments: Passed when requested.
Anticipation: Layered closure requires strict needle and sponge counts.

Step 12 – De-air heart and remove cross clamp
Instruments: None additional.
Anticipation: Maintain absolute stillness during de-airing. Be ready for immediate requests without prompting.

Step 13 – Wean from bypass and assess ventricular function
Instruments: None additional.
Anticipation: Surgeon may request pacing wires or additional sutures as pressures normalize.

Step 14 – Hemostasis and chest tube placement
Instruments: Chest tubes passed from back table when requested.
Anticipation: Confirm tube size and number before opening.

Step 15 – Sternal closure
Instruments: Sternal wires and wire driver passed from back table when requested.
Anticipation: Heavy instruments introduced only at this phase. Ensure counts are correct and communicated clearly.

Step 16 – Soft tissue and skin closure
Instruments: Brought from back table when requested.
Anticipation: Closure may proceed quickly after a long case—stay disciplined with instrument flow.

Step 17 – Dressing application and line security
Instruments: Dressing supplies.
Anticipation: Secure chest tubes, pacing wires, and lines prior to drape removal.

Mayo Stand Suggestion:

- #7 Knife Handle with #15 blade
- Potts-Smith Scissors (45° vascular)
- Metzenbaum Scissors
- Debakey Forceps
- Gerald Forceps (without teeth)
- Right-Angle Clamp (Mixter)
- Atraumatic Bulldog Clamp
- Castroviejo Needle driver
- Debakey Needle driver
- Frazier Suction Tip (6–10 Fr)
- Nerve Hook
- Pledget Forceps

Video Assisted Thoracic Surgery (VATS)

Step 1 – Patient positioning and verification
Instruments: Lateral decubitus positioning aids, axillary roll, padding.
Anticipation: Confirm operative side and planned procedure (diagnostic vs resection). Verify double-lumen tube placement with anesthesia before prep.

Step 2 – Chest preparation and sterile draping
Instruments: Prep supplies, thoracoscopic drapes.
Anticipation: Prep from axilla to iliac crest and midline anteriorly. Maintain room for conversion to open thoracotomy.

Step 3 – Mark port sites
Instruments: Skin marker.
Anticipation: Port placement is procedure-specific. Keep marker available for adjustments before incision.

Step 4 – Initial port incision
Instruments: Scalpel handle with #10 or #15 blade, Adsons forceps with teeth.
Anticipation: Incisions are small but vascular. Be ready with mosquito hemostats immediately.

Step 5 – Blunt dissection and trocar placement
Instruments: Trocar passed from back table when requested.
Anticipation: Confirm trocar size before opening. Protect lung during entry.

Step 6 – Insert thoracoscope and establish visualization
Instruments: Thoracoscope and camera system ().
Anticipation: Verify white balance and image clarity prior to insertion.

Step 7 – Place additional working ports
Instruments: Scalpel handle with blade as requested.
Anticipation: Port number varies. Open trocars sequentially only as requested.

Step 8 – Perform thoracoscopic procedure
Instruments: Staplers, graspers, dissectors passed from back table when requested.
Anticipation: Instrument needs change rapidly. Stay focused on surgeon's visual cues rather than verbal requests.

Step 9 – Specimen removal
Instruments: Specimen retrieval bag passed from back table when requested.
Anticipation: Open bag only when specimen is ready to be removed. Confirm specimen labeling.

Step 10 – Inspect lung and achieve hemostasis
Instruments: Managed .
Anticipation: Surgeon checks for air leaks. Be ready for reinforcement sutures if request.

Step 11 – Place chest tube(s)
Instruments: Chest tube passed from back table when requested.
Anticipation: Confirm size and number before opening.

Step 12 – Remove trocars and close port sites
Instruments: Brought from back table when requested.
Anticipation: Begin closing counts early. Closure instruments move forward only after surgeon commits.

Video Assisted Thoracic Surgery (VATS)

Step 13 – Apply sterile dressing
Instruments: Dressing supplies.
Anticipation: Secure chest tube and maintain line organization before drapes come down.

Mayo Stand Suggestion:

- #3 Knife Handle with #10 blade
- Metzenbaum Scissors
- Long Metzenbaum Scissors
- Endoscopic Right-Angle Dissector
- Endoscopic Grasper (atraumatic)
- Endoscopic Lung Grasper
- Endoscopic Scissors
- Endoscopic Clip Applier
- Endoscopic Stapler (with appropriate reload)
- Frazier Suction Tip
- Yankauer Suction
- Foerster Sponge Forceps

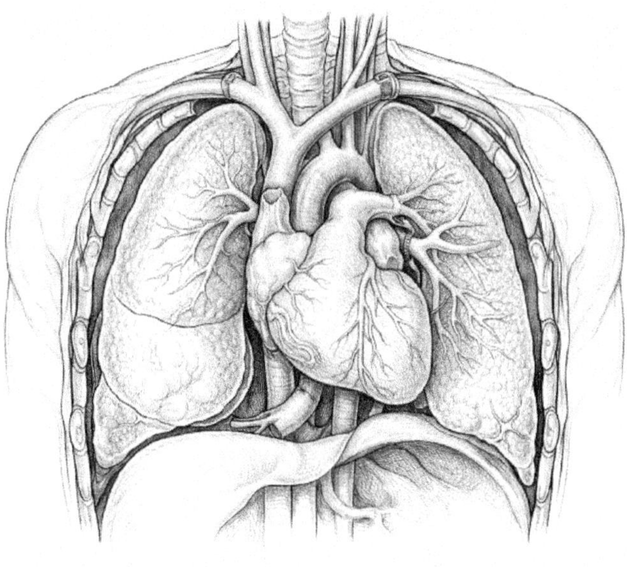

Section X:

Peripheral Vascular Procedures

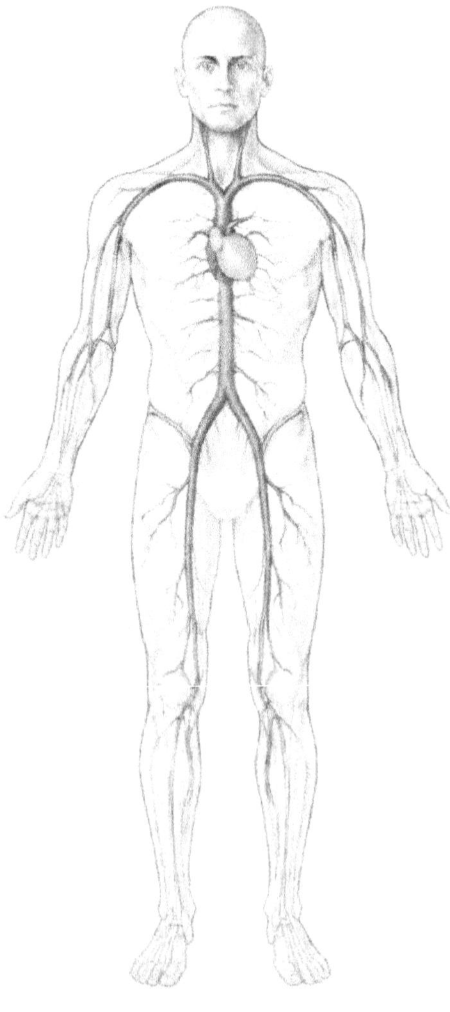

Abdominal Aortic Aneurysm with Graft

Step 1 – Patient positioning and verification
Instruments: Supine positioning aids, padding, arm boards.
Anticipation: Confirm aneurysm location (infrarenal vs suprarenal), graft type (tube vs bifurcated), and availability of appropriate vascular clamp sizes.

Step 2 – Abdominal preparation and wide sterile draping
Instruments: Prep supplies, vascular drapes.
Anticipation: Prep from nipple line to mid-thighs for possible femoral access. Keep groins accessible.

Step 3 – Midline abdominal incision
Instruments: Scalpel handle with #10 blade, Adsons forceps with teeth.
Anticipation: Incision is long and vascular. Be ready with mosquito hemostats immediately.

Step 4 – Enter abdominal cavity and expose retroperitoneum
Instruments: Metzenbaum scissors, 2 mosquito hemostats.
Anticipation: Follow clamp–cut rhythm. Protect bowel and maintain moist lap control.

Step 5 – Mobilize bowel and expose aorta
Instruments: Handheld retractor passed from back table when requested.
Anticipation: Bowel protection is critical. Keep moist laps available and countable.

Step 6 – Isolate proximal and distal aorta and iliac arteries
Instruments: Passed from back table when requested.
Anticipation: Dissection is deliberate. Be prepared for multiple vessel loop requests without opening early.

Step 7 – Systemic heparinization and apply vascular clamps
Instruments: Vascular clamps passed from back table when requested.
Anticipation: Clamp timing is critical. Maintain a quiet field and do not clutter the Mayo.

Step 8 – Open aneurysm sac
Instruments: Scalpel handle with #15 blade, Metzenbaum scissors.
Anticipation: Expect back-bleeding. Suction is managed ; anticipate clamp adjustments.

Step 9 – Remove thrombus and debris
Instruments: Passed from back table when requested.
Anticipation: Have specimen containers ready if thrombus is sent to pathology.

Step 10 – Anastomose proximal graft to aorta
Instruments: Graft, sutures, needle driver passed from back table when requested.
Anticipation: Do not open graft until surgeon confirms size and configuration. Organize sutures carefully.

Step 11 – Anastomose distal graft to aorta or iliac arteries
Instruments: Passed from back table when requested.
Anticipation: Distal anastomosis sequence varies—confirm side before passing graft limbs.

Step 12 – Release clamps and inspect for bleeding
Instruments: Mosquito hemostats if needed.
Anticipation: Be ready for additional sutures immediately after reperfusion.

Abdominal Aortic Aneurysm with Graft

Step 13 – Close aneurysm sac over graft
Instruments: Passed from back table when requested.
Anticipation: Sac closure protects graft—suture organization matters.

Step 14 – Irrigate and achieve hemostasis
Instruments: Managed .
Anticipation: Ensure all laps are accounted for before abdominal closure.

Step 15 – Layered abdominal closure
Instruments: Brought from back table when requested.
Anticipation: Begin closing counts early. Closure instruments move forward only when surgeon commits.

Step 16 – Apply sterile dressing
Instruments: Dressing supplies.
Anticipation: Ensure drains (if placed) are secured and visible.

Mayo Stand Suggestion:

- Knife with #10 blade
- Metzenbaum Scissors
- Potts-Smith Scissors
- Debakey Forceps
- Gerald Forceps (without teeth)
- Right-Angle Clamp (Mixter)
- Satinsky Partial-Occlusion Clamp
- Debakey Aortic Cross-Clamp
- Atraumatic Bulldog Clamp
- Debakey Needle driver
- Castroviejo Needle driver
- Frazier Suction Tip

Angioplasty

Step 1 – Patient positioning and verification
Instruments: Supine positioning aids, padding.
Anticipation: Confirm target vessel, access site (femoral, radial, brachial), and whether stenting is planned. Verify contrast availability and imaging readiness.

Step 2 – Access site preparation and sterile draping
Instruments: Prep supplies, vascular drapes.
Anticipation: Prep widely to allow alternative access if initial site fails.

Step 3 – Establish vascular access (percutaneous or cutdown)
Instruments:
- Percutaneous: Access needle and sheath
- Cutdown: Scalpel handle with #10 blade, Adsons forceps with teeth, Metzenbaum scissors, 2 mosquito hemostats

Anticipation: Clarify approach before opening cutdown instruments. Do not stage both methods simultaneously.

Step 4 – Insert guidewire into vessel
Instruments: Guidewire passed from back table when requested.
Anticipation: Maintain strict wire control. Never allow wire to be set down or contaminated.

Step 5 – Advance introducer sheath
Instruments: Introducer sheath passed from back table.
Anticipation: Confirm sheath size before opening. Maintain wire position at all times.

Angioplasty

Step 7 – Inflate balloon to dilate vessel
Instruments: Inflation device
Anticipation: Inflation timing is controlled by surgeon. Monitor sterile tubing organization.

Step 8 – Deflate and remove balloon
Instruments: None additional.
Anticipation: Maintain wire access in case repeat dilation is required.

Step 9 – Deploy stent if indicated
Instruments: Stent delivery system passed from back table when requested.
Anticipation: Confirm stent size, length, and deployment mechanism before opening.

Step 10 – Confirm vessel patency via imaging
Instruments: Imaging managed .
Anticipation: Avoid movement during imaging acquisition.

Step 11 – Remove sheath and achieve hemostasis
Instruments: Closure device or manual pressure supplies
Anticipation: Hemostasis method varies. Confirm closure plan before opening devices.

Step 12 – Apply sterile dressing
Instruments: Dressing supplies.
Anticipation: Secure dressing firmly to prevent bleeding at access site.

Mayo Stand Suggestion:

- Knife with #11 blade
- Mosquito Hemostat
- Right-Angle Clamp
- Debakey Forceps
- Gerald Forceps (without teeth)
- Introducer Needle
- Guidewire
- Vascular Sheath with Dilator
- Angioplasty Balloon Catheter
- Torque Device
- Contrast Syringe (luer-lock)
- Frazier Suction Tip

Angioscopy

Step 1 – Patient positioning and verification
Instruments: Supine positioning aids, padding.
Anticipation: Confirm target vessel, access site (femoral, brachial, or open vessel), and whether angioscopy is diagnostic or adjunct to another vascular procedure.

Step 2 – Access site preparation and sterile draping
Instruments: Prep supplies, vascular drapes.
Anticipation: Prep widely to allow alternative access or conversion to open exposure if needed.

Step 3 – Establish vascular access (percutaneous or open)
Instruments:
- Percutaneous: introducer needle and sheath
- Open: scalpel handle with #10 blade, Adsons forceps with teeth, Metzenbaum scissors, 2 mosquito hemostats

Anticipation: Clarify approach before opening instruments. Do not stage open and percutaneous tools together.

Step 4 – Insert guidewire and introducer sheath
Instruments: Guidewire and sheath passed from back table when requested.
Anticipation: Maintain strict wire control. Never allow wire to be released or set down.

Step 5 – Flush angioscope and tubing
Instruments: Angioscope system
Anticipation: Ensure all tubing is flushed and air-free before insertion to prevent embolism.

Step 6 – Insert angioscope into vessel
Instruments: Angioscope
Anticipation: Protect optics and avoid torque on the scope. Maintain a quiet field.

Step 7 – Clear blood field for visualization
Instruments: Saline flush system
Anticipation: Visualization depends on adequate flushing. Manage tubing to avoid tangling or contamination.

Step 8 – Inspect vessel lumen or graft interior
Instruments: None additional.
Anticipation: Surgeon may pause frequently. Avoid unnecessary movement or instrument handling.

Step 9 – Perform adjunct procedure if indicated
Instruments: Passed from back table when requested.
Anticipation: Angioscopy often accompanies thrombectomy or angioplasty—be prepared for rapid workflow shift.

Step 10 – Withdraw angioscope and sheath
Instruments: None additional.
Anticipation: Maintain wire access if additional intervention is planned.

Step 11 – Achieve hemostasis at access site
Instruments: Closure device or manual pressure supplies
Anticipation: Confirm hemostasis method before opening devices.

Step 12 – Apply sterile dressing
Instruments: Dressing supplies.
Anticipation: Secure dressing firmly and monitor for bleeding.

Mayo Stand Suggestion:

- #3 Knife Handle with #11 blade
- Introducer Needle (vascular access needle)
- Guidewire (J-tip or hydrophilic wire)
- Vascular Sheath with Dilator
- Angioscope (fiberoptic or digital)
- Angioscopy Catheter
- Irrigation Tubing (heparinized saline)
- Luer-Lock Syringe (for flushing)
- Debakey Forceps
- Gerald Forceps (without teeth)
- Mosquito Hemostat
- Frazier Suction Tip

Aortofemoral Bypass

Step 1 – Patient positioning and verification
Instruments: Supine positioning aids, padding, arm boards.
Anticipation: Confirm graft type and size (bifurcated), laterality of femoral exposure, and availability of appropriate vascular clamp sizes.

Step 2 – Abdominal and bilateral groin preparation and draping
Instruments: Prep supplies, vascular drapes.
Anticipation: Prep from nipple line to mid-thighs. Both groins must remain sterile and accessible throughout the case.

Step 3 – Midline abdominal incision
Instruments: Scalpel handle with #10 blade, Adsons forceps with teeth.
Anticipation: Long incision with significant bleeding potential. Be ready with mosquito hemostats immediately.

Step 4 – Enter abdominal cavity and expose retroperitoneum
Instruments: Metzenbaum scissors, 2 mosquito hemostats.
Anticipation: Follow clamp-cut rhythm. Protect bowel and keep moist laps controlled and counted.

Step 5 – Mobilize bowel and expose abdominal aorta
Instruments: Handheld retractor passed from back table when requested.
Anticipation: Bowel protection is critical. Maintain moist laps.

Step 6 – Expose bilateral femoral arteries via groin incisions
Instruments: Passed from back table when requested.
Anticipation: Two operative fields require heightened count awareness and organization.

Step 7 – Isolate proximal aorta and distal femoral arteries
Instruments: Vessel loops and vascular clamps passed from back table when requested.
Anticipation: Dissection is deliberate. Do not open loops or clamps prematurely.

Step 8 – Systemic heparinization and apply vascular clamps
Instruments: Vascular clamps passed from back table.
Anticipation: Clamp timing is critical. Maintain a quiet field and confirm clamp placement sequence.

Step 9 – Anastomose proximal graft to aorta
Instruments: Graft, sutures, needle driver passed from back table when requested.
Anticipation: Do not open graft until surgeon confirms orientation and size.

Step 10 – Tunnel graft limbs to groins
Instruments: Passed from back table when requested.
Anticipation: Ensure graft limbs remain untwisted and protected during tunneling.

Step 11 – Anastomose graft limbs to femoral arteries
Instruments: Sutures and needle driver passed from back table when requested.
Anticipation: Confirm right vs left limb before passing sutures.

Step 12 – Release clamps and assess flow
Instruments: Mosquito hemostats if needed.
Anticipation: Be prepared for immediate hemostasis after reperfusion.

Aortofemoral Bypass

Step 13 – Close retroperitoneum and abdominal incision
Instruments: Passed from back table when requested.
Anticipation: Ensure all laps are accounted for before abdominal closure.

Step 14 – Close groin incisions
Instruments: Brought from back table when requested.
Anticipation: Two closure sites require strict count discipline.

Step 15 – Apply sterile dressings
Instruments: Dressing supplies.
Anticipation: Secure dressings at groin sites to prevent contamination.

Mayo Stand Suggestion:

- Knife with #10 blade
- Metzenbaum Scissors
- Potts-Smith Scissors
- Debakey Forceps
- Gerald Forceps (without teeth)
- Right-Angle Clamp (Mixter)
- Debakey Aortic Cross-Clamp
- Satinsky Partial-Occlusion Clamp
- Atraumatic Bulldog Clamp
- Debakey Needle driver
- Castroviejo Needle driver
- Frazier Suction Tip

Arteriovenous Fistula and Shunt

Step 1 – Patient positioning and verification
Instruments: Supine positioning aids, arm board, padding.
Anticipation: Confirm access type (radiocephalic, brachiocephalic, brachiobasilic, or graft), operative extremity, and availability of vein mapping results if referenced.

Step 2 – Extremity preparation and sterile draping
Instruments: Prep supplies, extremity drape.
Anticipation: Prep from mid upper arm to hand. Ensure tourniquet availability if surgeon uses one, but do not apply unless directed.

Step 3 – Skin incision over planned access site
Instruments: Scalpel handle with #15 blade, Adsons forceps with teeth.
Anticipation: Incision is small but vascular. Be ready with mosquito hemostats immediately.

Step 4 – Dissect through subcutaneous tissue and identify vein
Instruments: Metzenbaum scissors, 2 mosquito hemostats.
Anticipation: Follow clamp–cut rhythm. Vein is fragile, anticipate gentle handling and minimal traction.

Step 5 – Isolate and mobilize vein
Instruments: Passed from back table when requested.
Anticipation: Surgeon may ask for vessel loops—do not open prematurely. Keep loops organized by color.

Step 6 – Identify and isolate artery
Instruments: Passed from back table when requested.
Anticipation: Arterial dissection is deliberate. Be ready to assist with retraction without crowding field.

Step 7 – Administer heparin and apply vascular clamps
Instruments: Vascular clamps passed from back table when requested.
Anticipation: Clamp timing is critical. Maintain a quiet field during clamping.

Arteriovenous Fistula and Shunt

Step 8 – Perform arteriotomy and venotomy
Instruments: Scalpel handle with #11 blade, Potts scissors passed from back table when requested.
Anticipation: Small vessel work requires precision—pass instruments cleanly and deliberately.

Step 9 – Create anastomosis (end to side or side to side)
Instruments: Sutures and needle driver passed from back table when requested.
Anticipation: Do not open sutures until surgeon confirms anastomosis type and vessel orientation.

Step 10 – Release clamps and assess thrill and bruit
Instruments: Mosquito hemostats if needed.
Anticipation: Immediate assessment of flow is expected. Be ready to pass additional sutures quickly if leaks are noted.

Step 11 – Place synthetic graft if shunt is used
Instruments: Graft material passed from back table when requested.
Anticipation: Confirm graft size and configuration before opening. Maintain strict graft sterility.

Step 12 – Achieve hemostasis and irrigate
Instruments: Managed .
Anticipation: Small bleeders are common. Be ready with clamps without cluttering the field.

Step 13 – Layered closure of incision
Instruments: Brought from back table when requested.
Anticipation: Begin closing counts early. Closure instruments move forward only when surgeon commits.

Step 14 – Apply sterile dressing
Instruments: Dressing supplies.
Anticipation: Dressing should not compress fistula. Ensure thrill remains palpable.

Mayo Stand Suggestion:

- Knife with #15 blade
- Metzenbaum Scissors
- Potts-Smith Scissors
- Debakey Forceps
- Gerald Forceps (without teeth)
- Right-Angle Clamp (Mixter)
- Vessel Loops
- Statinsky Partial-Occlusion Clamp
- Atraumatic Bulldog Clamp
- Debakey Needle Driver
- Castroviejo Needle Driver
- Frazier Suction Tip

Carotid Endarterectomy

Step 1 – Patient positioning and verification
Instruments: Supine positioning aids, shoulder roll, head ring or donut.
Anticipation: Confirm operative side and shunt plan (routine vs selective).

Step 2 – Neck preparation and sterile draping
Instruments: Prep supplies, head and neck vascular drapes.
Anticipation: Prep from ear to sternum and midline to lateral neck. Maintain clear access to mandible and clavicle.

Step 3 – Longitudinal neck incision along anterior SCM
Instruments: Scalpel handle with #10 blade, Adsons forceps with teeth.
Anticipation: Incision is vascular. Be ready with mosquito hemostats immediately.

Carotid Endarterectomy

Step 4 – Dissection through platysma and deep cervical fascia
Instruments: Metzenbaum scissors, 2 mosquito hemostats, Adsons forceps.
Anticipation: Follow clamp–cut rhythm. Protect marginal mandibular nerve and ansa cervicalis.

Step 5 – Expose carotid sheath and identify vessels
Instruments: Passed from back table when requested.
Anticipation: Surgeon will identify common, internal, and external carotid arteries. Be ready for vessel loop requests without opening early.

Step 6 – Isolate carotid arteries and place vessel loops
Instruments: Vessel loops passed from back table.
Anticipation: Color-coded loops may be used—track placement carefully.

Step 7 – Systemic heparinization and apply vascular clamps
Instruments: Vascular clamps passed from back table when requested.
Anticipation: Clamp order matters (ICA first). Maintain quiet field during clamping.

Step 8 – Arteriotomy of carotid artery
Instruments: Scalpel handle with #11 blade, Potts scissors
Anticipation: Precise arteriotomy—pass instruments deliberately and cleanly.

Step 9 – Insert carotid shunt if indicated
Instruments: Shunt passed from back table when requested.
Anticipation: Shunt use depends on monitoring and surgeon preference. Do not open unless clearly requested.

Step 10 – Remove atherosclerotic plaque (endarterectomy)
Instruments: Endarterectomy dissector passed from back table.
Anticipation: Plaque removal is delicate. Avoid crowding the field and protect intima.

Step 11 – Inspect distal endpoint and irrigate lumen
Instruments: Managed .
Anticipation: Surgeon may request additional fine instruments

Step 12 – Patch angioplasty or primary closure
Instruments: Patch material, sutures, needle driver passed from back table when requested.
Anticipation: Do not open patch until surgeon confirms need and size.

Step 13 – Remove shunt and release clamps
Instruments: Mosquito hemostats if needed.
Anticipation: Release sequence is critical. Be prepared for immediate hemostasis.

Step 14 – Achieve hemostasis and place drain if ordered
Instruments: Drain passed from back table if requested.
Anticipation: Drains are common, confirm type before opening.

Step 15 – Layered neck closure
Instruments: Brought from back table when requested.
Anticipation: Begin closing counts early. Closure instruments.

Step 16 – Apply sterile dressing
Instruments: Dressing supplies.
Anticipation: Avoid compressive dressings that could compromise airway or carotid flow.

Carotid Endarterectomy

Mayo Stand Suggestion:

- Knife with #15 blade
- Knife with #11 blade
- 2 curved mosquitos
- 4 curved hemostats
- 2 straight hemostats
- 2 right angles
- 2 curved Oschner
- 2 angled vascular clamps
- 1 Satinsky Vascular clamp
- 2 curved vascular clamps
- Adsons Brown toothed forcep
- Russian forcep
- 2 Weitlaner
- 2 small Richardson
- Jameson Scissors
- Tenotomy Scissors
- Potts-Smith Scissors
- Metzenbaum Scissors

Embolectomy or Thrombectomy

Step 1 – Patient positioning and verification
Instruments: Supine positioning aids, padding.
Anticipation: Confirm affected extremity, target vessel, and whether procedure is open or adjunct to endovascular intervention. Fogarty catheter sizes should be available but unopened.

Step 2 – Extremity preparation and sterile draping
Instruments: Prep supplies, extremity drape.
Anticipation: Prep widely to allow proximal or distal extension if thrombus migrates.

Step 3 – Skin incision over target vessel
Instruments: Scalpel handle with #15 blade, Adsons forceps with teeth.
Anticipation: Incision is small but vascular. Be ready with mosquito hemostats immediately.

Step 4 – Dissection to expose vessel
Instruments: Metzenbaum scissors, 2 mosquito hemostats.
Anticipation: Follow clamp-cut rhythm. Protect surrounding nerves and veins.

Step 5 – Isolate vessel and apply vessel loops
Instruments: Vessel loops passed from back table when requested.
Anticipation: Track loop placement carefully. Do not open extra loops.

Step 6 – Systemic heparinization and apply vascular clamps
Instruments: Vascular clamps passed from back table when requested.
Anticipation: Clamp timing is critical. Maintain quiet field.

Step 7 – Perform arteriotomy
Instruments: Scalpel handle with #11 blade, Potts scissors.
Anticipation: Small arteriotomy requires precision—pass instruments cleanly.

Step 8 – Insert Fogarty catheter and remove clot
Instruments: Fogarty catheter passed from back table when requested.
Anticipation: Balloon size varies—confirm size before opening. Maintain sterile catheter control.

Step 9 – Repeat passes proximally and distally
Instruments: Additional Fogarty catheters if requested.
Anticipation: Expect multiple passes. Have additional sizes available but unopened.

Step 10 – Flush vessel and assess back bleeding
Instruments: Managed .
Anticipation: Adequate back bleeding indicates patency—be ready for additional catheter passes.

Embolectomy or Thrombectomy

Step 11 – Close arteriotomy
Instruments: Sutures and needle driver passed from back table when requested.
Anticipation: Confirm suture type before opening. Needle counts are critical.

Step 12 – Release clamps and inspect flow
Instruments: Mosquito hemostats if needed.
Anticipation: Immediate bleeding control may be needed after reperfusion.

Step 13 – Achieve hemostasis and irrigate
Instruments: Managed .
Anticipation: Small bleeders are common. Avoid cluttering the field.

Step 14 – Layered closure of incision
Instruments: Brought from back table when requested.
Anticipation: Begin closing counts early. Closure instruments move forward only after surgeon commits.

Step 15 – Apply sterile dressing
Instruments: Dressing supplies.
Anticipation: Dressing should allow postoperative vascular assessment.

Mayo Stand Suggestion:

- Knife with #11 blade
- Metzenbaum Scissors
- Potts-Smith Scissors
- Debakey Forceps
- Gerald Forceps (without teeth)
- Right-Angle Clamp (Mixter)
- Atraumatic Bulldog Clamp
- Fogarty Balloon Catheter
- Debakey Needle driver
- Castroviejo Needle driver
- Frazier Suction Tip
- Vessel Loops

Femoropopliteal Bypass

Step 1 – Patient positioning and verification
Instruments: Supine positioning aids, padding, leg support.
Anticipation: Confirm operative extremity, graft choice (reversed saphenous vein vs PTFE), and whether above-knee or below-knee popliteal target is planned.

Step 2 – Lower extremity preparation and sterile draping
Instruments: Prep supplies, extremity drape.
Anticipation: Prep from groin to foot. Ensure knee remains accessible for distal exposure.

Step 3 – Proximal groin incision over common femoral artery
Instruments: Scalpel handle with #10 blade, Adsons forceps with teeth.
Anticipation: Incision is vascular. Be ready with mosquito hemostats immediately.

Step 4 – Dissection to expose femoral artery
Instruments: Metzenbaum scissors, 2 mosquito hemostats.
Anticipation: Follow clamp–cut rhythm. Protect femoral vein and nerve.

tep 5 – Distal incision to expose popliteal artery
Instruments: Scalpel handle with #10 or #15 blade, Adsons forceps with teeth.
Anticipation: Exposure varies by target level. Be prepared for deeper retraction requests.

Femoropopliteal Bypass

Step 6 – Dissection and isolation of popliteal artery
Instruments: Metzenbaum scissors, mosquito hemostats as needed.
Anticipation: Below-knee exposure is tight—maintain a clean, uncluttered field.

Step 7 – Harvest vein graft if autogenous conduit is used
Instruments: Passed from back table when requested.
Anticipation: Vein harvest may occur simultaneously—coordinate instrument flow carefully.

Step 8 – Systemic heparinization and apply vascular clamps
Instruments: Vascular clamps passed from back table when requested.
Anticipation: Clamp sequence matters. Maintain a quiet field during clamping.

Step 9 – Perform proximal anastomosis to femoral artery
Instruments: Graft or vein, sutures, needle driver passed from back table when requested.
Anticipation: Confirm graft orientation (reversed vs non-reversed vein) before opening.

Step 10 – Tunnel graft to distal incision
Instruments: Passed from back table when requested.
Anticipation: Ensure graft remains untwisted and protected during tunneling.

Step 11 – Perform distal anastomosis to popliteal artery
Instruments: Sutures and needle driver passed from back table when requested.
Anticipation: Distal vessels are smaller—be ready for fine suture handling.

Step 12 – Release clamps and assess distal flow
Instruments: Mosquito hemostats if needed.
Anticipation: Immediate bleeding control may be needed after reperfusion.

Step 13 – Achieve hemostasis and irrigate wounds
Instruments: Managed .
Anticipation: Ensure all bleeding is controlled before closure.

Step 14 – Layered closure of incisions
Instruments: Brought from back table when requested.
Anticipation: Two operative sites require strict count discipline.

Step 15 – Apply sterile dressings
Instruments: Dressing supplies.
Anticipation: Dressings should allow postoperative vascular checks.

Mayo Stand Suggestion:

- Knife with #15 blade
- Knife with #11 blade
- 2 curved mosquitos
- 4 curved hemostats
- 1 Kelly hemostats
- 2 right angles
- 2 curved Oschner
- 2 Bulldogs
- 1 angled vascular clmaps
- 2 curved vascular clamps
- 2 Satinsky vascular clamps
- 2 Debakeys
- 2 Weitlaner
- 2 small Richardson
- Jameson Scissors
- Mayo Scissors
- Potts-Smith Scissors
- Metzenbaum Scissors

Inferior Vena Cava Filter Placement (Jugular Vein Access)

Step 1 – Patient positioning and verification
Instruments: Supine positioning aids, shoulder roll, head turned slightly opposite access side.
Anticipation: Confirm right vs left internal jugular access, filter type (permanent vs retrievable), and imaging availability. Verify contrast and flush solutions are ready.

Step 2 – Neck preparation and sterile draping
Instruments: Prep supplies, head and neck vascular drapes.
Anticipation: Prep from mandible to upper chest. Maintain a wide sterile field for imaging and catheter manipulation.

Step 3 – Localize jugular vein and mark access site
Instruments: Skin marker.
Anticipation: Ultrasound may be used . Maintain clear access to neck without crowding.

Step 4 – Skin incision at access site (if cutdown used)
Instruments: Scalpel handle with #11 blade, Adsons forceps with teeth.
Anticipation: Incision is small but vascular. Be ready with mosquito hemostats immediately.

Step 5 – Percutaneous venous access and guidewire insertion
Instruments: Access needle and guidewire passed from back table when requested.
Anticipation: Maintain strict wire control. Never allow the wire to be released or contaminated.

Step 6 – Advance introducer sheath into jugular vein
Instruments: Introducer sheath passed from back table.
Anticipation: Confirm sheath size before opening. Maintain wire position at all times.

Step 7 – Perform venography to confirm IVC anatomy
Instruments: Imaging equipment managed .
Anticipation: Avoid movement during imaging. Be ready to pass flush syringes if requested.

Step 8 – Advance filter delivery system to IVC
Instruments: IVC filter delivery system passed from back table when requested.
Anticipation: Confirm correct orientation and deployment level (below renal veins) before opening device.

Step 9 – Deploy IVC filter
Instruments: None additional.
Anticipation: Deployment is precise and irreversible for permanent filters—maintain a quiet field.

Step 10 – Confirm filter position with imaging
Instruments: Imaging managed .
Anticipation: Be prepared for repositioning or retrieval if placement is suboptimal.

Step 11 – Remove sheath and achieve hemostasis
Instruments: Closure device or manual pressure supplies ().
Anticipation: Hemostasis method varies: confirm before opening closure devices.

Step 12 – Apply sterile dressing
Instruments: Dressing supplies.
Anticipation: Dressing should allow visual assessment for bleeding.

Inferior Vena Cava Filter Placement (Jugular Vein Access)

Mayo Stand Suggestion:

- Knife with #11 blade
- Introducer Needle
- Guidewire (J-tip or hydrophilic)
- Vascular Sheath with Dilator
- IVC Filter Delivery System
- Heparinized saline flush
- Debakey Forceps
- Gerald Forceps (without teeth)
- Mosquito Hemostat
- Torque Device
- Contrast Syringe
- Frazier Suction Tip

Insertion of Long Term Indwelling Central Venous Catheter

Step 1 – Patient positioning and verification
Instruments: Supine positioning aids, shoulder roll, head turned away from insertion side.
Anticipation: Confirm catheter type (tunneled catheter vs implanted port), access vein (IJ or subclavian), laterality, and fluoroscopy availability.

Step 2 – Chest and neck preparation and sterile draping
Instruments: Prep supplies, head and chest vascular drapes.
Anticipation: Prep from jawline to mid-chest. Maintain a wide sterile field for tunneling and imaging.

Step 3 – Localize vein and mark insertion site
Instruments: Skin marker.
Anticipation: Ultrasound may be used . Keep probe cover ready but unopened until requested.

Step 4 – Skin incision at venous access site
Instruments: Scalpel handle with #11 blade, Adsons forceps with teeth.
Anticipation: Small but vascular incision—be ready with mosquito hemostats immediately.

Step 5 – Percutaneous venous access and guidewire insertion
Instruments: Access needle and guidewire passed from back table when requested.
Anticipation: Maintain strict wire control. Never release or set down the wire.

Step 6 – Create subcutaneous tunnel (for tunneled catheter or port)
Instruments: Tunneler passed from back table when requested.
Anticipation: Confirm exit site before tunneling. Protect catheter sterility during passage.

Step 7 – Dilate tract and place introducer sheath
Instruments: Dilators and sheath passed from back table when requested.
Anticipation: Dilator size sequence matters—pass only one at a time.

Step 8 – Advance catheter or port catheter into vein
Instruments: Catheter system passed from back table when requested.
Anticipation: Confirm catheter length before insertion to ensure tip placement at cavoatrial junction.

Step 9 – Confirm catheter position with imaging
Instruments: Imaging equipment managed .
Anticipation: Avoid movement during imaging. Be prepared to reposition catheter if needed.

Step 10 – Secure catheter or port
Instruments: Sutures and needle driver passed from back table when requested.
Anticipation: Do not bring sutures forward until surgeon commits to securement phase.

Insertion of Long Term Indwelling Central Venous Catheter

Step 11 – Flush catheter lumens and cap ports
Instruments: Flush supplies passed from back table.
Anticipation: Maintain sterile technique. Confirm number of lumens before flushing.

Step 12 – Achieve hemostasis and close incisions
Instruments: Passed from back table when requested.
Anticipation: Incisions are small but bleeding can occur, be ready with clamps.

Step 13 – Apply sterile dressing
Instruments: Dressing supplies.
Anticipation: Dressing must allow catheter stabilization and site visualization.

Mayo Stand Suggestion:

- Knife with #15 blade
- Introducer Needle
- Guidewire (J-tip)
- Dilator
- Tunneled Central Venous Catheter
- Peel-Away Sheath
- Mosquito Hemostat
- Debakey Forceps
- Gerald Forceps (without teeth)
- Mayo-Hegar Needle driver
- Frazier Suction Tip
- Suture Scissors

Vein Ligation and Stripping (Unilateral)

Step 1 – Patient positioning and verification
Instruments: Supine positioning aids, padding, leg support.
Anticipation: Confirm operative leg, extent of stripping planned (groin to knee vs ankle), and whether stab phlebectomies are included.

Step 2 – Lower extremity preparation and sterile draping
Instruments: Prep supplies, extremity drape.
Anticipation: Prep from groin to foot. Entire limb must remain accessible.

Step 3 – Groin incision over saphenofemoral junction
Instruments: Scalpel handle with #10 blade, Adsons forceps with teeth.
Anticipation: Groin incision is vascular, be ready with mosquito hemostats immediately.

Step 4 – Dissection to identify great saphenous vein
Instruments: Metzenbaum scissors, 2 mosquito hemostats.
Anticipation: Follow clamp–cut rhythm. Protect femoral artery and vein.

Step 5 – Ligation of tributaries at saphenofemoral junction
Instruments: Passed from back table when requested.
Anticipation: Multiple small tributaries, be prepared for rapid clamp–tie sequence.

Step 6 – Proximal ligation and division of great saphenous vein
Instruments: Passed from back table when requested.
Anticipation: Confirm ligature placement before division. Specimen readiness matters.

Step 7 – Distal incision and identification of vein
Instruments: Scalpel handle with #15 blade, Adsons forceps with teeth.
Anticipation: Distal incision is smaller but still vascular—anticipate clamps.

Step 8 – Insert vein stripper
Instruments: Vein stripper passed from back table when requested.
Anticipation: Confirm stripper type and direction before passing.

Step 9 – Secure stripper and perform vein stripping
Instruments: None additional.
Anticipation: Stripping is forceful—ensure surrounding field is protected and clear.

Step 10 – Perform stab phlebectomies if planned
Instruments: Passed from back table when requested.
Anticipation: Multiple small incisions—maintain instrument organization and count awareness.

Step 11 – Achieve hemostasis along stripping tract
Instruments: Mosquito hemostats if needed.
Anticipation: Bleeding may track along vein bed—be ready for compression and ligation.

Step 12 – Layered closure of incisions
Instruments: Brought from back table when requested.
Anticipation: Multiple small closures require strict needle and sponge counts.

Step 13 – Apply compression dressing or wrap
Instruments: Dressing and compression supplies.
Anticipation: Dressing must provide uniform compression without compromising circulation.

Mayo Stand Suggestion:

- Knife with #15 blade
- Knife with #10 blade
- Adsons forceps with teeth
- Metzenbaum scissors
- 2 mosquito hemostats
- Vein stripper
- Vessel loops
- Ligatures
- Senn retractor
- Army Navy
- Small Richardson

Section XI:

Neurosurgery Procedures

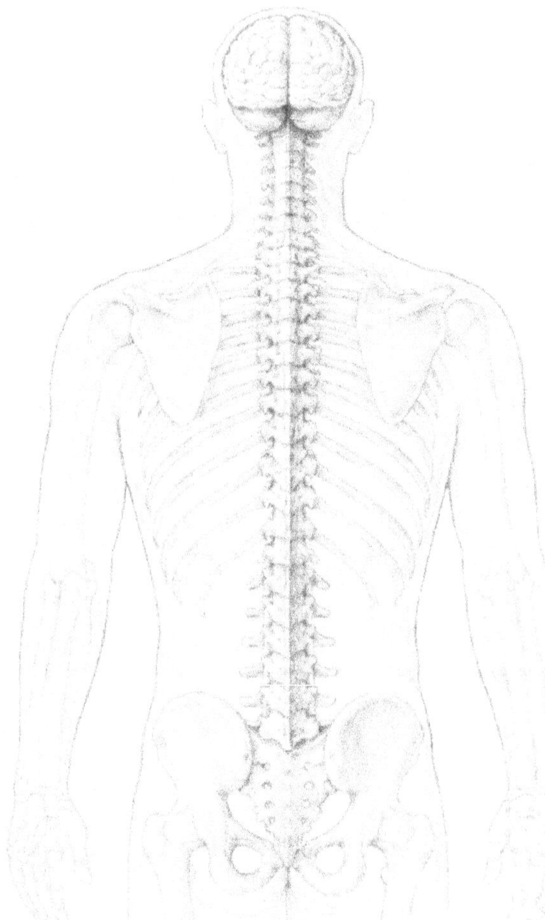

Anterior Cervical Discectomy and Fusion (ACDF): Cloward Technique

Step 1 – Patient positioning and verification
Instruments: Supine positioning aids, shoulder roll, head donut, arm tuck.
Anticipation: Confirm operative level(s), graft type (Cloward dowel), and fluoroscopy availability. Ensure neck positioning allows imaging without obstruction.

Step 2 – Neck preparation and sterile draping
Instruments: Prep supplies, head and neck drapes.
Anticipation: Prep from mandible to sternum and laterally to SCM. Keep imaging field unobstructed.

Step 3 – Transverse anterior cervical incision
Instruments: Scalpel handle with #15 blade, Adsons forceps with teeth.
Anticipation: Incision is superficial but vascular. Be ready with mosquito hemostats immediately.

Step 4 – Dissection through platysma and along natural tissue planes
Instruments: Metzenbaum scissors, 2 mosquito hemostats, Adsons forceps.
Anticipation: Follow clamp-cut rhythm. Protect marginal mandibular nerve and avoid unnecessary traction.

Step 5 – Retract trachea and esophagus medially, carotid laterally
Instruments: Handheld retractor passed from back table when requested.
Anticipation: Retraction is dynamic. Be prepared to adjust exposure frequently without cluttering the field.

Step 6 – Identify target disc level using fluoroscopy
Instruments: Spinal needle passed from back table if requested.
Anticipation: Confirm correct level before any disc work. Maintain quiet field during imaging.

Step 7 – Incise anterior longitudinal ligament and annulus
Instruments: Scalpel handle with #15 blade.
Anticipation: Precise incision; pass blade cleanly and deliberately.

Step 8 – Perform discectomy and endplate preparation
Instruments: Passed from back table when requested.
Anticipation: Instrument needs change rapidly (curettes, rongeurs). Open only what is requested and maintain organization.

Step 9 – Drill vertebral bodies for Cloward dowel
Instruments: Drill system passed from back table when requested.
Anticipation: Confirm dowel size before drilling. Protect surrounding soft tissue.

Step 10 – Insert Cloward dowel graft
Instruments: Graft and inserter passed from back table when requested.
Anticipation: Maintain graft sterility. Do not open dowel until surgeon confirms size.

Step 11 – Confirm graft placement with fluoroscopy
Instruments: Imaging managed .
Anticipation: Avoid movement during imaging confirmation.

Step 12 – Release retractor and inspect hemostasis
Instruments: Mosquito hemostats if needed.
Anticipation: Bleeding often occurs on release—be ready for immediate control.

Anterior Cervical Discectomy and Fusion (ACDF): Cloward Technique

Step 13 – Layered closure of platysma and skin
Instruments: Brought from back table when requested.
Anticipation: Begin closing counts early. Closure instruments move forward only when surgeon commits.

Step 14 – Apply sterile dressing and cervical collar if ordered
Instruments: Dressing supplies.
Anticipation: Ensure dressing does not interfere with collar placement.

Mayo Stand Suggestion:

- Knife with #15 blade
- Knife with #10 blade
- Adsons forceps with teeth
- Bayonet without teeth
- Penfield #3, #4
- Cushing without teeth
- Cushing with Teeth
- 2 curved hemostats
- 2 curved Oschners
- Freer Elevator
- Weitlaner
- Army Navy
- Pituitary Rongeur
- Kerrison Punch

Anterior Thoracic Decompression

Step 1 – Patient positioning and verification
Instruments: Lateral decubitus positioning aids, axillary roll, padding.
Anticipation: Confirm operative level(s), laterality, and approach (thoracotomy vs thoracoscopy). Verify imaging availability and spinal level markers.

Step 2 – Chest preparation and wide sterile draping
Instruments: Prep supplies, thoracic/spine drapes.
Anticipation: Prep from axilla to iliac crest and midline anteriorly. Maintain room for conversion to open thoracotomy if needed.

Step 3 – Thoracotomy incision or thoracoscopic port incisions
Instruments: Scalpel handle with #10 blade, Adsons forceps with teeth.
Anticipation: Incision is muscular and vascular. Be ready with mosquito hemostats immediately.

Step 4 – Dissection through chest wall musculature
Instruments: Metzenbaum scissors, 2 mosquito hemostats, Adsons forceps.
Anticipation: Follow clamp-cut rhythm. Protect intercostal neurovascular bundle.

Step 5 – Enter pleural space and expose thoracic spine
Instruments: Rib spreader or thoracoscopic access passed from back table when requested.
Anticipation: Exposure is critical. Keep Mayo minimal and avoid premature instrument staging.

Step 6 – Retract lung and identify target vertebral level
Instruments: Passed from back table when requested.
Anticipation: Lung retraction is dynamic. Maintain clear communication and field awareness.

Step 7 – Confirm spinal level with imaging
Instruments: Spinal needle or marker passed from back table if requested.
Anticipation: Do not proceed until level confirmation is complete. Maintain quiet field during imaging.

Step 8 – Remove rib head or vertebral body as needed
Instruments: Drill system, rongeurs passed from back table when requested.
Anticipation: Bone work requires controlled instrument flow—open only what is requested.

Anterior Thoracic Decompression

Step 9 – Decompress spinal cord and nerve roots
Instruments: Curettes and dissectors passed from back table when requested.
Anticipation: Precision work—anticipate instrument changes without clutter.

Step 10 – Place graft or cage if fusion is performed
Instruments: Graft or cage system passed from back table when requested.
Anticipation: Maintain implant sterility. Do not open until surgeon confirms size and plan.

Step 11 – Achieve hemostasis and inspect decompression
Instruments: Mosquito hemostats if needed.
Anticipation: Bleeding may increase after decompression; respond quickly but calmly.

Step 12 – Re-expand lung and place chest tube if ordered
Instruments: Chest tube passed from back table when requested.
Anticipation: Confirm tube size and number before opening.

Step 13 – Close thoracotomy or port sites
Instruments: Brought from back table when requested.
Anticipation: Begin closing counts early. Closure instruments move forward only after surgeon commits.

Step 14 – Apply sterile dressing
Instruments: Dressing supplies.
Anticipation: Secure chest tube and maintain line organization before drapes come down.

Mayo Stand Suggestion:

- Knife Handle with #10 blade
- Metzenbaum Scissors
- Long Metzenbaum Scissors
- Penfield #4
- Nerve Hook
- Pituitary Rongeur
- Kerrison Rongeur (1–2 mm)
- Cobb Elevator
- Debakey Forceps
- Mayo-Hegar Needle Driver
- Frazier Suction Tip
- Foerster Sponge Forceps

Carpal Tunnel Release

Step 1 – Patient positioning and verification
Instruments: Supine positioning aids, arm board, hand table.
Anticipation: Confirm operative hand, tourniquet use, and whether procedure is open vs endoscopic.

Step 2 – Upper extremity preparation and sterile draping
Instruments: Prep supplies, extremity drape.
Anticipation: Prep from mid-forearm to fingertips. Keep fingers exposed if surgeon checks motion intraoperatively.

Step 3 – Apply tourniquet (if used)
Instruments: Tourniquet ().
Anticipation: Confirm inflation timing with surgeon. Tourniquet is usually inflated after exsanguination.

Step 4 – Longitudinal or curvilinear palmar incision
Instruments: Scalpel handle with #15 blade, Adsons forceps with teeth.
Anticipation: Small incision but vascular skin—have mosquito hemostats ready immediately.

Carpal Tunnel Release

Step 5 – Dissection through subcutaneous tissue
Instruments: Metzenbaum scissors, 2 mosquito hemostats.
Anticipation: Follow clamp-cut rhythm. Protect palmar cutaneous branch of the median nerve.

Step 6 – Identify palmar fascia and transverse carpal ligament
Instruments: Metzenbaum scissors, Adsons forceps.
Anticipation: Exposure is narrow; anticipate small retractor from back table if requested.

Step 7 – Divide transverse carpal ligament
Instruments: Metzenbaum scissors or blade passed when requested.
Anticipation: Median nerve lies immediately beneath; pass instruments deliberately and avoid crowding the field.

Step 8 – Inspect median nerve and confirm decompression
Instruments: None additional.
Anticipation: Surgeon may visually confirm full release proximally and distally—do not rush closure.

Step 9 – Achieve hemostasis
Instruments: Mosquito hemostats if needed.
Anticipation: Bleeding is usually minimal but may increase after tourniquet release.

Step 10 – Release tourniquet and reassess field
Instruments: None additional.
Anticipation: Expect reactive bleeding—be ready with clamps without cluttering the Mayo.

Step 11 – Skin closure
Instruments: Sutures and needle driver passed from back table when requested.
Anticipation: Skin closure is often simple interrupted—confirm suture type before opening.

Step 12 – Apply sterile dressing and splint if ordered
Instruments: Dressing supplies, splint materials if used.
Anticipation: Dressing should allow finger movement and not compress median nerve.

Mayo Stand Suggestion:

- Knife Handle with #15 blade
- 2 curved hemostats
- Adsons with teeth
- small Metzenbaum
- small Gelpi
- small Weitlaner

Craniectomy for Stereotactic Procedures

Step 1 – Patient positioning and verification
Instruments: Supine or semi-sitting positioning aids, headrest or Mayfield fixation ().
Anticipation: Confirm target coordinates, imaging modality used for planning (CT/MRI), and whether a frame-based or frameless stereotactic system is planned.

Step 2 – Head preparation and sterile draping
Instruments: Prep supplies, cranial drapes.
Anticipation: Prep entire scalp widely even though incision is small. Maintain unobstructed access to navigation equipment.

Craniectomy for Stereotactic Procedures

Step 3 – Attach stereotactic frame or register navigation system
Instruments: Navigation system ().
Anticipation: This is a high-focus step. Maintain a quiet field and avoid introducing unnecessary instruments.

Step 4 – Mark incision and burr hole site
Instruments: Skin marker.
Anticipation: Verify location matches imaging coordinates before incision.

Step 5 – Scalp incision
Instruments: Scalpel handle with #10 blade, Adsons forceps with teeth.
Anticipation: Scalp is highly vascular; be ready with mosquito hemostats immediately.

Step 6 – Dissection through galea and periosteum
Instruments: Metzenbaum scissors, 2 mosquito hemostats, Adsons forceps.
Anticipation: Clamp-cut rhythm is common. Bleeding control is critical early.

Step 7 – Create burr hole or small craniectomy
Instruments: Drill and perforator passed from back table when requested.
Anticipation: Confirm drill bit size before passing. Protect dura and maintain irrigation control ().

Step 8 – Open dura
Instruments: Dural scissors and forceps passed from back table when requested.
Anticipation: Precise dural opening—anticipate cottonoids and fine instruments without crowding the field.

Step 9 – Introduce stereotactic instrument (biopsy needle, electrode, catheter)
Instruments: Stereotactic instrument passed from back table when requested.
Anticipation: Absolute sterility and accuracy matter. Introduce only after confirmation of trajectory.

Step 10 – Perform stereotactic procedure
Instruments: None additional.
Anticipation: Surgeon may pause frequently to confirm depth and position—maintain stillness and readiness.

Step 11 – Remove stereotactic instrument and inspect tract
Instruments: Cottonoids passed from back table if requested.
Anticipation: Be alert for bleeding on withdrawal.

Step 12 – Close dura if indicated
Instruments: Sutures and needle driver passed from back table when requested.
Anticipation: Not all cases require dural closure; wait for surgeon commitment.

Step 13 – Replace bone flap or cover burr hole
Instruments: Burr hole cover or plate passed from back table if used.
Anticipation: Confirm fixation method before opening hardware.

Step 14 – Layered scalp closure
Instruments: Brought from back table when requested.
Anticipation: Scalp closure often proceeds quickly; counts must already be in progress.

Craniectomy for Stereotactic Procedures

Step 15 – Apply sterile dressing
Instruments: Dressing supplies.
Anticipation: Dressing should not disrupt stereotactic landmarks if postoperative imaging is planned.

Mayo Stand Suggestion:

- Knife with #15 blade
- Metzenbaum Scissors
- Freer or Penfield #1
- High-Speed Drill with Burr
- Dural Hook
- Bayonet Forceps
- Gerald Forceps (with teeth)
- Kerrison Rongeur (1–2 mm)
- Pituitary Rongeur
- Mayo-Hegar Needle Driver
- Frazier Suction Tip
- Bipolar Forceps

Cranioplasty

Step 1 – Patient positioning and verification
Instruments: Supine positioning aids, headrest or Mayfield fixation ().
Anticipation: Confirm defect location, implant type (autologous vs synthetic), fixation method.

Step 2 – Scalp preparation and sterile draping
Instruments: Prep supplies, cranial drapes.
Anticipation: Prep entire scalp widely even if reopening prior incision. Maintain access for implant handling.

Step 3 – Reopen previous scalp incision
Instruments: Scalpel handle with #10 blade, Adsons forceps with teeth.
Anticipation: Scar tissue may bleed unpredictably—be ready with mosquito hemostats immediately.

Step 4 – Dissect through scalp layers to expose cranial defect
Instruments: Metzenbaum scissors, 2 mosquito hemostats, Adsons forceps.
Anticipation: Follow clamp–cut rhythm. Protect dura beneath defect edges.

Step 5 – Elevate scalp flap and expose margins of skull defect
Instruments: Handheld retractor passed from back table when requested.
Anticipation: Exposure must be adequate for implant seating—anticipate retractors adjustments.

Step 6 – Prepare defect edges and underlying dura
Instruments: Passed from back table when requested.
Anticipation: Surgeon may request rongeurs or burr smoothing; open only on request.

Step 7 – Prepare implant or bone flap
Instruments: Implant system passed from back table when requested.
Anticipation: Maintain strict implant sterility. Do not open until surgeon confirms size and orientation.

Step 8 – Place implant or bone flap into cranial defect
Instruments: Passed from back table when requested.
Anticipation: Implant positioning may require adjustments; avoid crowding field.

Step 9 – Secure implant with plates, screws, or wires
Instruments: Fixation system and driver passed from back table when requested.
Anticipation: Confirm screw length and plate type before opening.

Cranioplasty

Step 10 – Inspect repair and achieve hemostasis
Instruments: Mosquito hemostats if needed.
Anticipation: Bleeding may occur along scalp edges, be ready without cluttering Mayo.

Step 11 – Replace scalp flap and layered closure
Instruments: Sutures and needle driver passed from back table when requested.
Anticipation: Scalp closure proceeds quickly; counts must already be in progress.

Step 12 – Apply sterile head dressing
Instruments: Dressing supplies.
Anticipation: Dressing should protect repair without excessive compression.

Mayo Stand Suggestion:

- Knife with #15 blade
- Metzenbaum Scissors
- Freer or Penfield #1
- High-Speed Drill with Burr
- Craniotome
- Bayonet Forceps
- Gerald Forceps (with teeth)
- Kerrison Rongeur
- Plates and Screws
- Mayo-Hegar Needle Driver
- Frazier Suction Tip
- Bipolar Forceps

Craniotomy

Step 1 – Patient positioning and verification
Instruments: Supine, lateral, or prone positioning aids; headrest or Mayfield fixation ().
Anticipation: Confirm operative site, laterality, patient positioning, and imaging/navigation plan. Verify head fixation pins and navigation accuracy before prep.

Step 2 – Scalp preparation and sterile draping
Instruments: Prep supplies, cranial drapes.
Anticipation: Prep entire scalp widely. Maintain access for navigation reference arrays and microscope positioning.

Step 3 – Mark incision and craniotomy site
Instruments: Skin marker.
Anticipation: Confirm incision corresponds to imaging and neuro navigation before incision.

Step 4 – Scalp incision
Instruments: Scalpel handle with #10 blade, Adsons forceps with teeth.
Anticipation: Scalp is highly vascular—be ready with mosquito hemostats immediately.

Step 5 – Dissection through galea and periosteum
Instruments: Metzenbaum scissors, 2 mosquito hemostats, Adsons forceps.
Anticipation: Clamp–cut rhythm common. Control bleeding early to maintain visualization.

Step 6 – Reflect scalp flap and expose skull
Instruments: Handheld retractor passed from back table when requested.
Anticipation: Flap edges may ooze—anticipate rapid clamp placement without crowding.

Step 7 – Burr hole placement
Instruments: Drill and perforator passed from back table when requested.
Anticipation: Confirm burr hole locations and drill bit type before passing.

Craniotomy

Step 8 – Create bone flap using craniotome
Instruments: Craniotome passed from back table when requested.
Anticipation: Maintain bone flap orientation. Be ready to manage bone dust control ().

Step 9 – Elevate and preserve bone flap
Instruments: Passed from back table when requested.
Anticipation: Bone flap may be stored sterilely or prepared for later replacement—confirm handling method.

Step 10 – Open dura
Instruments: Dural scissors and forceps passed from back table when requested.
Anticipation: Precise dural opening—anticipate cottonoids and dural tack-up sutures.

Step 11 – Intracranial procedure performed
Instruments: Passed from back table when requested.
Anticipation: This phase is variable—monitor surgeon cues closely and introduce instruments deliberately.

Step 12 – Achieve hemostasis and irrigate
Instruments: Mosquito hemostats if needed.
Anticipation: Bleeding may increase during closure prep—respond quickly but calmly.

Step 13 – Close dura
Instruments: Sutures and needle driver passed from back table when requested.
Anticipation: Confirm dural substitute use before opening any materials.

Step 14 – Replace bone flap and secure
Instruments: Plates, screws, and driver passed from back table when requested.
Anticipation: Maintain strict count of cranial hardware.

Step 15 – Layered scalp closure
Instruments: Brought from back table when requested.
Anticipation: Scalp closure proceeds quickly—counts must already be correct and communicated.

Step 16 – Apply sterile head dressing
Instruments: Dressing supplies.
Anticipation: Dressing should protect incision without excessive compression.

Mayo Stand Suggestion:

- Knife with #15 blade
- Knife with #10 blade
- Knife with #11 blade
- 4-6 Dandy
- 2 curved hemostats
- Adsons toothed forceps
- Bayonet without teeth
- Cushing with teeth
- Vein retractors
- Cushing
- Weitlaner
- Frazier Suction Tip

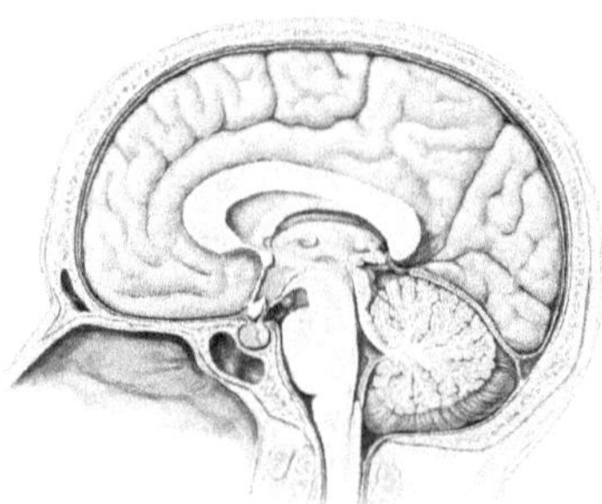

Craniotomy for Aneurysm Repair

Step 1 – Patient positioning and verification
Instruments: Supine or lateral positioning aids, headrest or Mayfield fixation ().
Anticipation: Confirm aneurysm location, laterality, clip inventory availability (sizes, angles), microscope readiness, and neuromonitoring setup.

Step 2 – Scalp preparation and sterile draping
Instruments: Prep supplies, cranial drapes.
Anticipation: Prep entire scalp widely. Maintain unobstructed access for microscope and navigation systems.

Step 3 – Mark incision and craniotomy site
Instruments: Skin marker.
Anticipation: Verify incision correlates with imaging and aneurysm projection before incision.

Step 4 – Scalp incision
Instruments: Scalpel handle with #10 blade, Adsons forceps with teeth.
Anticipation: Scalp bleeding is significant—have mosquito hemostats ready immediately and manage clamps efficiently.

Step 5 – Dissection through galea and periosteum
Instruments: Metzenbaum scissors, 2 mosquito hemostats, Adsons forceps.
Anticipation: Clamp-cut rhythm is continuous. Keep clamps organized and ready.

Step 6 – Reflect scalp flap and expose skull
Instruments: Handheld retractor passed from back table when requested.
Anticipation: Exposure must remain stable to prevent rebleeding from flap edges.

Step 7 – Burr hole placement and craniotomy creation
Instruments: Drill and craniotome passed from back table when requested.
Anticipation: Confirm burr hole locations and craniotome footplate position before passing.

Step 8 – Elevate bone flap and secure
Instruments: Passed from back table when requested.
Anticipation: Maintain bone flap orientation and protect sterile storage if temporarily removed.

Step 9 – Open dura and place dural tack-up sutures
Instruments: Dural scissors, forceps, sutures passed from back table when requested.
Anticipation: Dural bleeding can obscure field; anticipate tack-up sutures early.

Step 10 – Microsurgical dissection to expose aneurysm
Instruments: Microsurgical instruments passed from back table when requested.
Anticipation: This is a high-focus phase. Keep Mayo minimal and avoid unnecessary motion.

Step 11 – Temporary clip placement if needed
Instruments: Temporary aneurysm clip and applier passed from back table when requested.
Anticipation: Temporary clips are time-sensitive; confirm size and orientation before opening.

Step 12 – Definitive aneurysm clip placement
Instruments: Selected permanent aneurysm clip and applier passed from back table when requested.
Anticipation: Maintain strict clip control and count. Do not open extra clips prematurely.

Craniotomy for Aneurysm Repair

Step 13 – Inspect clip placement and aneurysm occlusion
Instruments: None additional.
Anticipation: Surgeon may reposition clips—be ready with alternative sizes quickly.

Step 14 – Achieve hemostasis and irrigate
Instruments: Mosquito hemostats if needed.
Anticipation: Bleeding risk remains high—respond calmly and efficiently.

Step 15 – Close dura (with graft if needed)
Instruments: Sutures, needle driver, dural substitute passed from back table when requested.
Anticipation: Confirm dural substitute type before opening.

Step 16 – Replace bone flap and secure
Instruments: Plates, screws, and driver passed from back table when requested.
Anticipation: Maintain meticulous hardware counts.

Step 17 – Layered scalp closure
Instruments: Brought from back table when requested.
Anticipation: Closure may proceed quickly—ensure counts are correct before final sutures.

Step 18 – Apply sterile head dressing
Instruments: Dressing supplies.
Anticipation: Dressing should protect incision without increasing intracranial pressure.

Mayo Stand Suggestion:

- Knife with #15 blade
- Knife with #10 blade
- Knife with #11 blade
- 4-6 Dandy
- 2 curved hemostats
- Adsons toothed forceps
- Bayonet without teeth
- Cushing with teeth
- Vein retractors
- Cushing
- Weitlaner
- Frazier Suction Tip

Craniosynostosis Repair

Step 1 – Patient positioning and verification
Instruments: Supine positioning aids, headrest or Mayfield fixation ().
Anticipation: Confirm type of craniosynostosis (sagittal, coronal, metopic, lambdoid), planned technique (strip vs vault remodeling), and blood products availability—blood loss can be significant in infants.

Step 2 – Scalp preparation and sterile draping
Instruments: Prep supplies, cranial drapes.
Anticipation: Prep entire scalp widely. Keep access for anesthesia lines and warming devices—temperature control is critical in pediatric cases.

Step 3 – Mark incision and cranial remodeling plan
Instruments: Skin marker.
Anticipation: Confirm markings match surgical plan and imaging before incision.

Step 4 – Bicoronal or linear scalp incision
Instruments: Scalpel handle with #10 blade, Adsons forceps with teeth.
Anticipation: Scalp is extremely vascular in infants—be ready with mosquito hemostats immediately and manage clamp rhythm efficiently.

Craniosynostosis Repair

Step 5 – Elevate scalp and periosteal flap
Instruments: Metzenbaum scissors, 2 mosquito hemostats, Adsons forceps.
Anticipation: Clamp-cut rhythm is continuous. Maintain organized clamp placement to avoid confusion.

Step 6 – Expose cranial sutures and skull
Instruments: Handheld retractor passed from back table when requested.
Anticipation: Exposure must be wide but gentle—avoid excessive traction on scalp flap.

Step 7 – Perform strip craniectomy or cranial vault osteotomies
Instruments: Power saws and osteotomes passed from back table when requested.
Anticipation: Bone removal is staged—open cutting instruments only when surgeon commits to that phase.

Step 8 – Remove fused sutures and reshape cranial segments
Instruments: Rongeurs and reshaping tools passed from back table when requested.
Anticipation: Bone segments are small and numerous—maintain strict accounting and organization.

Step 9 – Reconstruct cranial vault and reposition bone segments
Instruments: Fixation system passed from back table when requested.
Anticipation: Confirm resorbable vs titanium fixation before opening hardware.

Step 10 – Secure bone segments and inspect symmetry
Instruments: Passed from back table when requested.
Anticipation: Surgeon may adjust positioning multiple times—avoid cluttering the field.

Step 11 – Achieve hemostasis and irrigate
Instruments: Mosquito hemostats if needed.
Anticipation: Bleeding control is critical—anticipate rapid responses without adding unnecessary instruments.

Step 12 – Replace scalp flap and layered closure
Instruments: Sutures and needle driver passed from back table when requested.
Anticipation: Closure may proceed quickly after a long case—counts must already be in progress.

Step 13 – Apply head dressing and protective wrap
Instruments: Dressing supplies.
Anticipation: Dressing should protect repair without excessive compression that could affect cerebral perfusion.

Mayo Stand Suggestion:

- Knife Handle with #10 blade
- Metzenbaum Scissors
- Periosteal Elevator (Freer or Penfield #1)
- Hudson Brace with Perforator or High-Speed Drill with Cranial Burr
- Craniotome
- Leksell Rongeur
- Kerrison Rongeur (1–2 mm)
- Bayonet Forceps
- Gerald Forceps (with teeth)

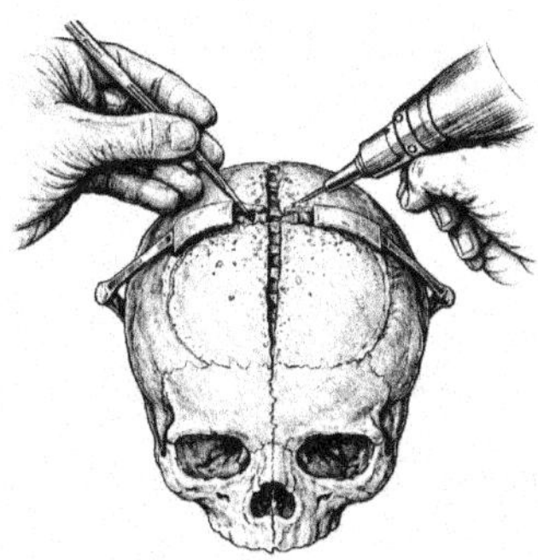

Lumbar Laminectomy for Discectomy with Spinal Fixation

Step 1 – Patient positioning and verification
Instruments: Prone positioning aids, chest rolls or Wilson frame, padding.
Anticipation: Confirm operative level(s), fixation plan (levels to be instrumented), and imaging availability. Ensure all implants are available but unopened.

Step 2 – Back preparation and sterile draping
Instruments: Prep supplies, spine drapes.
Anticipation: Prep widely to allow extension of exposure. Maintain fluoroscopy access without breaking sterility.

Step 3 – Midline posterior lumbar incision
Instruments: Scalpel handle with #10 blade, Adsons forceps with teeth.
Anticipation: Incision is long and vascular—be ready with mosquito hemostats immediately.

Step 4 – Dissection through subcutaneous tissue and fascia
Instruments: Metzenbaum scissors, 2 mosquito hemostats, Adsons forceps.
Anticipation: Follow clamp-cut rhythm. Control bleeding early to maintain visualization.

Step 5 – Subperiosteal muscle dissection to expose lamina
Instruments: Passed from back table when requested.
Anticipation: Exposure widens progressively—anticipate retractors adjustments without cluttering Mayo.

Step 6 – Confirm spinal level with fluoroscopy
Instruments: Spinal needle or marker passed from back table if requested.
Anticipation: Level confirmation is critical—do not proceed until confirmed.

Step 7 – Perform laminectomy and decompression
Instruments: Rongeurs, Kerrisons, drill system passed from back table when requested.
Anticipation: Bone removal proceeds in stages—open cutting instruments only when surgeon commits.

Step 8 – Identify and protect nerve roots
Instruments: Passed from back table when requested.
Anticipation: Nerve protection is critical, maintain calm, deliberate instrument flow.

Step 9 – Perform discectomy
Instruments: Disc instruments
Anticipation: Disc material may be removed in multiple passes—stay organized and responsive.

Step 10 – Prepare pedicles for fixation
Instruments: Pedicle awls, probes, taps passed from back table when requested.
Anticipation: Implant sequence matters—do not open screws or rods prematurely.

Step 11 – Insert pedicle screws
Instruments: Pedicle screws and drivers passed from back table when requested.
Anticipation: Maintain strict implant counts and laterality awareness.

Step 12 – Place rods and secure fixation
Instruments: Rods, set screws, and drivers passed from back table when requested.
Anticipation: Rod contouring may occur—be ready with additional lengths if needed.

Lumbar Laminectomy for Discectomy with Spinal Fixation

Step 13 – Confirm fixation and decompression with imaging
Instruments: Imaging managed .
Anticipation: Avoid movement during imaging confirmation.

Step 14 – Achieve hemostasis and irrigate
Instruments: Mosquito hemostats if needed.
Anticipation: Bleeding often increases after decompression—respond quickly without clutter.

Step 15 – Place drain if ordered
Instruments: Drain passed from back table when requested.
Anticipation: Confirm drain type and exit site before opening.

Step 16 – Layered closure of fascia, subcutaneous tissue, and skin
Instruments: Brought from back table when requested.
Anticipation: Begin closing counts early. Closure instruments move forward only when surgeon commits.

Step 17 – Apply sterile dressing
Instruments: Dressing supplies.
Anticipation: Dressing must accommodate drain tubing if present.

Mayo Stand Suggestion:

- Knife with #15 blade
- Knife with #10 blade
- 2 long straight hemostat
- small Metzenbaum
- Micro scissors
- Adsons toothed forceps
- Bayonet without teeth
- Cushing with teeth
- Gelpi
- Meyerding
- Weitlander
- Adsons
- nerve root retractors

Microdecompression Endoscopic Spinal Discectomy

Step 1 – Patient positioning and verification
Instruments: Prone positioning aids, Wilson frame or chest rolls, padding.
Anticipation: Confirm operative level and side, endoscopic system readiness, and fluoroscopy availability. Ensure correct endoscope and working channel are present but unopened.

Step 2 – Back preparation and sterile draping
Instruments: Prep supplies, minimally invasive spine drapes.
Anticipation: Prep widely to allow fluoroscopic adjustments without contamination.

Step 3 – Localize operative level with fluoroscopy
Instruments: Spinal needle or marker passed from back table if requested.
Anticipation: Level confirmation is critical—do not proceed until verified.

Step 4 – Small paramedian skin incision
Instruments: Scalpel handle with #15 blade, Adsons forceps with teeth.
Anticipation: Incision is small but vascular, have mosquito hemostats ready immediately.

Step 5 – Dilate soft tissue and place tubular retractors
Instruments: Sequential dilators and tubular retractors passed from back table when requested.
Anticipation: Dilators are passed in sequence—open only the next size requested.

Microdecompression Endoscopic Spinal Discectomy

Step 6 – Insert endoscope and establish visualization
Instruments: Endoscope and camera system
Anticipation: Verify white balance and image clarity before insertion. Protect optics at all times.

Step 7 – Perform laminotomy and medial facetectomy if needed
Instruments: Kerrison rongeurs, drill system passed from back table when requested.
Anticipation: Bone removal is incremental, do not stage multiple cutting instruments.

Step 8 – Identify and protect nerve root
Instruments: Passed from back table when requested.
Anticipation: Nerve manipulation is minimal maintain calm, deliberate instrument flow.

Step 9 – Remove herniated disc fragments
Instruments: Disc forceps and curettes passed from back table when requested.
Anticipation: Disc removal may require repeated passes; stay organized and responsive.

Step 10 – Inspect decompression endoscopically
Instruments: None additional.
Anticipation: Surgeon confirms nerve mobility—do not rush closure.

Step 11 – Achieve hemostasis and irrigate
Instruments: Mosquito hemostats if needed.
Anticipation: Bleeding control is critical in a confined working channel.

Step 12 – Remove tubular retractors and close fascia/skin
Instruments: Brought from back table when requested.
Anticipation: Closure is minimal but precise—counts must still be correct.

Step 13 – Apply sterile dressing
Instruments: Dressing supplies.
Anticipation: Dressing should not restrict mobility or cause pressure.

Mayo Stand Suggestion:

- Knife Handle with #15 blade
- Metzenbaum Scissors
- Sequential Dilators
- Endoscopic Working Cannula
- Endoscope (spinal endoscope)
- Pituitary Rongeur (endoscopic)
- Kerrison Rongeur (1–2 mm)
- Nerve Hook
- Penfield #4
- Endoscopic Grasper
- Frazier Suction Tip
- Bipolar Forceps

Posterior Cervical Decompression

Step 1 – Patient positioning and verification
Instruments: Prone positioning aids, Mayfield head fixation (), chest rolls, padding.
Anticipation: Confirm operative levels, laterality, and whether fusion or instrumentation is planned

Step 2 – Posterior neck preparation and sterile draping
Instruments: Prep supplies, spine drapes.
Anticipation: Prep from occiput to upper thoracic spine. Maintain access for imaging and neuromonitoring leads.

Step 3 – Midline posterior cervical incision
Instruments: Scalpel handle with #10 blade, Adsons forceps with teeth.
Anticipation: Cervical incisions are vascular—be ready with mosquito hemostats immediately.

Posterior Cervical Decompression

Step 4 – Dissection through subcutaneous tissue and fascia
Instruments: Metzenbaum scissors, 2 mosquito hemostats, Adsons forceps.
Anticipation: Follow clamp-cut rhythm. Control bleeding early to preserve visualization.

Step 5 – Subperiosteal muscle dissection to expose laminae
Instruments: Passed from back table when requested.
Anticipation: Exposure is incremental—anticipate retractors adjustments

Step 6 – Confirm operative levels with imaging
Instruments: Spinal needle or marker passed from back table if requested.
Anticipation: Level confirmation is critical—do not proceed until verified.

Step 7 – Perform cervical laminectomy or laminoplasty
Instruments: Kerrison rongeurs and drill system passed from back table when requested.
Anticipation: Bone removal proceeds, open cutting instruments only when surgeon commits.

Step 8 – Decompress spinal cord and nerve roots
Instruments: Passed from back table when requested.
Anticipation: Neural elements are vulnerable—maintain calm, deliberate instrument flow.

Step 9 – Place instrumentation if fusion is planned
Instruments: Instrumentation system passed from back table when requested.
Anticipation: Do not open screws or rods until surgeon confirms fixation plan.

Step 10 – Inspect decompression and achieve hemostasis
Instruments: Mosquito hemostats if needed.
Anticipation: Bleeding often increases after decompression—respond quickly without clutter.

Step 11 – Place drain if ordered
Instruments: Drain passed from back table when requested.
Anticipation: Confirm drain type and exit site before opening.

Step 12 – Layered closure of fascia, muscle, and skin
Instruments: Brought from back table when requested.
Anticipation: Begin closing counts early. Closure instruments move forward only when surgeon commits.

Step 13 – Apply sterile dressing and cervical support if ordered
Instruments: Dressing supplies.
Anticipation: Ensure dressing does not interfere with postoperative immobilization devices.

Mayo Stand Suggestion:

- Knife Handle with #10 blade
- Metzenbaum Scissors
- Cobb Elevator
- Penfield #4
- Nerve Hook
- Kerrison Rongeur (1–2 mm)
- Leksell Rongeur
- High-Speed Drill (with matchstick or diamond burr)
- Adsons Forceps (with teeth)
- Mayo-Hegar Needle Driver

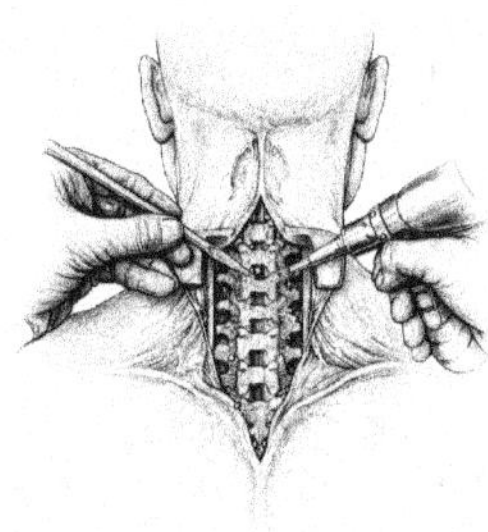

Rhizotomy

Step 1 – Patient positioning and verification
Instruments: Prone positioning aids, chest rolls or frame, padding.
Anticipation: Confirm indication (pain vs spasticity), target nerve roots, laterality, and whether procedure is open vs percutaneous.

Step 2 – Back preparation and sterile draping
Instruments: Prep supplies, spine drapes.
Anticipation: Prep widely to allow exposure extension if needed.

Step 3 – Midline posterior incision
Instruments: Scalpel handle with #10 blade, Adsons forceps with teeth.
Anticipation: Incision may be small but vascular, be ready with mosquito hemostats immediately.

Step 4 – Dissection through fascia and muscle
Instruments: Metzenbaum scissors, 2 mosquito hemostats, Adsons forceps.
Anticipation: Clamp–cut rhythm common. Control bleeding early to maintain visualization.

Step 5 – Expose lamina and perform limited laminectomy or laminotomy
Instruments: Kerrison rongeurs or drill system passed when requested.
Anticipation: Bone removal is limited, open cutting instruments only when surgeon commits.

Step 6 – Identify target nerve root(s)
Instruments: Passed from back table when requested.
Anticipation: Accurate identification is critical, maintain quiet field and controlled instrument flow.

Step 7 – Section or ablate nerve root(s)
Instruments: Passed from back table when requested.
Anticipation: Timing matters, be ready with required instruments immediately once nerve is identified.

Step 8 – Inspect field and confirm adequate rhizotomy
Instruments: None additional.
Anticipation: Surgeon may reassess multiple roots, stay alert for repeat passes.

Step 9 – Achieve hemostasis
Instruments: Mosquito hemostats if needed.
Anticipation: Bleeding may increase after nerve section, respond quickly without clutter.

Step 10 – Layered closure of fascia and skin
Instruments: Brought from back table when requested.
Anticipation: Begin closing counts early.

Step 11 – Apply sterile dressing
Instruments: Dressing supplies.
Anticipation: Dressing should not place pressure on operative site.

Mayo Stand Suggestion:

- Knife Handle with #10 blade
- Metzenbaum Scissors
- Cobb Elevator
- Penfield #4
- Nerve Hook
- Kerrison Rongeur (1–2 mm)
- Pituitary Rongeur
- Bayonet Forceps
- Adsons Forceps (with teeth)
- Mayo-Hegar Needle driver
- Frazier Suction Tip
- Bipolar Forceps

Transsphenoidal Hypophysectomy

Step 1 – Patient positioning and verification
Instruments: Supine positioning aids head donut or Mayfield fixation
Anticipation: Confirm nasal approach unilateral vs bilateral endoscopic vs microscopic technique and navigation readiness. Verify pituitary instrument tray and sellar reconstruction materials are available.

Step 2 – Nasal and facial preparation and sterile draping
Instruments: Prep supplies head and facial drapes
Anticipation: Prep includes upper lip nose and face. Maintain clear access for endoscope microscope and navigation arrays.

Step 3 – Nasal cavity exposure
Instruments: Nasal speculum Hardy or Cottle passed from back table when requested
Anticipation: Exposure is tight and delicate. Be ready to exchange speculums quickly without cluttering the field.

Step 4 – Incision of nasal septum or mucosa
Instruments: Scalpel handle with #15 blade, Adsons forceps with teeth
Anticipation: Small incision but vascular mucosa. Have mosquito hemostats available.

Step 5 – Submucosal dissection to sphenoid rostrum
Instruments: Freer elevator, Cottle elevator, Metzenbaum scissors
Anticipation: Elevators are used repeatedly. Keep tips clean and oriented correctly to avoid mucosal tears.

Step 6 – Open sphenoid sinus
Instruments: Kerrison rongeur, sphenoid punch, drill system passed from back table when requested
Anticipation: Bone removal is incremental. Confirm instrument size before passing to avoid excessive bone removal.

Step 7 – Remove sphenoid sinus septations
Instruments: Takayama or pituitary rongeur, Kerrison rongeur
Anticipation: Septations may bleed. Anticipate quick clamp passes without crowding the field.

Step 8 – Open sellar floor
Instruments: High speed drill with diamond burr, Kerrison rongeur
Anticipation: Precision drilling phase. Keep Mayo minimal and avoid unnecessary movement.

Step 9 – Open dura over pituitary gland
Instruments: Microscissors, bayonet forceps, nerve hook
Anticipation: Dural opening is delicate. Be ready with cottonoids

Step 10 – Tumor removal
Instruments: Pituitary curettes various angles ring curettes suction curette
Anticipation: Tumor is removed in stages. Anticipate instrument changes based on tumor consistency and depth.

Step 11 – Inspect sellar cavity and confirm decompression
Instruments: Endoscope or microscope
Anticipation: Surgeon may pause frequently to inspect. Maintain quiet field and readiness.

Transsphenoidal Hypophysectomy

Step 12 – Reconstruct sellar floor
Instruments: Fat graft, fascia lata, titanium mesh, fibrin sealant when requested
Anticipation: Confirm reconstruction method before opening graft materials to avoid waste.

Step 13 – Nasal packing or splint placement
Instruments: Merocel or Vaseline gauze packing
Anticipation: Confirm type and laterality of packing. Account for all packing material.

Step 14 – Remove speculum and inspect nasal cavity
Instruments: None additional
Anticipation: Be alert for bleeding after removal of retraction.

Step 15 – Apply external dressing if ordered
Instruments: Dressing supplies

Mayo Stand Suggestion:

- Knife Handle with #10 blade
- Knife Handle with #11 blade
- Knife Handle with #15 blade
- 2 curved hemostats
- Debakey forceps
- Cushing with teeth
- Bayonet without teeth
- bivalve nasal speculum
- small Metzenbaums
- small straight Mayos
- Angled sickle scissors

Ulnar Nerve Transposition

Step 1 – Patient positioning and verification
Instruments: Supine positioning aids arm board or hand table
Anticipation: Confirm operative arm transposition type planned subcutaneous intramuscular or submuscular. Verify tourniquet use and padding of pressure points.

Step 2 – Upper extremity preparation and sterile draping
Instruments: Prep supplies extremity drape
Anticipation: Prep from mid upper arm to hand. Keep elbow freely movable for nerve assessment.

Step 3 – Apply tourniquet if used
Instruments: Tourniquet
Anticipation: Confirm inflation timing with surgeon. Tourniquet is often inflated after exsanguination.

Step 4 – Curvilinear incision over medial elbow
Instruments: Scalpel handle with #15 blade, Adsons forceps with teeth
Anticipation: Incision crosses flexion crease. Be ready with mosquito hemostats immediately due to superficial veins.

Step 5 – Dissection through subcutaneous tissue
Instruments: Metzenbaum scissors 2 mosquito hemostats
Anticipation: Clamp cut rhythm common. Protect medial antebrachial cutaneous nerve branches.

Step 6 – Identify ulnar nerve in cubital tunnel
Instruments: Passed from back table when requested
Anticipation: Once nerve is visualized the pace slows. Keep field uncluttered and instruments deliberate.

Ulnar Nerve Transposition

Step 7 – Release Osborne ligament and surrounding fascia
Instruments: Metzenbaum scissors or blade passed when requested
Anticipation: Release must be complete proximally and distally. Anticipate retraction adjustments without crowding Mayo.

Step 8 – Mobilize ulnar nerve proximally and distally
Instruments: Vessel loops passed from back table when requested
Anticipation: Vessel loop color and placement matter. Keep loop organized and visible.

Step 9 – Create new nerve bed anterior to medial epicondyle
Instruments: Passed from back table when requested
Anticipation: Depth varies by technique. Be ready for deeper exposure if submuscular transposition is chosen.

Step 10 – Transpose ulnar nerve to new position
Instruments: None additional
Anticipation: Ensure nerve lies without tension through elbow range of motion.

Step 11 – Secure nerve in transposed position
Instruments: Sutures passed from back table when requested
Anticipation: Confirm fixation method before opening sutures. Avoid premature needle driver placement.

Step 12 – Release tourniquet and reassess hemostasis
Instruments: Mosquito hemostats if needed
Anticipation: Bleeding may increase after release. Be ready to assist without cluttering the field.

Step 13 – Layered closure of subcutaneous tissue and skin
Instruments: Brought from back table when requested
Anticipation: Begin closing counts early. Closure proceeds efficiently once nerve is secured.

Step 14 – Apply sterile dressing and splint if ordered
Instruments: Dressing supplies splint materials if used
Anticipation: Dressing should avoid pressure over transposed nerve.

Mayo Stand Suggestion:

- Knife Handle with #15 blade
- Metzenbaum Scissors
- Tenotomy Scissors
- Adsons Forceps (with teeth)
- Adsons Forceps (without teeth)
- Debakey Forceps
- Right-Angle Clamp (Mixter)
- Nerve Hook
- Penfield #4
- Mayo-Hegar Needle driver
- Frazier Suction Tip
- Bipolar Forceps

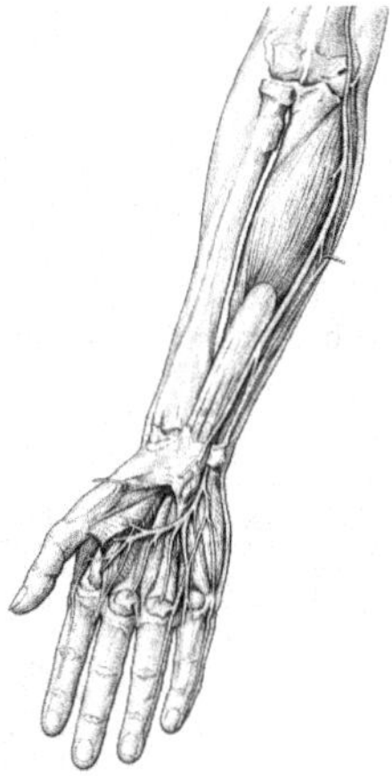

Ventriculoscopy

Step 1 – Patient positioning and verification
Instruments: Supine positioning aids, head donut or Mayfield fixation
Anticipation: Confirm indication (ETV, biopsy, cyst fenestration), laterality, burr hole location, and neuronavigation availability. Verify correct neuroendoscope system is present.

Step 2 – Scalp preparation and sterile draping
Instruments: Prep supplies, cranial drapes
Anticipation: Prep entire scalp widely even though incision is small. Maintain access for navigation arrays and camera equipment.

Step 3 – Mark incision and burr hole site
Instruments: Skin marker
Anticipation: Confirm burr hole location corresponds to ventricular trajectory and imaging before incision.

Step 4 – Scalp incision
Instruments: Scalpel handle with #10 blade, Adsons forceps with teeth
Anticipation: Scalp bleeding is common—have mosquito hemostats ready immediately and manage clamp placement efficiently.

Step 5 – Dissection through galea and periosteum
Instruments: Metzenbaum scissors, 2 mosquito hemostats, Adsons forceps
Anticipation: Clamp-cut rhythm is brief but important to control early bleeding.

Step 6 – Create burr hole
Instruments: Perforator drill bit passed from back table when requested
Anticipation: Confirm perforator type and size before passing. Protect dura immediately after penetration.

Step 7 – Open dura
Instruments: Dural scissors, bayonet forceps passed from back table
Anticipation: Dural opening is small and precise. Anticipate cottonoids for protection.

Step 8 – Insert ventricular introducer or peel away sheath
Instruments: Ventricular introducer, peel away sheath passed from back table
Anticipation: Maintain absolute sterility and trajectory control. Do not advance without surgeon cue.

Step 9 – Introduce neuroendoscope into ventricle
Instruments: Rigid or flexible neuroendoscope
Anticipation: Protect optics. Confirm white balance and focus before insertion.

Step 10 – Perform intraventricular procedure
Instruments:

- Fogarty balloon catheter (for ETV)
- Endoscopic biopsy forceps
- Endoscopic scissors or graspers
- (passed from back table when requested)

Anticipation: Instrument changes are frequent and delicate. Pass only one instrument at a time and keep tips protected.

Ventriculoscopy

Step 11 – Inspect ventricular anatomy and confirm outcome
Instruments: None additional
Anticipation: Surgeon may pause for visualization—maintain quiet field and avoid unnecessary motion.

Step 12 – Withdraw endoscope and inspect tract
Instruments: Cottonoids passed from back table if requested
Anticipation: Bleeding may occur on withdrawal—be ready without cluttering the field.

Step 13 – Close dura if indicated
Instruments: Sutures and needle driver passed from back table when requested
Anticipation: Not all cases require dural closure. Wait for surgeon commitment.

Step 14 – Close scalp incision
Instruments: Brought from back table when requested
Anticipation: Closure is usually quick; counts must already be correct.

Step 15 – Apply sterile dressing
Instruments: Dressing supplies
Anticipation: Dressing should not interfere with postoperative imaging or ICP monitoring

Mayo Stand Suggestion:

- #3 Knife Handle with #15 blade
- Metzenbaum Scissors
- Periosteal Elevator (Penfield #1 or Freer)
- High-Speed Drill (with cranial burr)
- Bayonet Forceps
- Ventriculoscope (rigid or flexible)
- Endoscopic Sheath with Obturator
- Endoscopic Grasper / Forceps
- Endoscopic Scissors

Ventriculoperitoneal Shunt Placement

Step 1 – Patient positioning and verification
Instruments: Supine positioning aids, head donut or Mayfield fixation
Anticipation: Confirm shunt side, valve type and pressure setting, antibiotic-impregnated tubing if ordered, and whether general surgery will assist with distal catheter placement.

Step 2 – Head, neck, chest, and abdomen preparation and draping
Instruments: Prep supplies, cranial and abdominal drapes
Anticipation: This is a multi-field procedure. Ensure wide prep from scalp to abdomen and maintain clear separation of cranial and abdominal work zones.

Step 3 – Mark cranial incision and burr hole site
Instruments: Skin marker
Anticipation: Confirm burr hole location corresponds to ventricular trajectory and imaging.

Step 4 – Scalp incision
Instruments: Scalpel handle with #10 blade, Adsons forceps with teeth
Anticipation: Scalp bleeding is common—have mosquito hemostats immediately available and manage clamps efficiently.

Step 5 – Dissection through galea and periosteum
Instruments: Metzenbaum scissors, 2 mosquito hemostats, Adsons forceps
Anticipation: Clamp-cut rhythm is brief but important to control bleeding before burr hole creation.

Ventriculoperitoneal Shunt Placement

Step 6 – Create burr hole
Instruments: Perforator drill bit passed from back table when requested
Anticipation: Confirm perforator type and size before passing. Protect dura immediately after penetration.

Step 7 – Open dura
Instruments: Dural scissors, bayonet forceps
Anticipation: Opening is small and precise. Anticipate cottonoids for cortical protection.

Step 8 – Insert ventricular catheter
Instruments: Ventricular catheter passed from back table when requested
Anticipation: Maintain strict sterility and trajectory control.

Step 9 – Confirm CSF flow
Instruments: None additional
Anticipation: Once CSF is confirmed, be ready to pass valve components promptly.

Step 10 – Attach valve and reservoir
Instruments: Shunt valve and reservoir system passed from back table when requested
Anticipation: Confirm valve type and pressure before opening. Orientation matters.

Step 11 – Tunnel distal catheter subcutaneously
Instruments: Shunt passer or tunneling device passed from back table
Anticipation: Maintain catheter sterility during tunneling. Protect tubing from kinking or contamination.

Step 12 – Abdominal incision and peritoneal access
Instruments: Passed from back table when requested
Anticipation: Distal placement may be done by neurosurgery or general surgery. Coordinate timing and instrument flow carefully.

Step 13 – Insert distal catheter into peritoneal cavity
Instruments: Distal catheter tubing passed from back table
Anticipation: Ensure adequate catheter length without tension.

Step 14 – Secure shunt components and inspect system
Instruments: Passed from back table when requested
Anticipation: Confirm all connections are tight before closure.

Step 15 – Layered closure of cranial and abdominal incisions
Instruments: Sutures and needle driver passed from back table when requested
Anticipation: This is a multi-site closure; counts must be meticulously coordinated.

Step 16 – Apply sterile dressings
Instruments: Dressing supplies
Anticipation: Dressings should allow inspection for CSF leak or abdominal bleeding.

Mayo Stand Suggestion:

- Knife with #15 blade
- Metzenbaum Scissors
- Periosteal Elevator (Penfield #1 or Freer)
- High-Speed Drill (with cranial burr)
- Bayonet Forceps
- Dural Hook
- Gerald Forceps (with teeth)
- Ventricular Catheter with Stylet
- Tunneling Tool (shunt passer)

Bibliography

Surgical Technology Core References

- Association of Surgical Technologists. Core Curriculum for Surgical Technology. AST.
- Association of Surgical Technologists. Surgical Technology for the Surgical Technologist: A Positive Care Approach. Cengage Learning.
- Berry, E. C., & Kohn, M. L. Berry & Kohn's Operating Room Technique. Elsevier.
- Rothrock, J. C. Alexander's Care of the Patient in Surgery. Elsevier.
- Phillips, N. Berry & Kohn's Operating Room Technique (instrumentation, sterile technique, intraoperative workflow). Elsevier.
- Association of periOperative Registered Nurses. Guidelines for Perioperative Practice. AORN.

General Surgery (Abdominal, GI, Hepatobiliary, Hernia)

- Brunicardi, F. C., et al. Schwartz's Principles of Surgery. McGraw Hill.
- Townsend, C. M., et al. Sabiston Textbook of Surgery: The Biological Basis of Modern Surgical Practice. Elsevier.
- Fischer, J. E., & Jones, D. B. Fischer's Mastery of Surgery. Wolters Kluwer.
- Cameron, J. L., & Cameron, A. M. Current Surgical Therapy. Elsevier.
- SAGES (Society of American Gastrointestinal and Endoscopic Surgeons). Clinical guidelines and statements (laparoscopy, cholecystectomy, hernia, reflux procedures).
- American College of Surgeons (ACS). Principles of safe surgery, perioperative standards, and patient safety resources.

Breast and Endocrine Surgery

- Bland, K. I., et al. The Breast: Comprehensive Management of Benign and Malignant Diseases. Elsevier.
- ACS (American College of Surgeons). Breast surgery principles and operative standards resources.
- ATA (American Thyroid Association). Thyroid disease management guidelines (thyroidectomy context and perioperative considerations).
- Doherty, G. M. Current Diagnosis & Treatment: Surgery. McGraw Hill (endocrine surgery overview).

Obstetrics and Gynecology

- Berek, J. S. Berek & Novak's Gynecology. Wolters Kluwer.
- Hoffman, B. L., et al. Williams Gynecology. McGraw Hill.
- Cunningham, F. G., et al. Williams Obstetrics. McGraw Hill.
- Rock, J. A., & Jones, H. W. Te Linde's Operative Gynecology. Wolters Kluwer.
- ACOG (American College of Obstetricians and Gynecologists). Practice bulletins and committee opinions (C section, hysteroscopy, D and C, sterilization, hysterectomy).

Ophthalmology

- AAO (American Academy of Ophthalmology). Basic and Clinical Science Course (BCSC) series.
- Yanoff, M., & Duker, J. S. Ophthalmology. Elsevier.
- Tasman, W., & Jaeger, E. A. Duane's Ophthalmology. Lippincott Williams & Wilkins (reference set).
- Jaffe, N. S., Jaffe, M. S., & Jaffe, G. F. Cataract Surgery and Its Complications. Elsevier (for cataract-related technique and instrumentation context).

Otolaryngology (ENT)

- Flint, P. W., et al. Cummings Otolaryngology: Head and Neck Surgery. Elsevier.
- Johnson, J. T., et al. Bailey's Head and Neck Surgery: Otolaryngology. Wolters Kluwer.
- KJ Lee. Essential Otolaryngology: Head & Neck Surgery. McGraw Hill.
- AAO-HNSF (American Academy of Otolaryngology–Head and Neck Surgery Foundation). Clinical guidance statements (tonsillectomy, sinus surgery, airway procedures).

Orthopedic Surgery

- Canale, S. T., & Beaty, J. H. Campbell's Operative Orthopaedics. Elsevier.
- Azar, F. M., et al. Orthopaedic Knowledge Update (OKU) series. AAOS.
- AAOS (American Academy of Orthopaedic Surgeons). Technique references, perioperative guidance, and orthopedic standards resources.
- Hoppenfeld, S., et al. Surgical Exposures in Orthopaedics: The Anatomic Approach. Wolters Kluwer (approaches and anatomy).

Bibliography

Neurosurgery and Spine

- Greenberg, M. S. Handbook of Neurosurgery. Thieme.
- Winn, H. R. (Ed.). Youmans & Winn Neurological Surgery. Elsevier.
- Schmidek, H. H., & Sweet, W. H. Schmidek and Sweet Operative Neurosurgical Techniques. Elsevier.
- Benzel, E. C. Spine Surgery: Techniques, Complication Avoidance, and Management. Elsevier.
- Barrow Neurological Institute and other academic neurosurgical operative references (for consensus approach patterns and instrumentation categories).

Cardiothoracic Surgery (Thoracic and Cardiac)

- Shields, T. W., et al. General Thoracic Surgery. Wolters Kluwer.
- Sellke, F. W., et al. Sabiston and Spencer Surgery of the Chest. Elsevier.
- Kirklin, J. W., & Barratt-Boyes, B. G. Cardiac Surgery. Elsevier.
- STS (Society of Thoracic Surgeons). Clinical practice guidelines (CABG, valve surgery, perioperative standards).
- AATS (American Association for Thoracic Surgery). Selected consensus statements and guidelines.

Vascular Surgery

- Cronenwett, J. L., & Johnston, K. W. (Eds.). Rutherford's Vascular Surgery and Endovascular Therapy. Elsevier.
- Moore, W. S. Vascular and Endovascular Surgery: A Comprehensive Review. Elsevier.
- SVS (Society for Vascular Surgery). Clinical practice guidelines (carotid disease, PAD, aneurysm management, access procedures).
- ACC/AHA (American College of Cardiology/American Heart Association). PAD and vascular disease guidelines (perioperative considerations and standards of care).

Safety, Sterile Technique, and Instrumentation Standards

- AORN. Guidelines for Perioperative Practice (sterile technique, counts, surgical attire, skin prep, positioning, specimen handling).
- CDC. Infection prevention guidance relevant to operative and sterile practice (hand hygiene and surgical site infection fundamentals).
- OSHA. Bloodborne pathogens standards (PPE and exposure control).
- Manufacturer Instructions for Use (IFUs) for specialty devices and implants (endoscopy systems, staplers, clip appliers, vascular grafts, energy devices, shunt systems, and orthopedic implants).

www.ingramcontent.com/pod-product-compliance
Lightning Source LLC
La Vergne TN
LVHW022202200926
848481LV00006B/1820

* 9 7 9 8 9 0 2 7 1 6 5 4 9 *